ATLAS OF NEUROANATOMY

WITH

RADIOLOGIC CORRELATION

AND

PATHOLOGIC ILLUSTRATION

ATLAS OF NEUROANATOMY

WITH

RADIOLOGIC CORRELATION

AND

PATHOLOGIC ILLUSTRATION

By

ARTHUR BROOKS DUBLIN, M.D.

Associate Professor of Radiology
Chief of Neuroradiology
University of California School of Medicine
Davis, California

And

WILLIAM BROOKS DUBLIN, M.A., M.D.

Chief of Neuropathology
Veterans Administration Medical Center
Martinez, California
Associate Clinical Professor of Pathology in
Neurological Surgery and Otorhinolaryngology
University of California School of Medicine
Davis, California

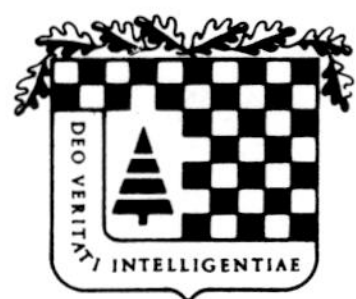

WARREN H. GREEN, INC.
St. Louis, Missouri, U.S.A.

Published by

WARREN H. GREEN, INC.
8356 Olive Boulevard
St. Louis, Missouri 63132, U.S.A.

© 1982 by WARREN H. GREEN, INC.

ISBN No. 87527-204-5

Printed in the United States of America

Outline

ATLAS OF NEUROANATOMY
WITH
RADIOLOGIC CORRELATION
AND
PATHOLOGIC ILLUSTRATION

Chapter One

Embryology

The proper study of neuroanatomy requires as prerequisite a clear understanding of the basic embryologic processes that effect the development of the brain. It is difficult to remember and identify the various subdivisions of the brain without such a basic foundation. A brief discussion of embryology accordingly appears to be in order.

The embryonic disc is composed of ectoderm and endoderm, the mesoderm developing in between. The nervous system arises from a specialized region of ectoderm; the latter raises two wave-like crests that fuse, forming the neural tube. By the end of the fourth embryonic week, three divisions of the neural tube can be identified as swellings that are destined to produce the mature brain structures. The divisions are the prosencephalon (forebrain), mesencephalon (midbrain), and rhombencephalon (hindbrain).

The prosencephalon divides into the telencephalon and diencephalon. The telencephalon gives rise to three major portions. The first of these is the rhinencephalon (literally, nosebrain), which includes the olfactory lobes, hippocampus, piriform lobes, fornix, septum pellucidum, parahippocampal gyrus, stria terminalis, and cingulate gyrus. The second, the corpus striatum, forms the internal capsule and basal ganglion. The basal ganglion consists of the globus pallidus and putamen (together constituting the lenticular nucleus), the caudate nucleus, amygdaloid body, and claustrum. The third region of the telencephalon is the suprastriatal area; it eventually develops into the cerebral cortex and associated underlying white matter. The diencephalon gives rise to the thalamus and hypothalamus, the central cavity becoming the third ventricle.

The mesencephalon forms the adult midbrain, and its central chamber becomes the cerebral aqueduct.

The rhombencephalon divides further into metencephalon and myelencephalon. The metencephalon gives rise to the pons and cerebellum, while the myelencephalon becomes the medulla. The cavity of the rhombencephalon becomes the fourth ventricle.

Some regions of junction between the major portions of the primitive brain are represented in the mature state. One such structure is the thalamostriate groove in the lateral wall of the lateral ventricle between caudate nucleus and thalamus; it represents a region of junction between telencephalon and diencephalon. Another example of primitive junctional relation is the lamina terminalis, the limiting membrane of the diencephalon; it becomes the anterior wall of the third ventricle.

The following illustrations will demonstrate roughly the embryonic derivation of the mature brain as visualized by computed tomography; it is hoped that they will be helpful in understanding the relationships of the divisions of the neural tube and their products.

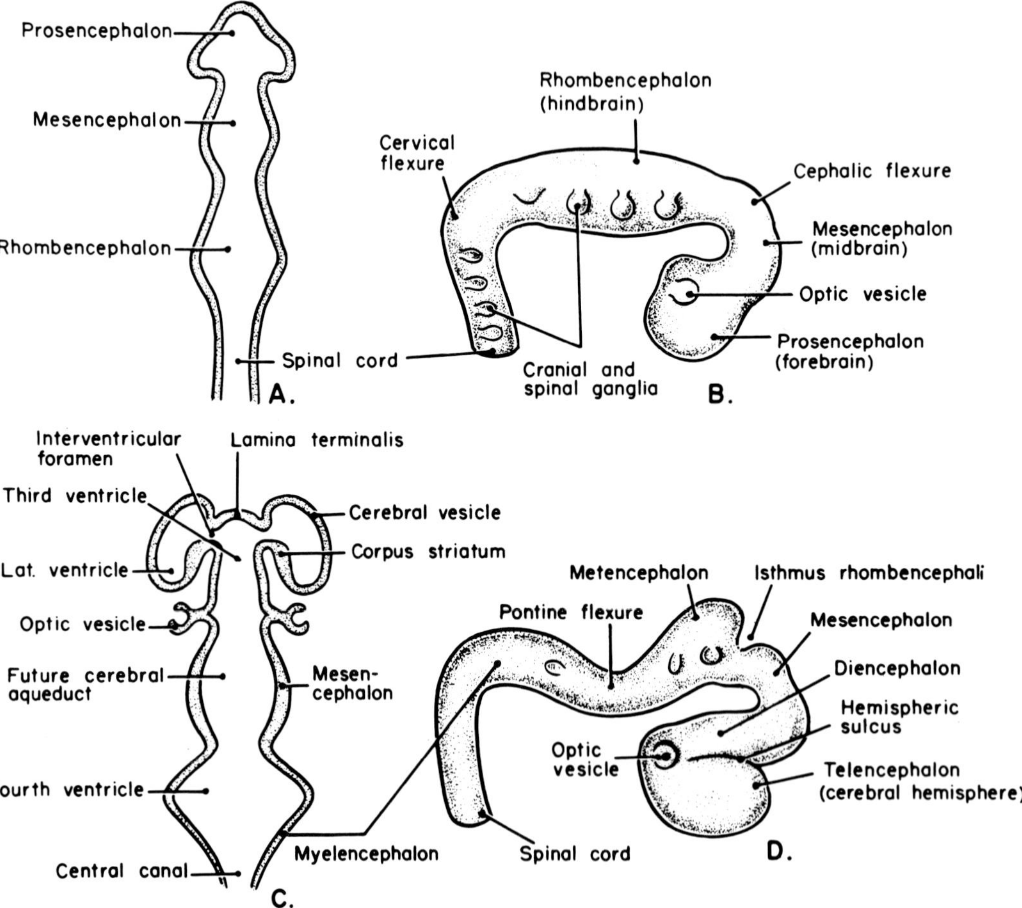

Figure 1-1. **Diagrams of the Developing Brain Vesicles and Ventricular System. A** and **B**, Three brain vesicle stage of a 4-week embryo. **C** and **D**, Five brain vesicle stage of a 6-week human embryo. After Truex, R. C. and Carpenter, M. B.: *Human Neuroanatomy,* Ed. VI, 1969, Williams and Wilkins, Baltimore (modified from Hochstetter, F.: *Beiträge zur Entwicklungsgeschichte des menschlichen Gehirns,* 1919, vol. I, F. Deuticke, Vienna, and from Langman, J.: *Medical Embryology,* Ed. II, 1969, Williams and Wilkins, Baltimore).

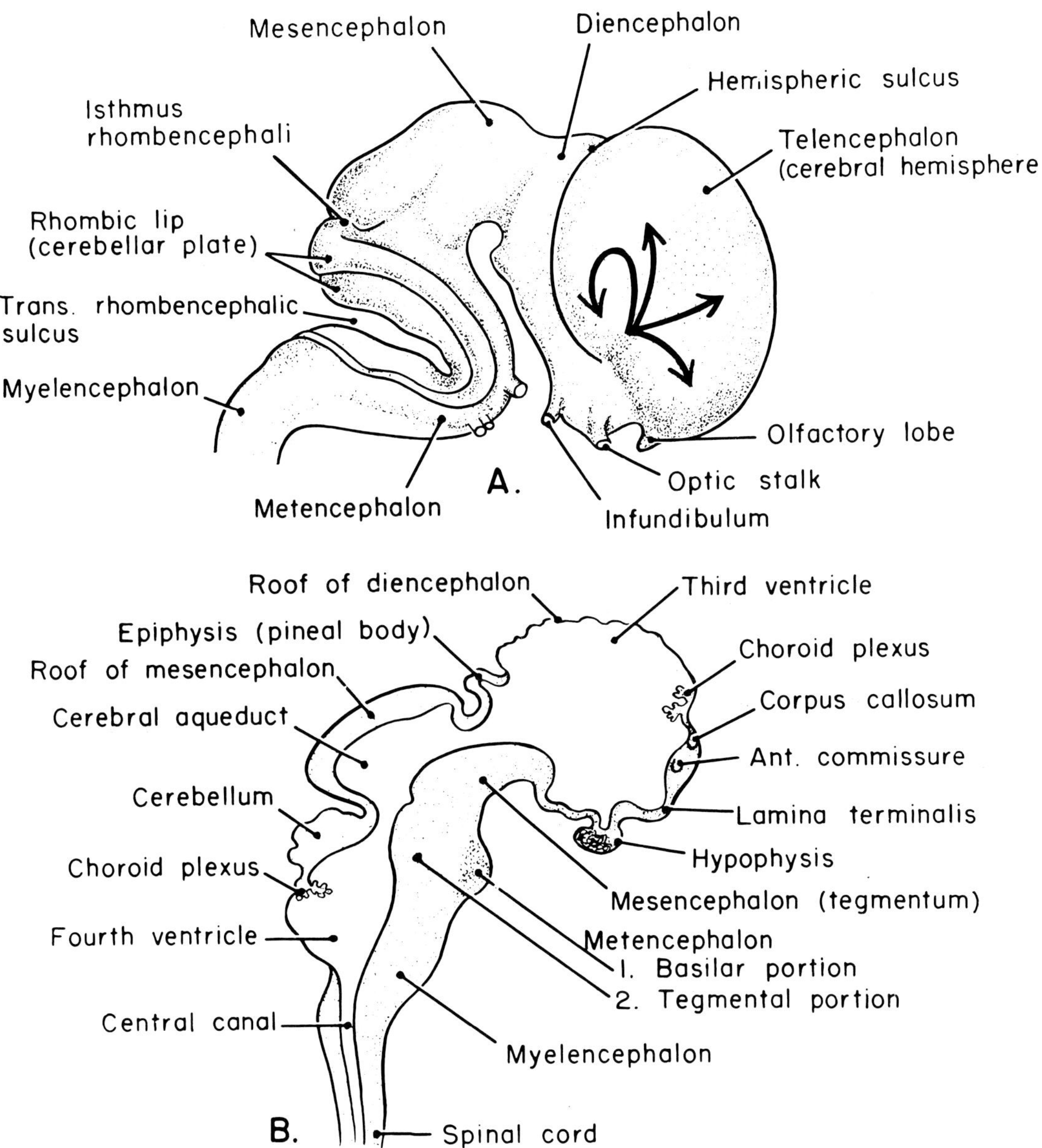

Figure 1-2. **Diagrams of the Developing Brain Vesicles and Ventricular System. A,** Lateral view of cerebral vesicle. Arrows indicate directions of growth and expansion of hemisphere. Note the relations of the developing cerebellum. Human embryo of 8 weeks. **B,** Sagittal section through brain of a human fetus of 12 weeks. After Truex and Carpenter (modified from Hochstetter) (see Fig. 1-1).

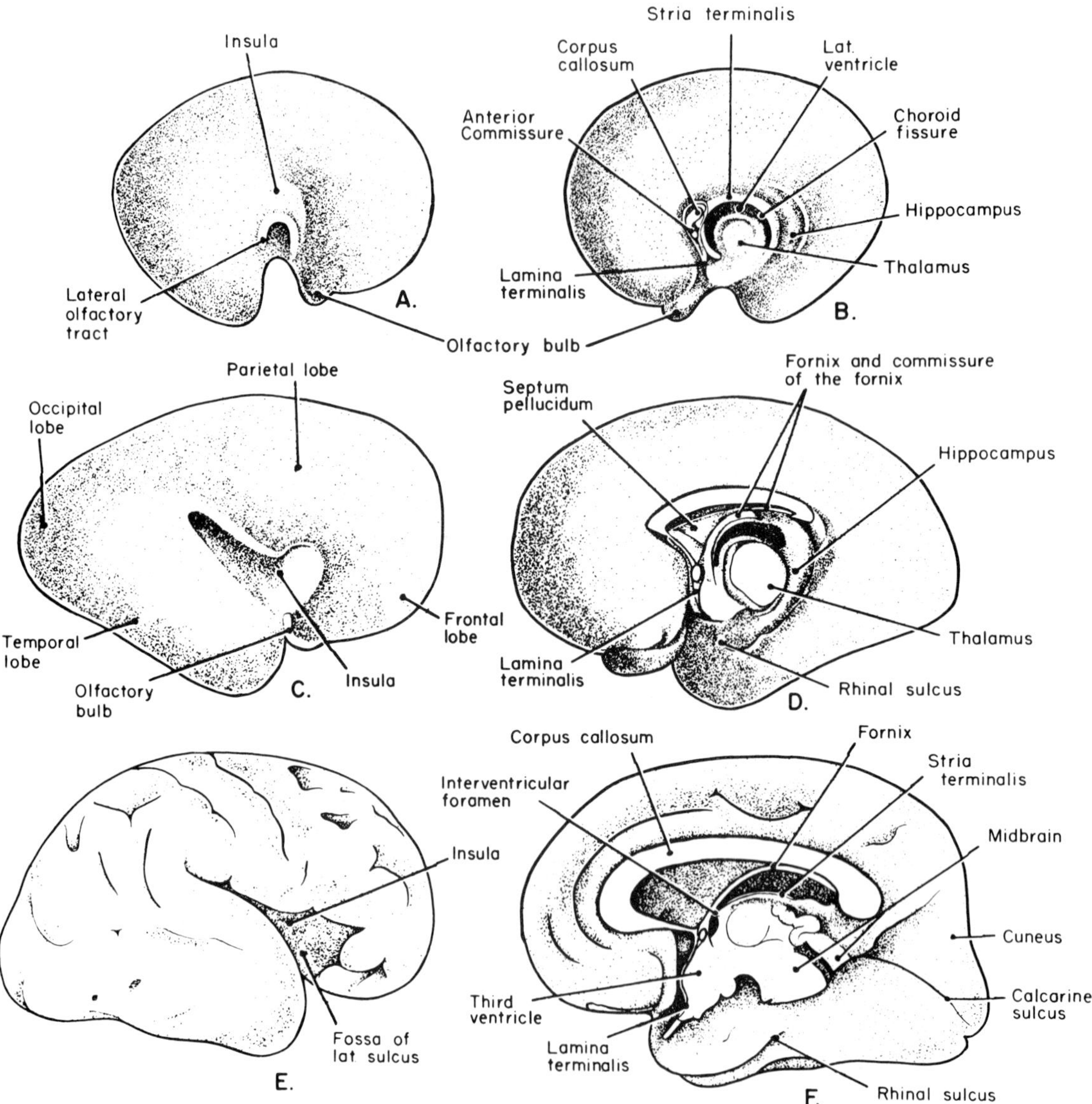

Figure 1-3. **Development of Human Cerebral Hemisphere. A** and **B,** Lateral and medial surfaces of the hemisphere in a fetus of 3 months. **C** and **D,** Lateral and medial surfaces of the hemisphere in a fetus at beginning of the fifth month. **E** and **F,** Lateral and medial surfaces of the hemisphere at the end of the seventh month. After Truex and Carpenter (see Fig. 1-1) (modified from Keibel, F. and Mall, F. P.: *Manual of Human Embryology,* 1912, Vol. II, J. B. Lippincott, Philadelphia).

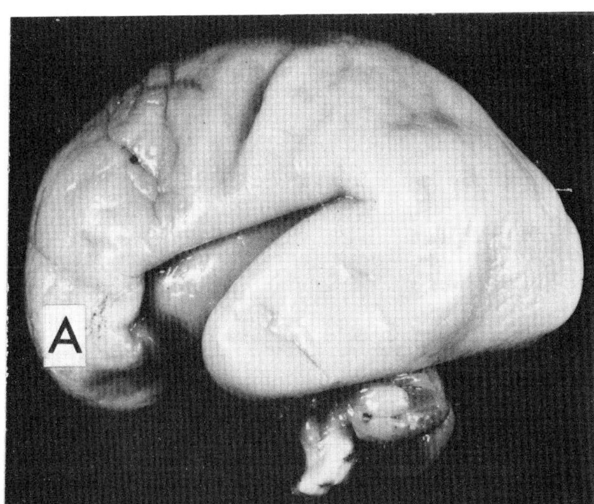

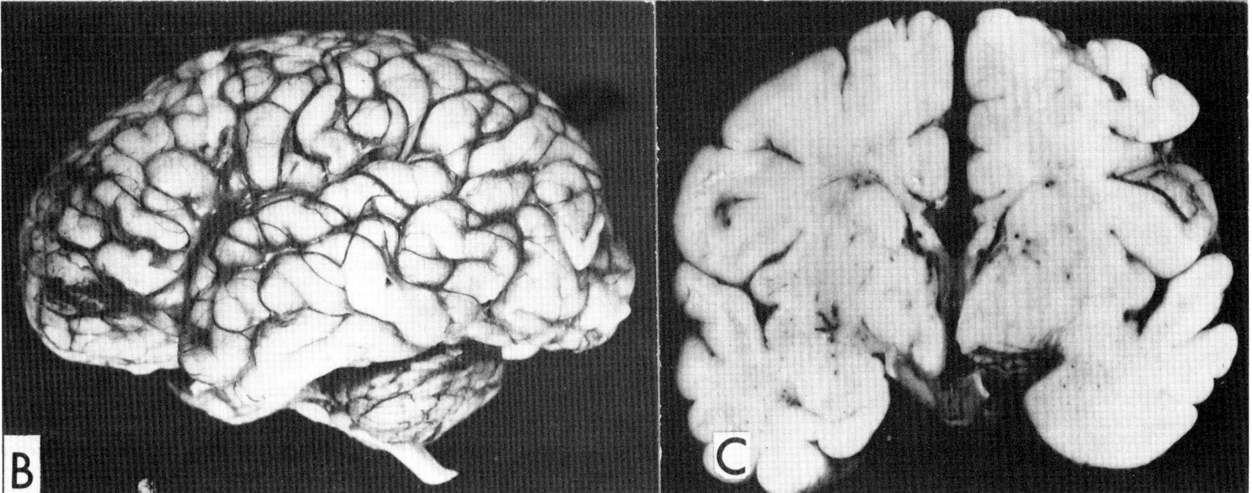

Figure 1-4. **A. Lateral View of Brain of 6¾ Months Fetus.** Fissures consist of little more than central and lateral; the latter is open.

B. Similar view of term fetus. Cerebellum is still comparatively small.

C. Coronal section of **B.** White matter is not distinct, and fissures are incompletely developed.

From Dublin, W. B.: *Fundamentals of Neuropathology,* Ed. I, 1954, Ed. II, 1967, Charles C Thomas. Springfield, Illinois.

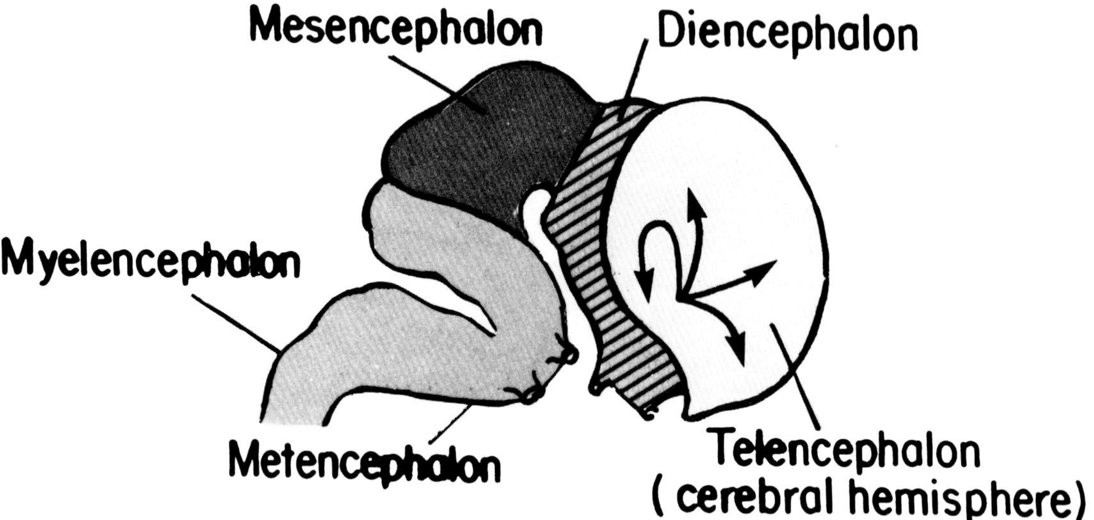

Figure 1-5-1. **Key for Embryology/CT Sections.** A schematic lateral view of the neural tube (approximately 25 mm) demonstrates the basic embryonic divisions of the brain and will be used as a key for Figures 1-5-2 through 1-5-8, with reference to the shades of gray employed in this illustration. Modified after Truex and Carpenter (see Figure 1-1).

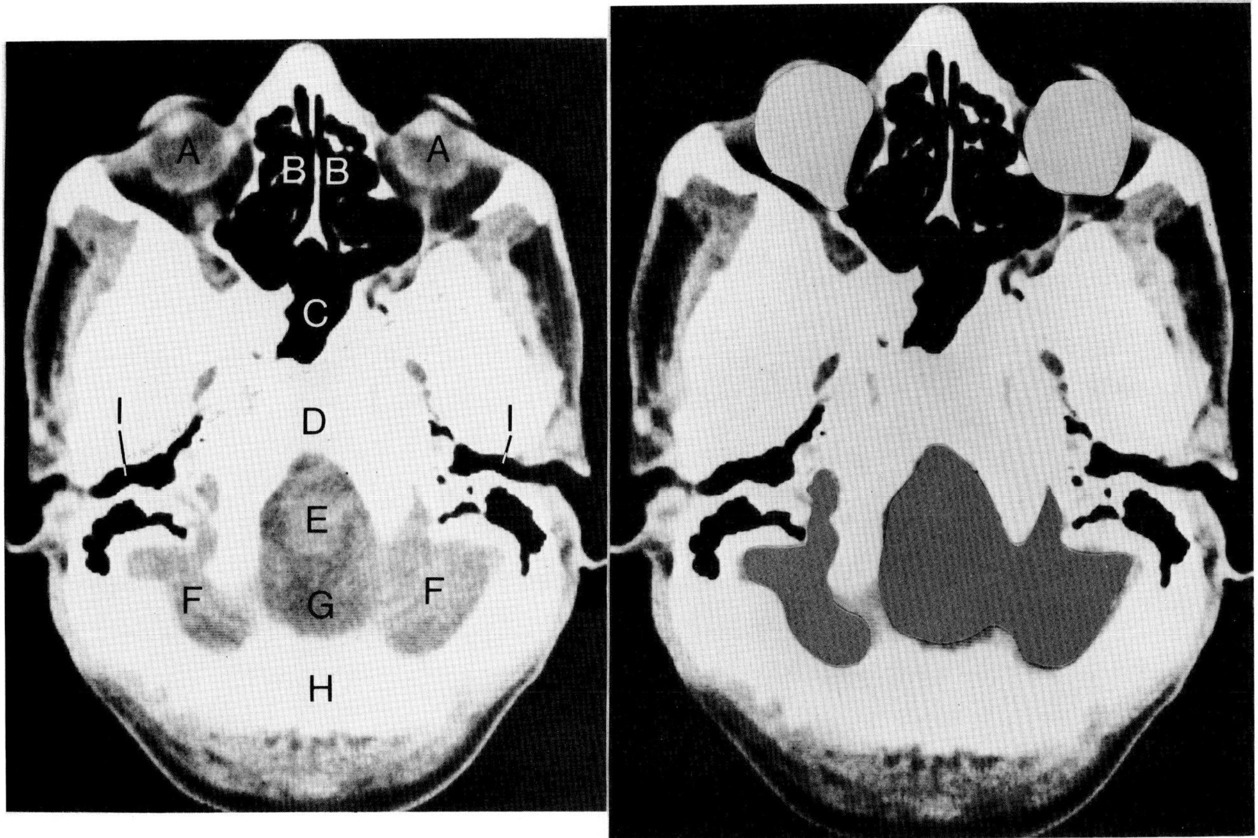

Figure 1-5-2. **Embroyonic Level #1.**
Figures 1-5-2 to 1-5-8 CTs are on the left and embryologic keys are on the
right. (See Figure 1-5-1 for shades representing the embryologic divisions.)
A. Optic globes.
B. Ethmoid sinuses.
C. Sphenoid sinus.
D. Clivus.
E. Medulla.
F. Cerebellum.
G. Cerebellomedullary cistern.
H. Occiput.
I. External auditory canals.

CT scans, Figures 1-5-2 through 1-5-8, courtesy Medical Systems Division,
General Electric Company, Milwaukee, Wisconsin.

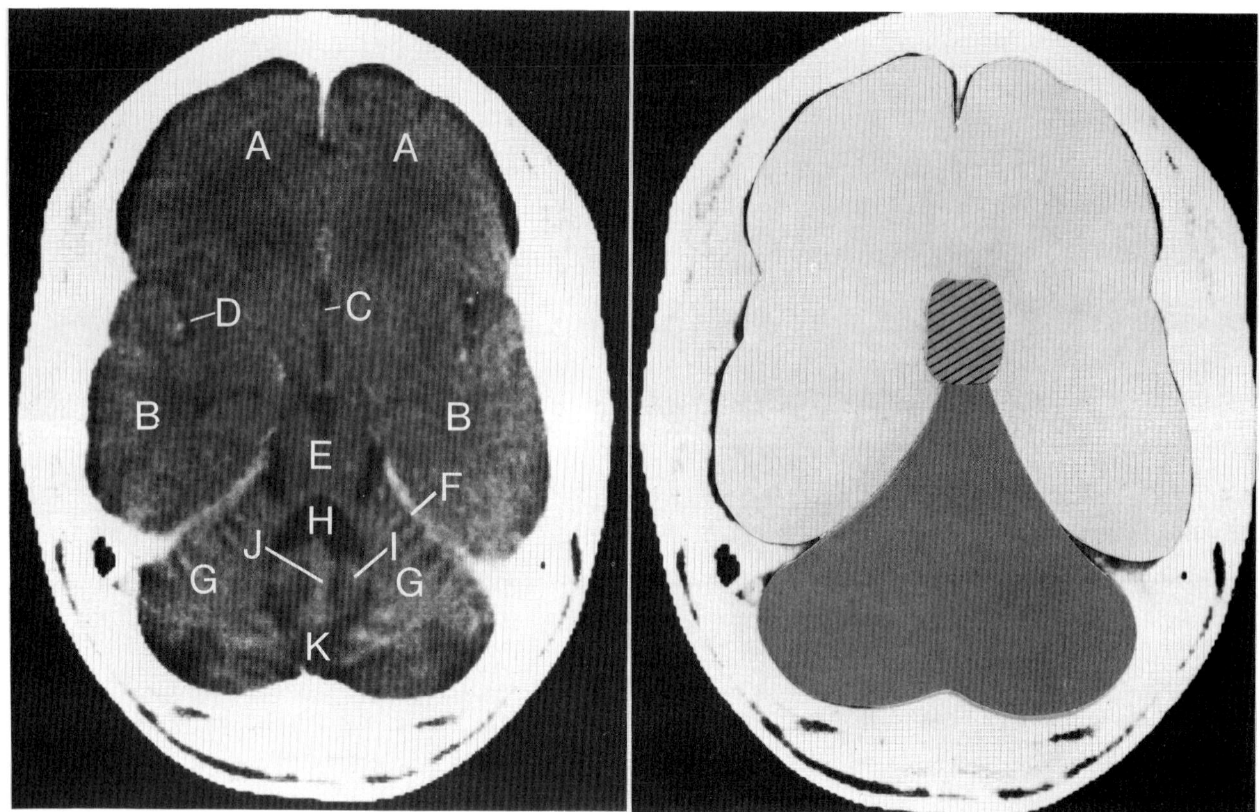

Figure 1-5-3. **Embryology Level #2.**

A. Frontal lobe.
B. Temporal lobes.
C. Inferior third ventricle.
D. Suprainsular cistern containing middle cerebral vessels.
E. Brain stem.
G. Cerebellar hemispheres.
H. Fourth ventricle.
I. Cerebellar tonsil.
J. Cerebellar vermis.
K. Cerebellomedullary cistern.

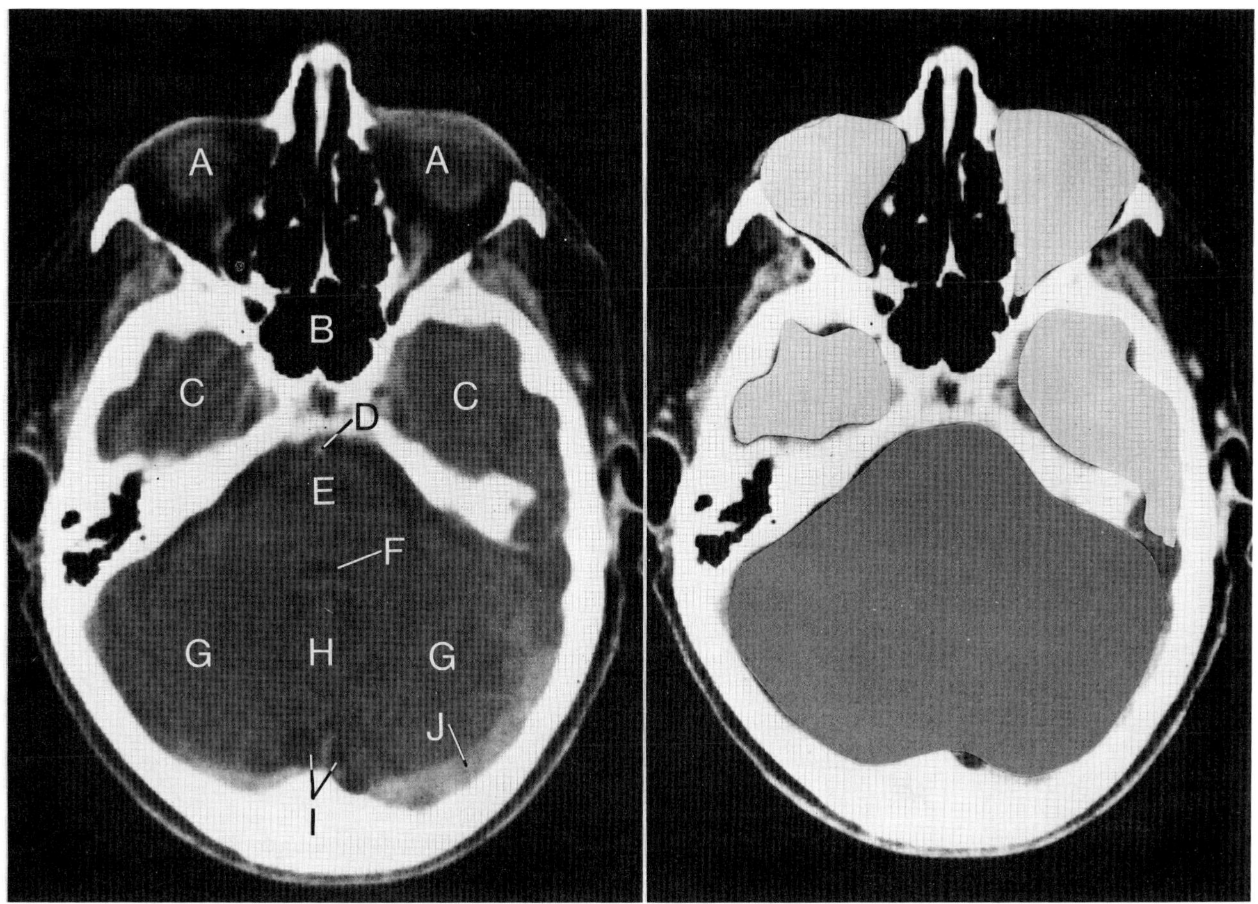

Figure 1-5-4. **Embryology Level #3.**
A. Optic globes.
B. Sphenoid sinus.
C. Temporal lobes.
D. Basilar artery.
E. Pons.
F. Fourth ventricle.
G. Cerebellar hemispheres.
H. Cerebellar vermis.
I. Cerebellomedullary cistern.
J. Transverse sinus.

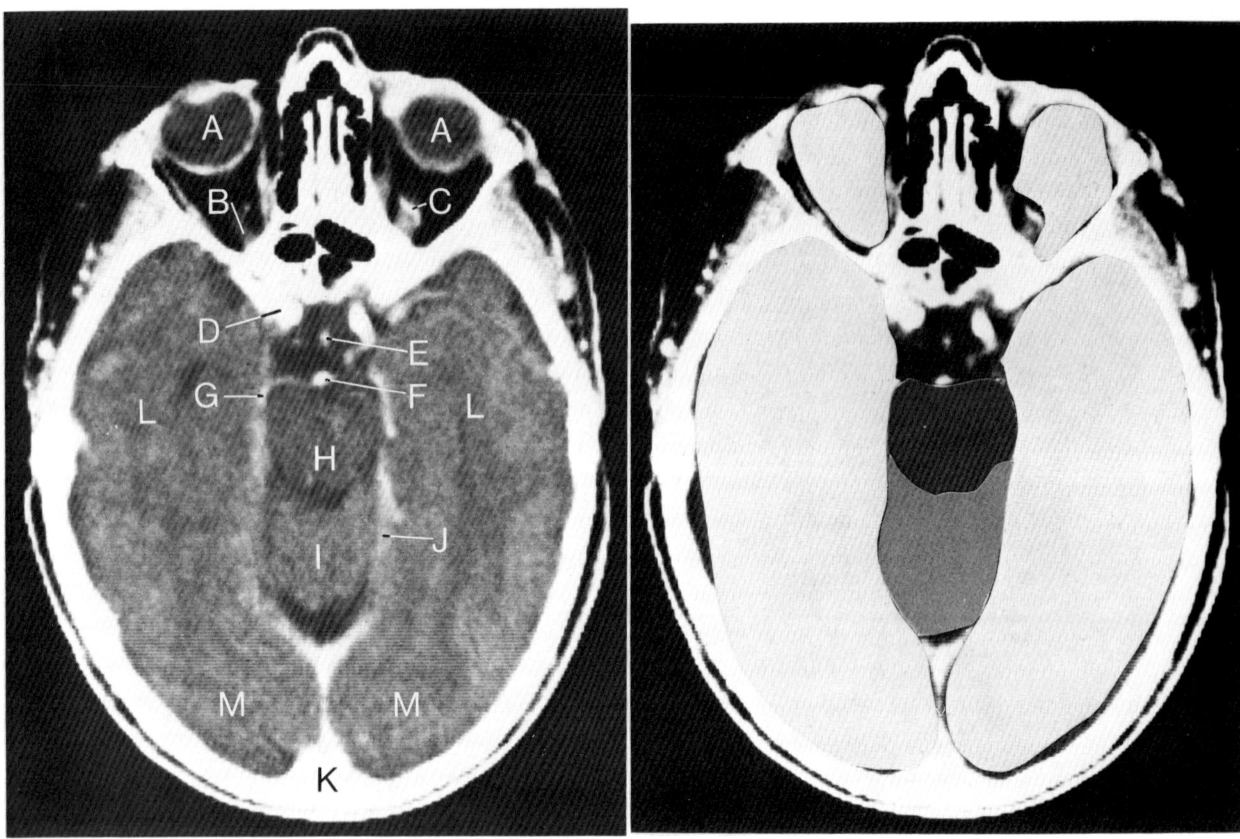

Figure 1-5-5. **Embryology Level #4.**

A. Optic globes.
B. Optic nerve.
C. Superior ophthalmic vein.
D. Anterior clinoid.
E. Pituitary stalk.
F. Basilar artery.
G. Posterior cerebral artery.
H. Upper pons, lower cerebral peduncules.
I. Cerebellum.
J. Tentorial edge.
K. Internal occipital protuberance.
L. Temporal lobes.
M. Occipital lobes.

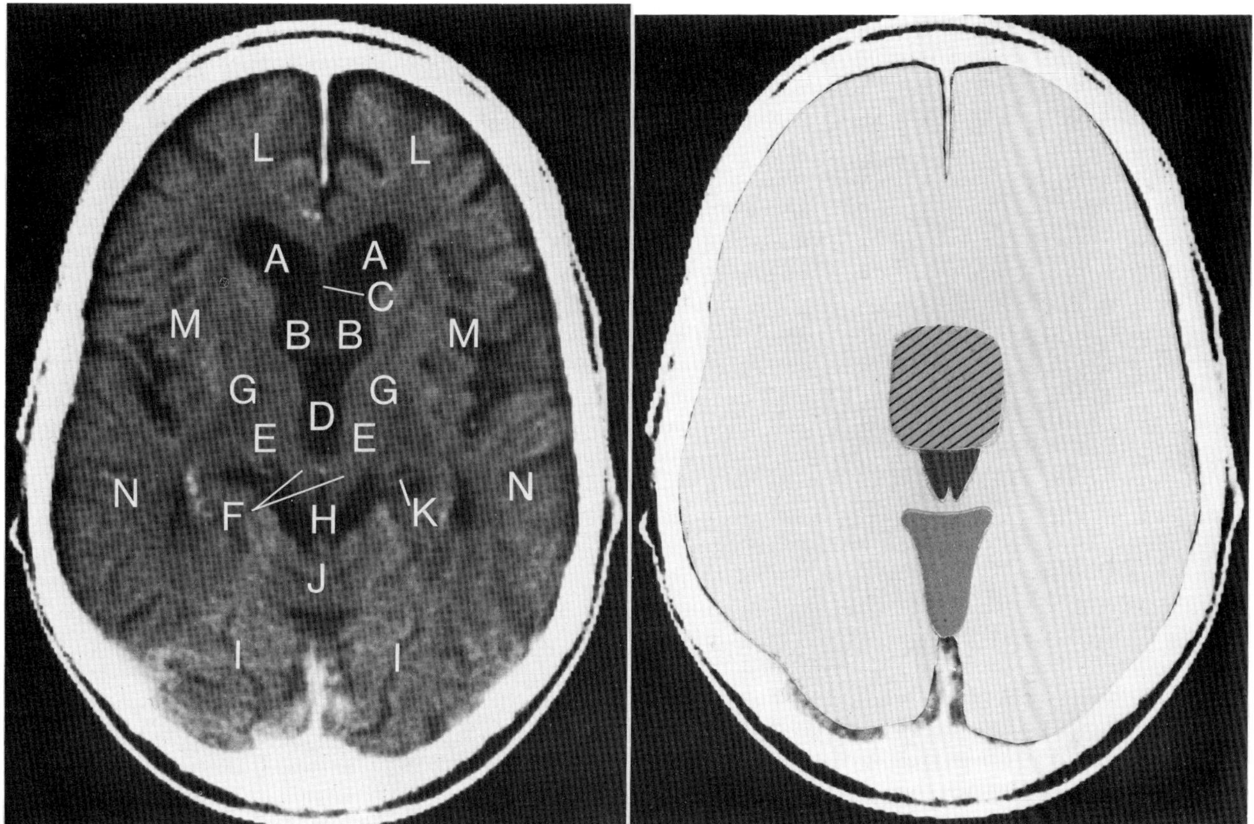

Figure 1-5-6. **Embryology Level #5.**
A. Anterior horns, lateral ventricles.
B. Anterior bodies, lateral ventricles.
C. Septum pellucidum.
D. Third ventricle.
E. Thalamus.
F. Quadrigeminal (collicular) plate.
G. Internal capsule.
H. Quadrigeminal cistern.
I. Occipital lobes with some superimposed tentorial blush.
J. Cerebellum.
K. Lateral atrial vein in the upper retropulvinar cistern.
L. Frontal lobes.
M. Insula, medial to suprainsular cistern.
N. Temporal lobes.

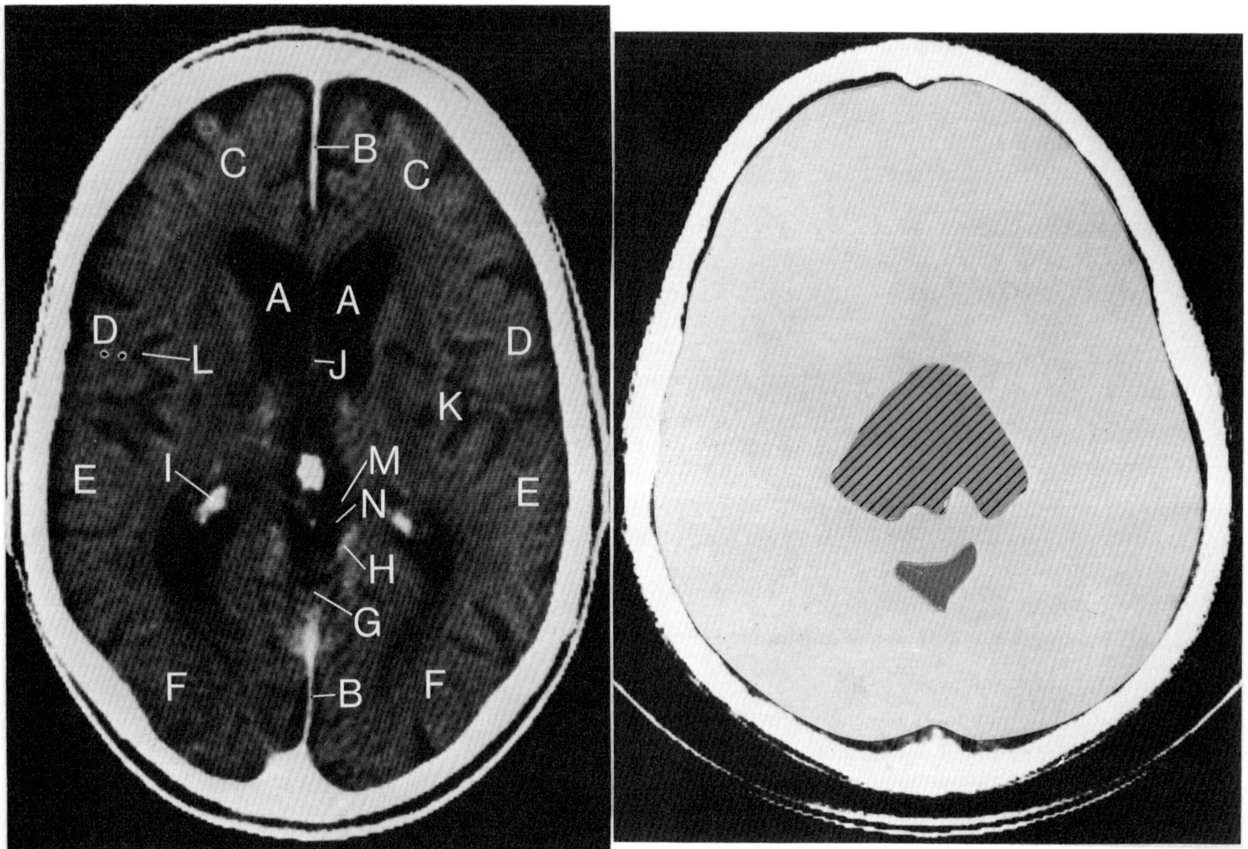

Figure 1-5-7. **Embryology Level #6.**

A. Anterior horns, lateral ventricles.
B. Falx cerebri.
C. Frontal lobes.
D. Parietal operculum.
E. Temporal lobes.
F. Occipital lobes.
G. Cerebellum.
H. Tentorium.
I. Calcified choroid plexus in the trigone of the lateral ventricle.
J. Septum pellucidum.
K. Insula.
L. Suprainsular cistern.
M. Basal vein.
N. Lateral atrial vein.

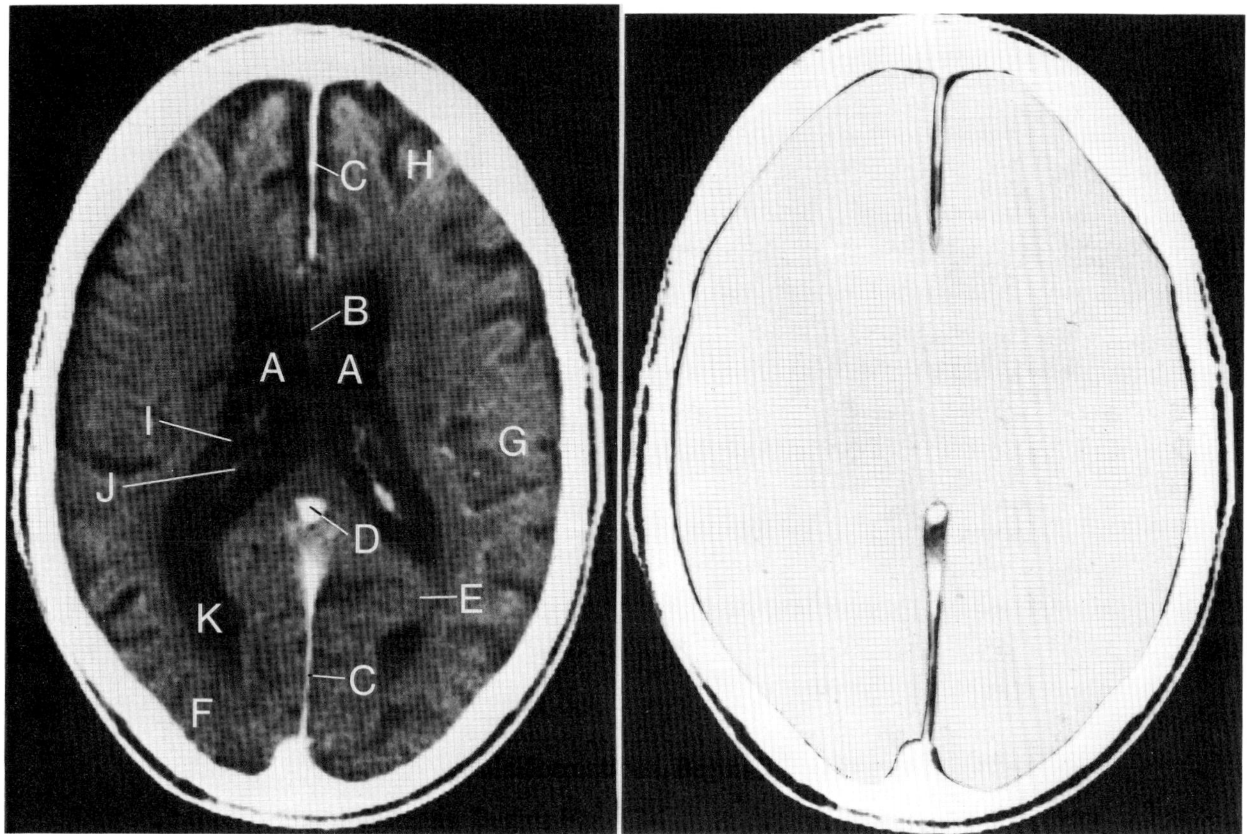

Figure 1-5-8. **Embryology Level #7.**
A. Body, lateral ventricle.
B. Septum pellucidum.
C. Falx cerebri.
D. Great cerebral vein.
E. Calcar avis.
F. Occipital lobe.
G. Parietal lobe.
H. Frontal lobe.
I. Thalamostriate vein.
J. Choroid plexus.
K. Occipital horn, lateral ventricle.

Chapter Two

Anatomy

SURFACE

→

Figure 2-1. **Basic View of Vertex of Brain.**

A. Frontal pole.

B. Longitudinal fissure.

C. Central sulcus. A superior cerebral vein extends along the sulcus.

D. Precentral gyrus (motor—Brodmann's area 4).

E. Postcentral gyrus (sensory—Brodmann's area 1). Note the variation in configuration of gyri and sulci, between the two hemispheres. Compare also with Figures 2-2, 8-9.

F. Another superior cerebral vein, with entry into a lacuna of sagittal sinus. See also Figure 8-2.

G. Pacchyonian granulation (fibrous hypertrophy of arachnoidal villi).

H. Occipital pole.

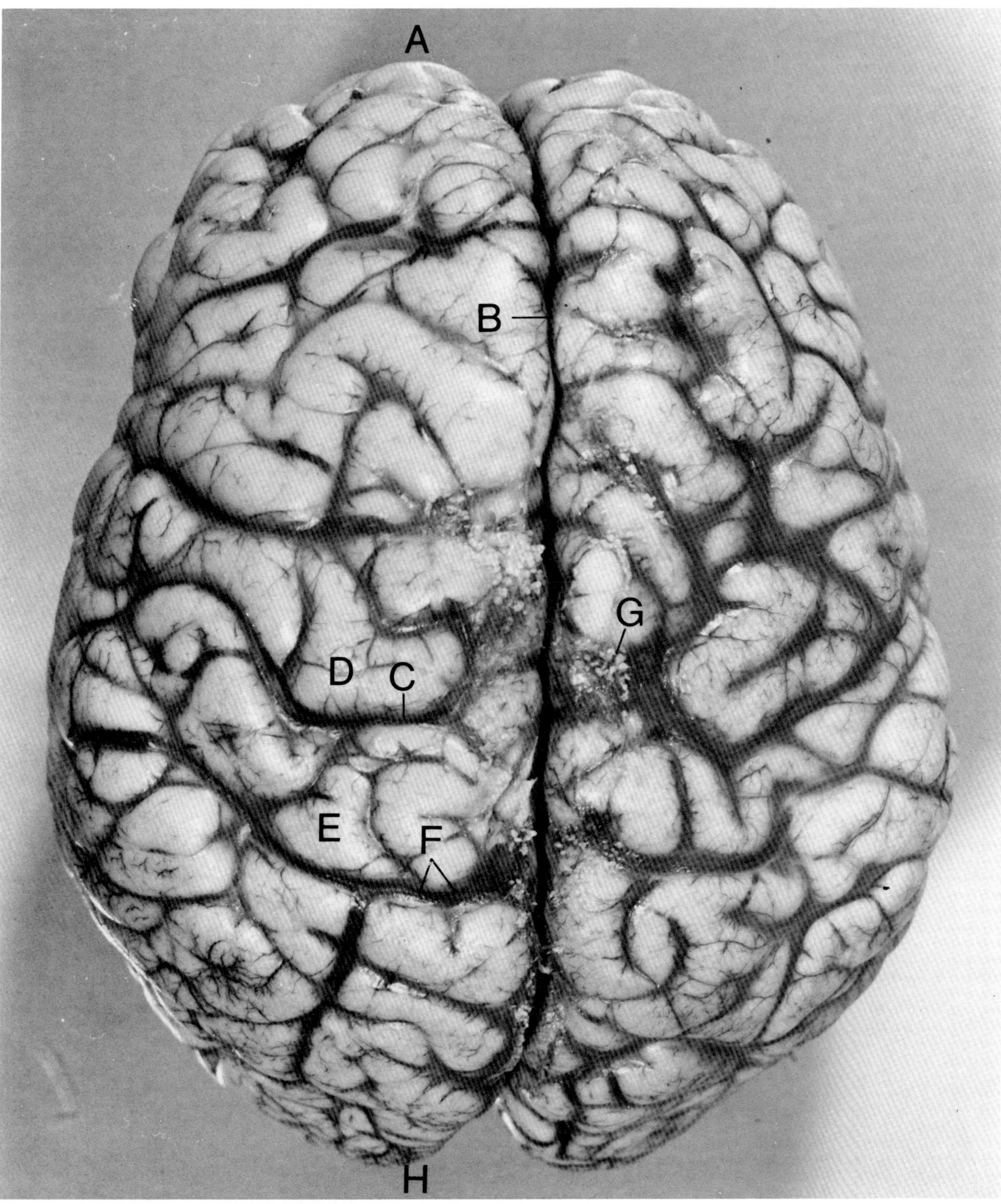
A
B
G
D
C
E
F
H

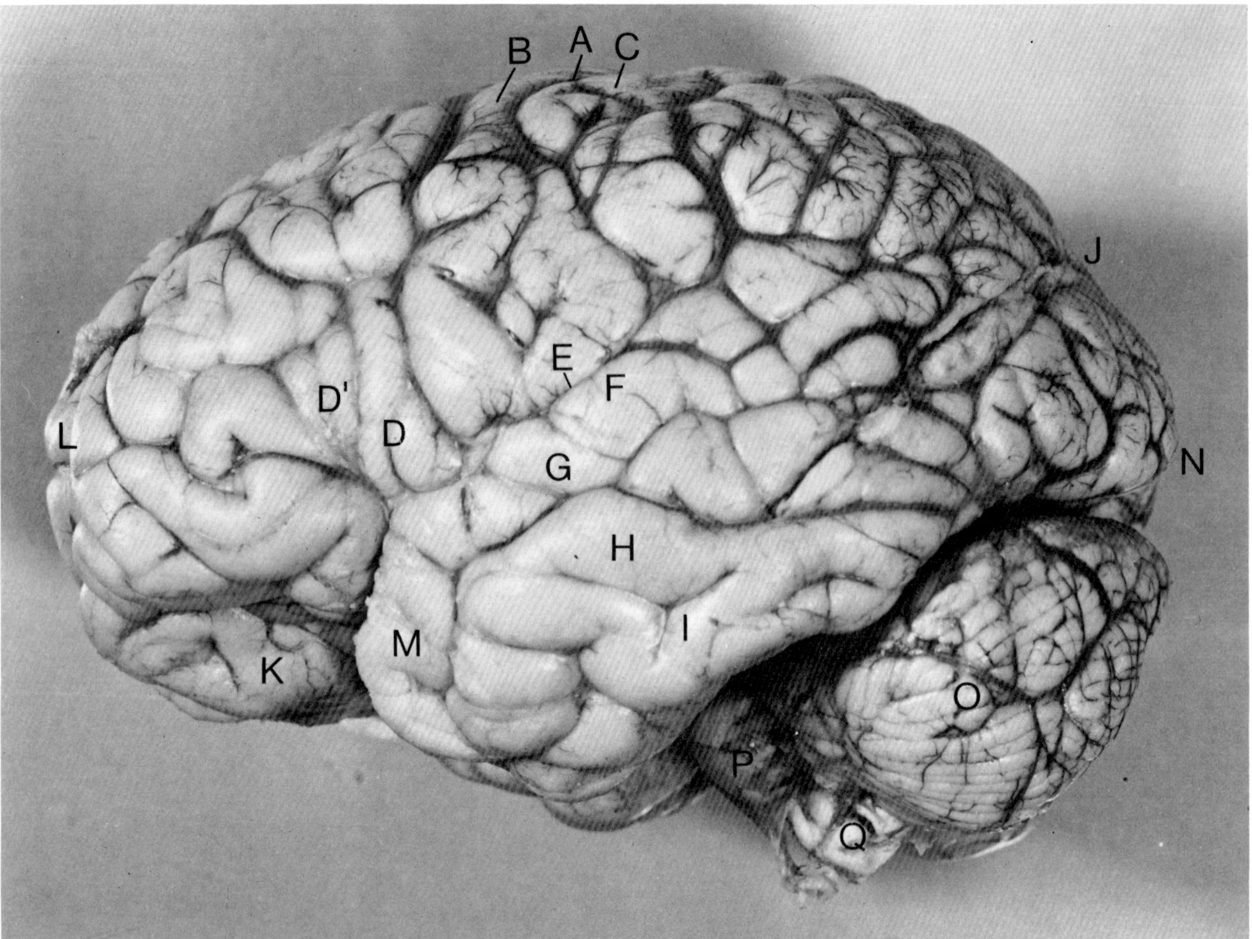

Figure 2-2. **Basic View of Lateral Surface of Brain.** The view of brain is slightly oblique, looking upward from below. The apparent area of temporal lobe is increased at expense of frontal and parietal lobes. The variability of pattern of gyri and sulci is well represented. (See also, and compare with, Fig. 2-3.)

A. Central sulcus (frontoparietal boundary).

B. Precentral gyrus (motor—Brodmann's area 4).

C. Postcentral gyrus (sensory—Brodmann's area 1).

D. Pars opercularis of inferior frontal gyrus; D', pars triangularis. (Portions of the pars opercularis and triangularis on the dominant side represent the motor speech area—Brodmann's area 44.)

E. Lateral sulcus.

F. Primary sensory acoustic area—Brodmann's area 41. Most of this area lies within, and on the floor of, the lateral sulcus. (See also Fig. 2-3.)

G. Superior temporal gyrus.

H. Middle temporal gyrus.

I. Inferior temporal gyrus.

J. Occipitoparietal boundary.

K. Orbital surface of frontal lobe.

L. Frontal pole

M. Temporal pole.

N. Occipital pole.

O. Cerebellar hemisphere.

P. Pons.

Q. Medulla.

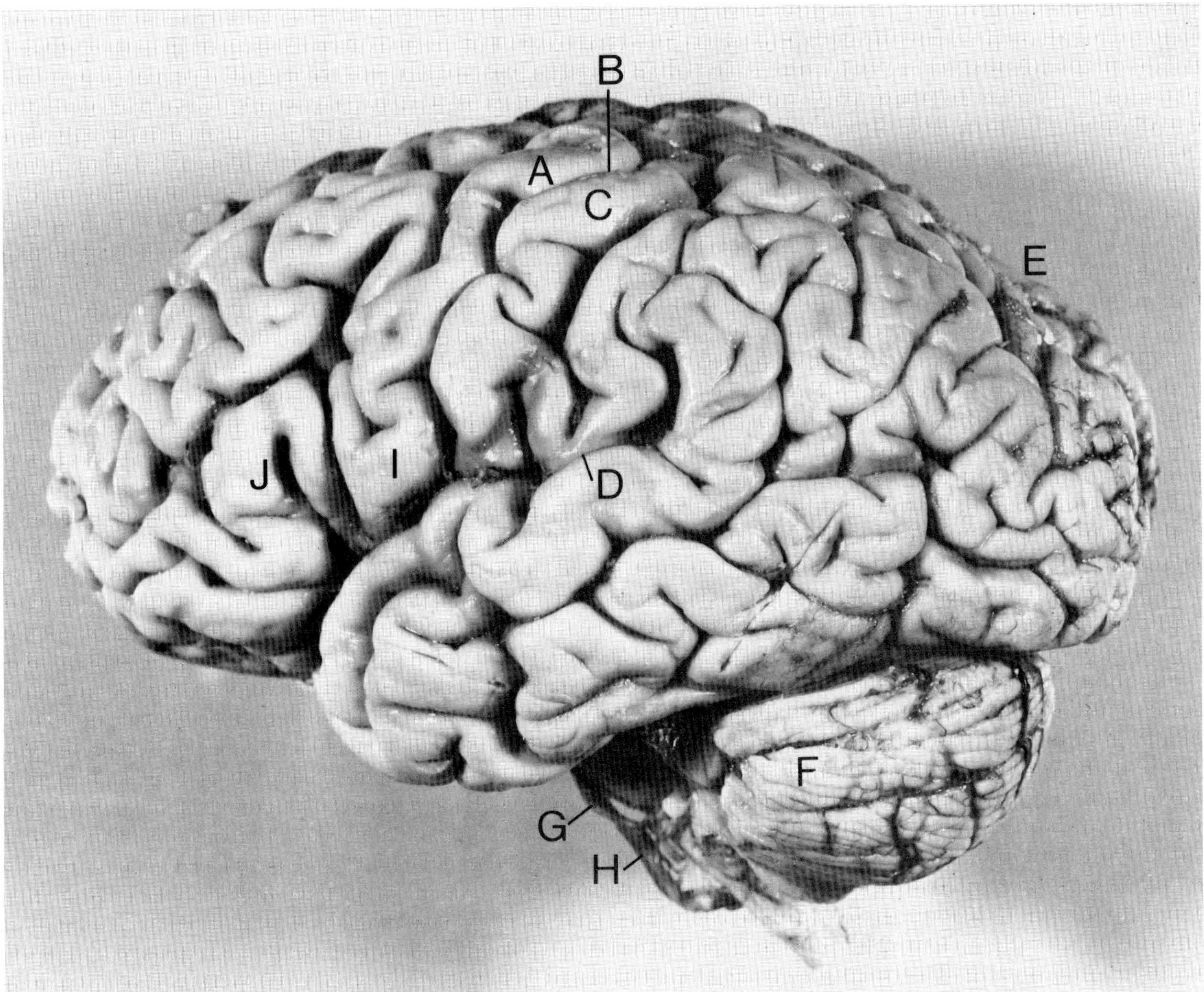

Figure 2-3. **Basic View of Lateral Surface of Brain** (subject other than that of Figure 2-2). Arachnoid has been removed. There is moderate convolutional atrophy, mainly frontal.

A. Precentral gyrus (motor).
B. Central sulcus—point of demarcation of frontal lobe from parietal.
C. Postcentral gyrus (sensory).
D. Lateral sulcus—point of demarcation of frontal and parietal lobes from temporal.
E. Point of demarcation of parietal and temporal lobes from occipital.
F. Cerebellar hemisphere.
G. Basilar artery.
H. Vertebral artery.
I. Pars opercularis of inferior frontal gyrus; J. pars triangularis. Portions of the pars opercularis and triangularis on the dominant side constitute the motor speech area—Brodmann's area 44.

$\longrightarrow$

Figure 2-4. **Basic View of Base of Brain.** See also Figure 6-1, especially for cranial nerves.

A. Anterior extremity of longitudinal fissure.
B. Orbital surface of frontal lobe.
C. Olfactory bulb.
D. Olfactory tract.
E. Optic nerve and chiasm.
F. Infundibulum.
G. Internal carotid artery.
H. Uncus.
I. Arachnoid covering interpeduncular fossa and cistern.
J. Oculomotor nerve.
K. Trigeminal nerve.
L. Basilar artery.
M. Pons.
N. Abducens nerve.
O. Parahippocampal gyrus.
P. Facial and auditory nerves.
Q. Medulla.
R. Glossopharyngeal, vagus, and spinal accessory nerves.
S. Hypoglossal nerve.
T. Cerebellar hemisphere.
U. Arachnoid covering cerebellomedullary cistern (cisterna magna).
V. Posterior inferior cerebellar artery, hemispheric branch.

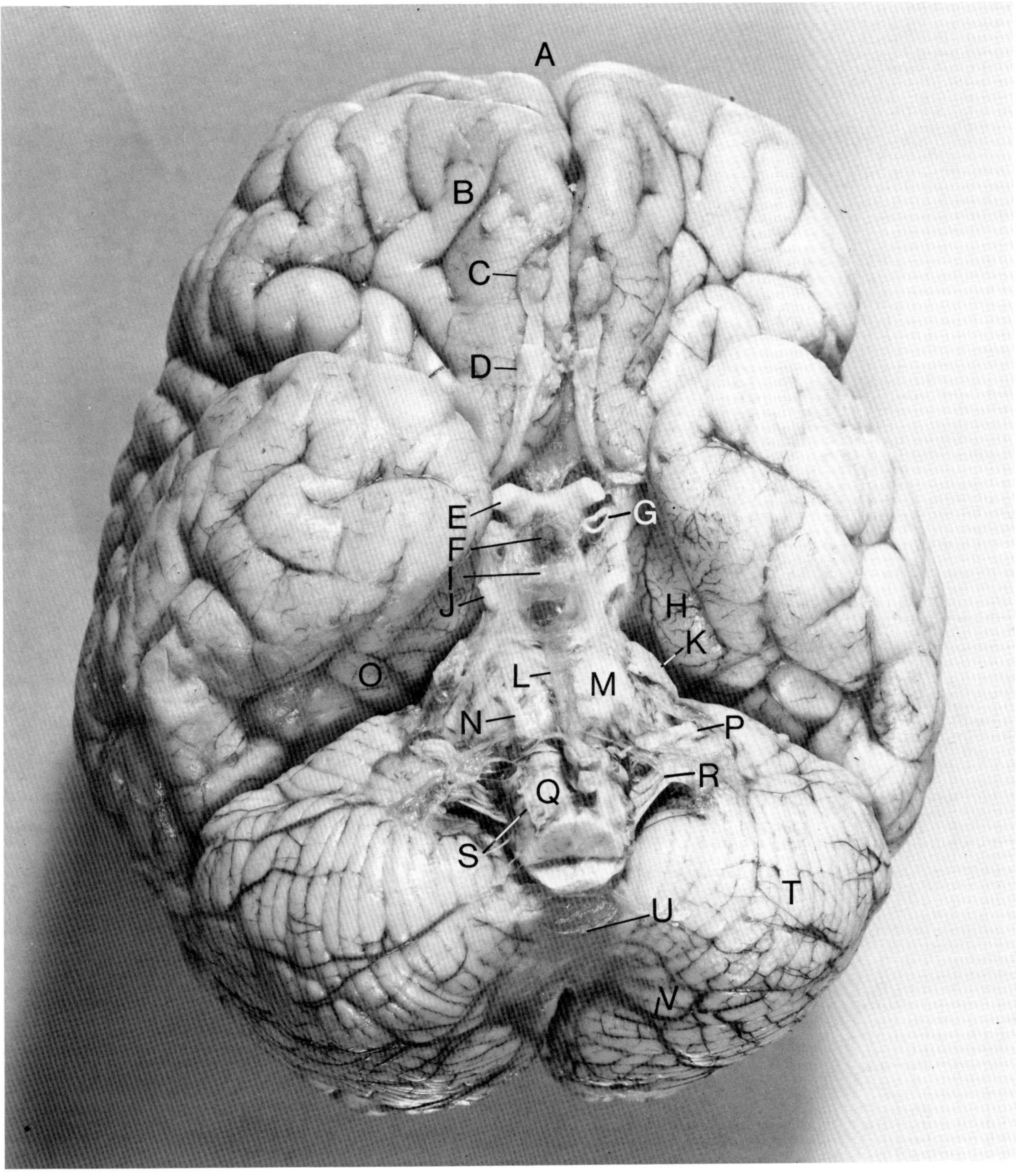
A
B
C
D
E
F
J
G
H
K
O
L
M
N
P
Q
R
S
U
T
V

Figure 2-5. **Operculum and Insula.**

A. A. Central sulcus.
   B. Lateral sulcus.
   C. Postcentral gyrus (parietal) (sensory—area 1 of Brodmann).
   D. Precentral gyrus (frontal) (motor—area 4 of Brodmann).
   E. Pars triangularis of inferior frontal gyrus. See Figures 2-2, 2-3.
   F. Superior temporal gyrus.

B. The upper (frontal and parietal) portions of the operculum, the latter being the part
   of the brain overlying the insula, have been removed, revealing the corresponding
   portion of the insula.
   A. Insula.
   B. Anterior oblique (customarily but incorrectly referred to as anterior tranverse—the
      gyrus extends anterolaterally) temporal gyrus—primary sensory acoustic area
      (41 of Brodmann).

C. The lower (temporal) portion of the operculum also has been removed.

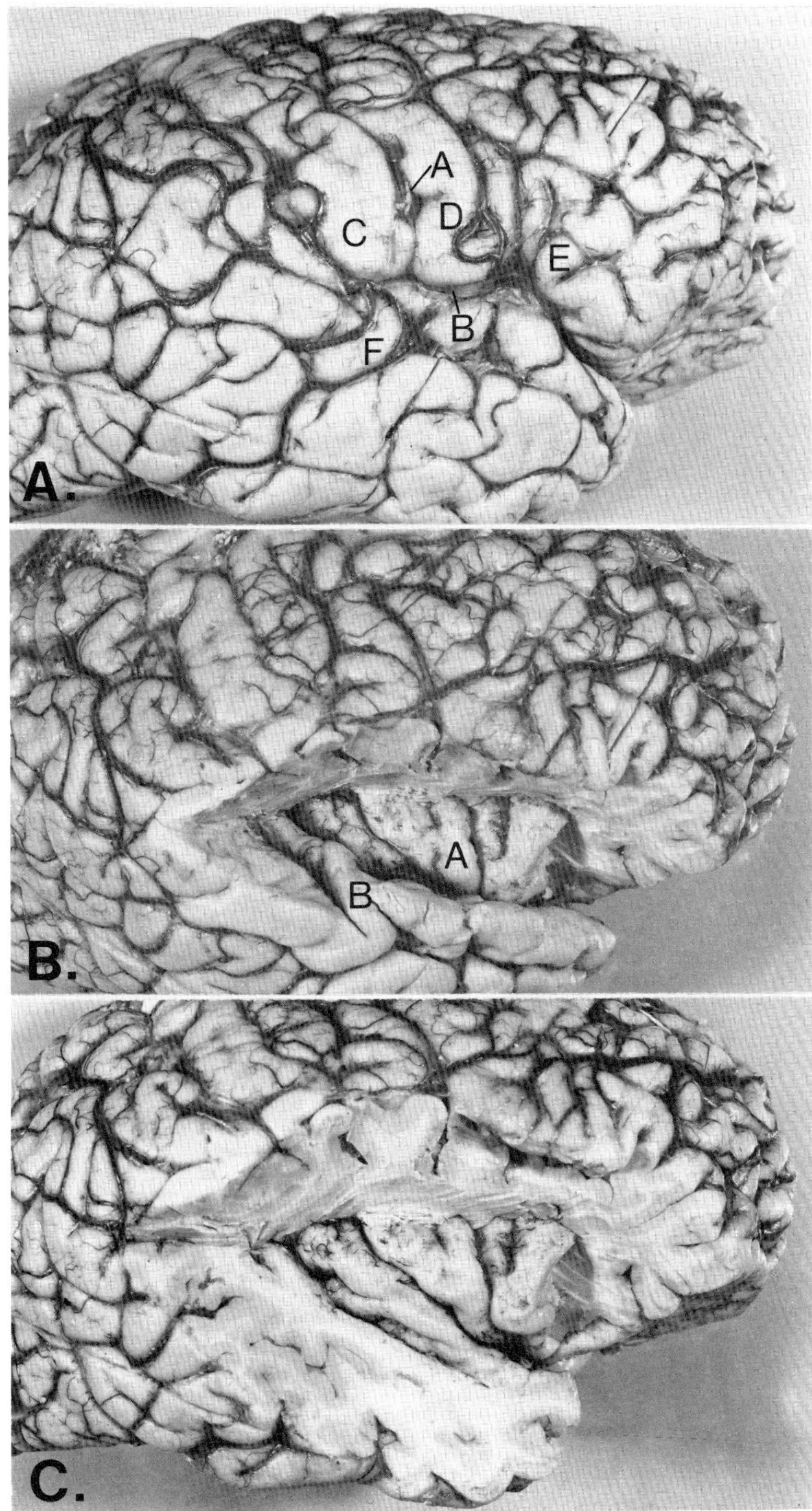

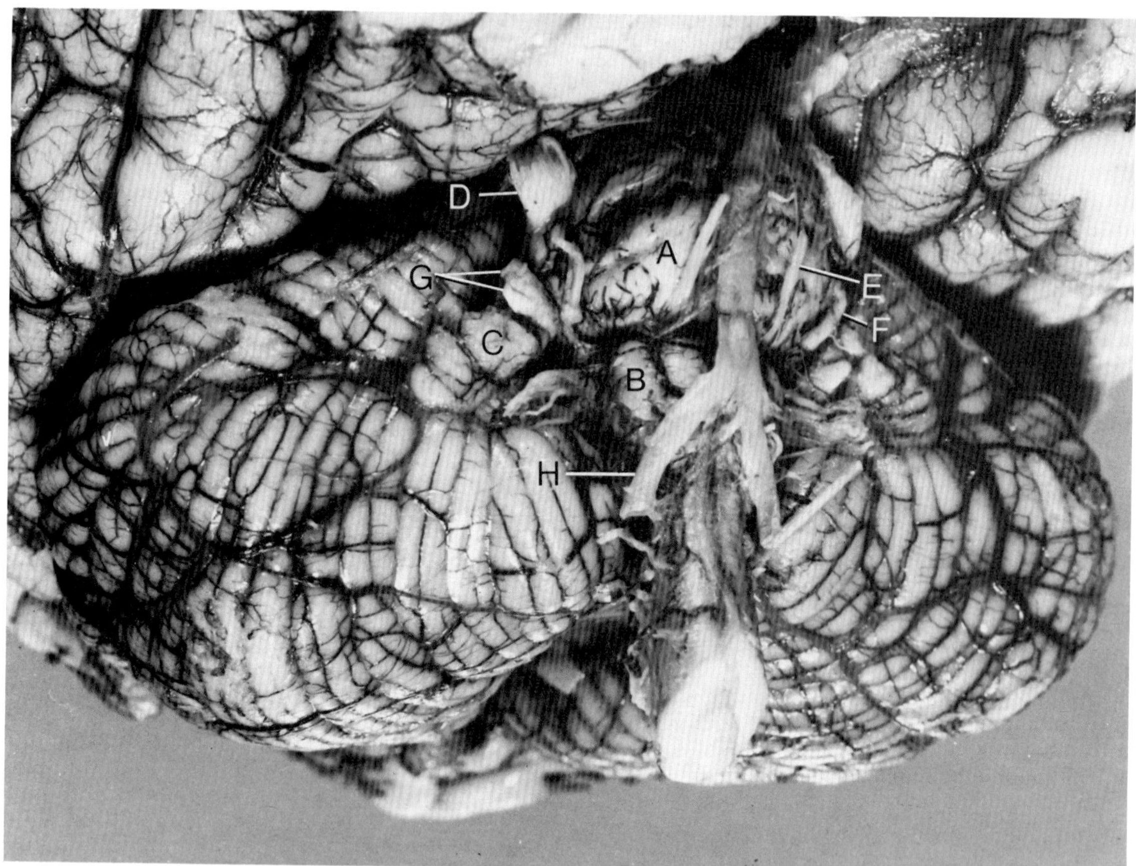

Figure 2-6. **Acoustic Recess.** (So-called "cerebellopontine angle." The recess is a three-dimensional structure.)

A. Pons.
B. Medulla.
C. Cerebellum (flocculus).
D. Trigeminal nerve.
E. Abducens nerve.
F. Facial nerve.
G. Auditory nerve.
H. Vertebral artery.

INTERIOR

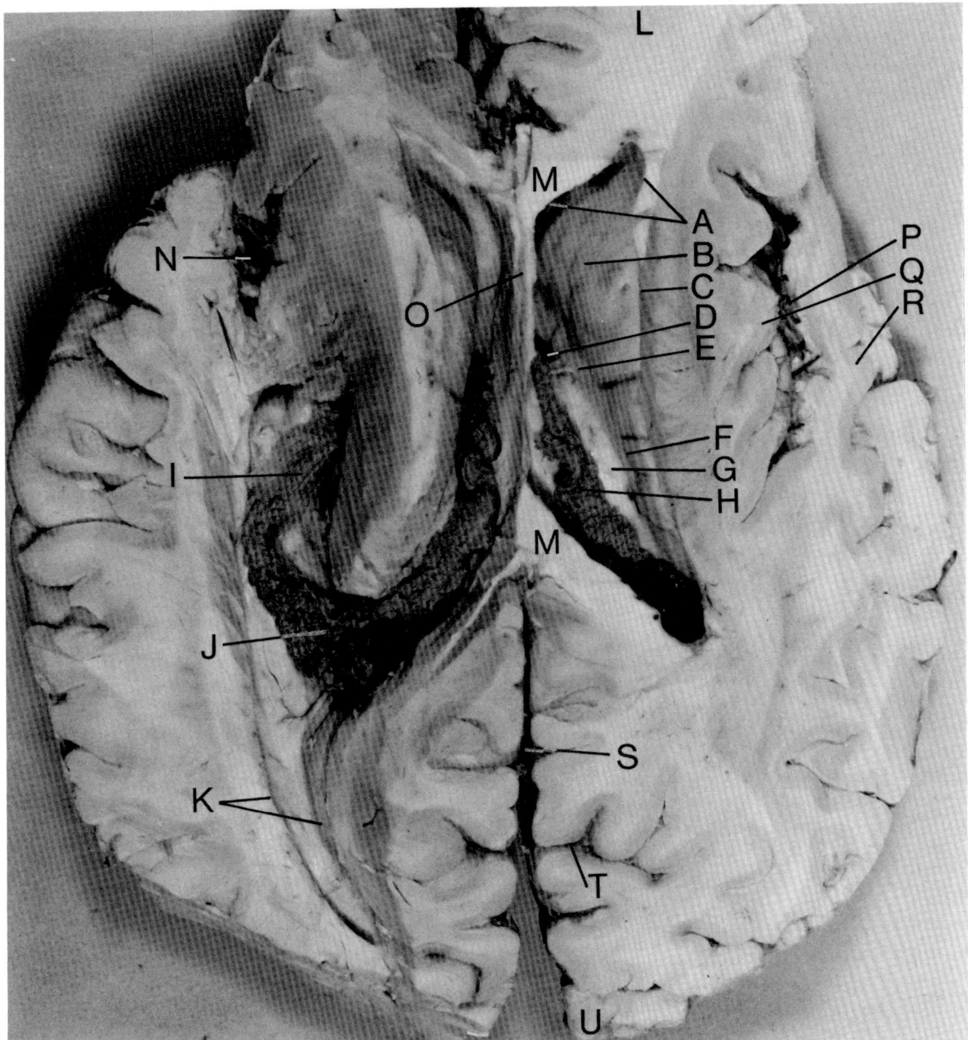

Figure 3-1. **The Lateral Ventricles. Horizontal View.**

A. Anterior horn, walls.

B. Caudate nucleus.

C. Body of lateral ventricle, lateral wall.

D. Interventricular foramen.

E. Thalamostriate vein, turning medially to join choroidal vein in choroid plexus, to form internal cerebral vein. Short final segment of thalamostriate vein is open.

F. Thalamostriate vein, more posteriorly, in thalamostriate groove.

G. Thalamus.

H. Choroid plexus in lateral ventricle.

I. Choroid plexus in temporal horn.

J. Choroid plexus in atrium.

K. Posterior horn walls.

L. Frontal lobe, near pole.

M. Corpus callosum.

N. Lateral sulcus, containing branches of middle cerebral artery.

O. Septum pellucidum.

P. Suprainsular sulcus, containing branches of middle cerebral artery.

Q. Insula.

R. Frontal operculum.

S. Longitudinal fissure.

T. Calcarine sulcus.

U. Occipital pole.

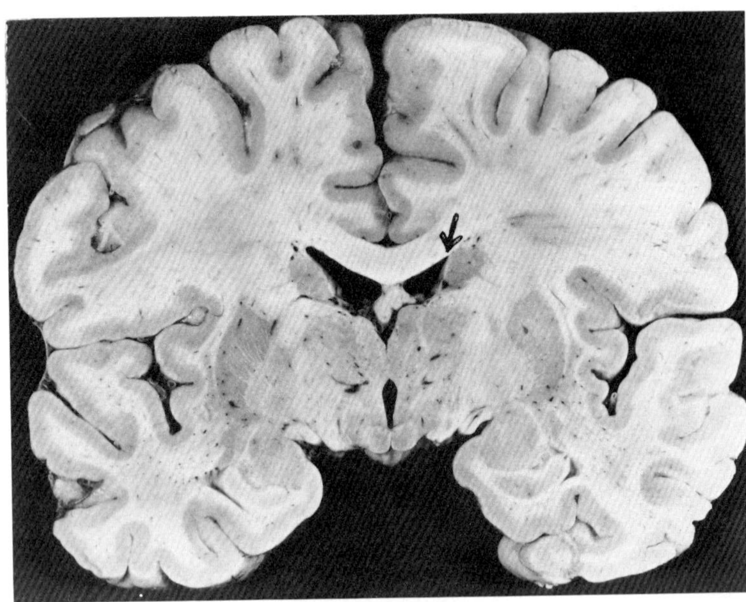

Figure 3-2-1. **Coarctation of Lateral Ventricle** (*arrow*). From Dublin, W. B.: *Fundamentals of Neuropathology,* Ed. II, 1967, Charles C. Thomas, Springfield, Illinois.

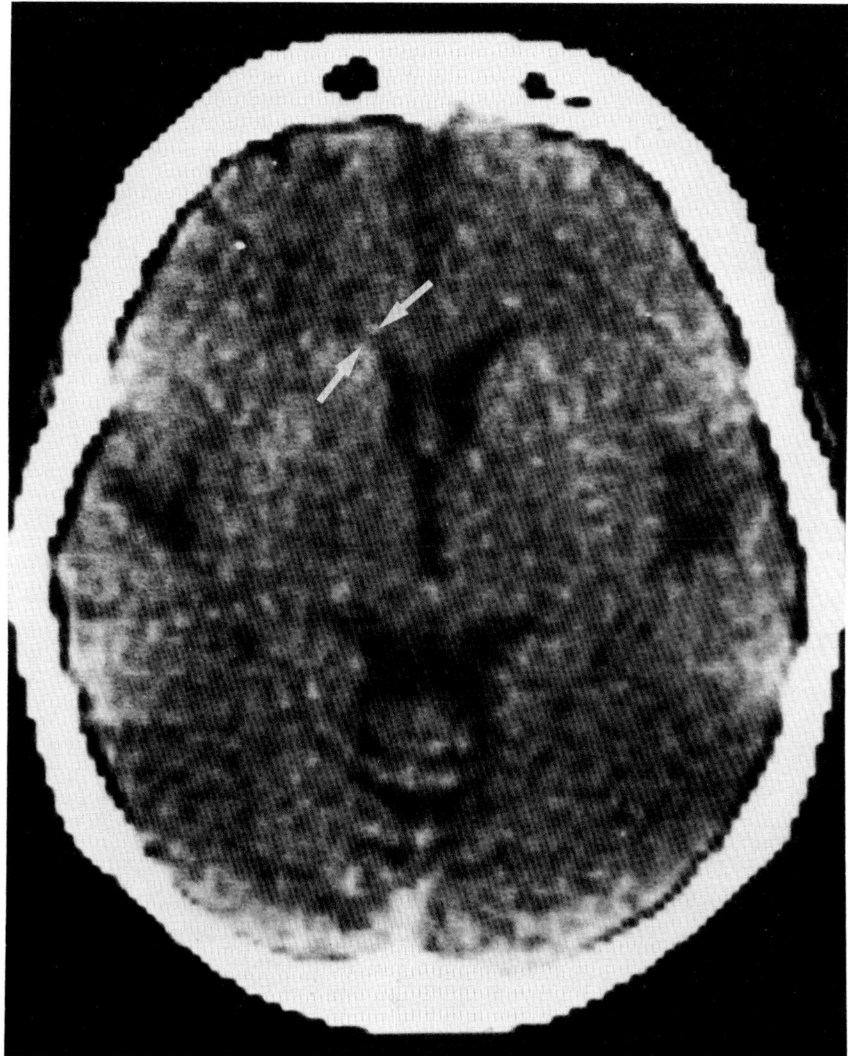

Figure 3-2-2. **Coarctation of Lateral Ventricle—Normal Variant.** Narrowing of one of the anterior horns of the lateral ventricles (arrows) is due to the coarctation or congenital failure of normal ventricular cavitation. This is usually most evident on perfectly centered CT scans, since some rotation of the patient's head may produce artifactual coarctations.

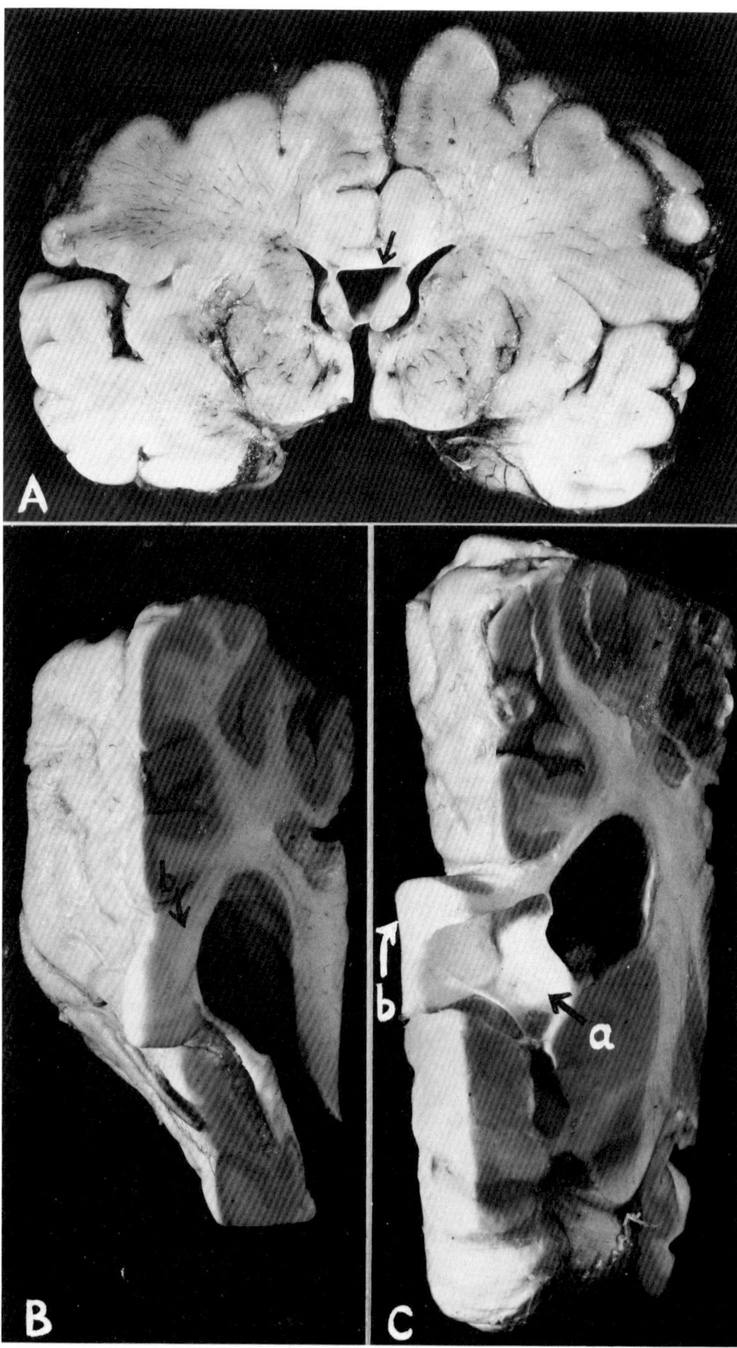

Figure 3-3-1. **Cavum Septi Pellucidi and Cavum Vergae.**
A. Cavum septi pellucidi (*arrow*).
B, C. Cavum Vergae (a). A 1 cm coronal section of brain separates the two sections. The portion of splenium of corpus callosum shown in **B** (b) fits (allowing for the interval section) to the posterior surface of the corresponding structure (b) shown in **C.**
From Dublin, W. B.: *Fundamentals of Neuropathology,* Ed. II, 1967, Charles C. Thomas, Springfield, Illinois.

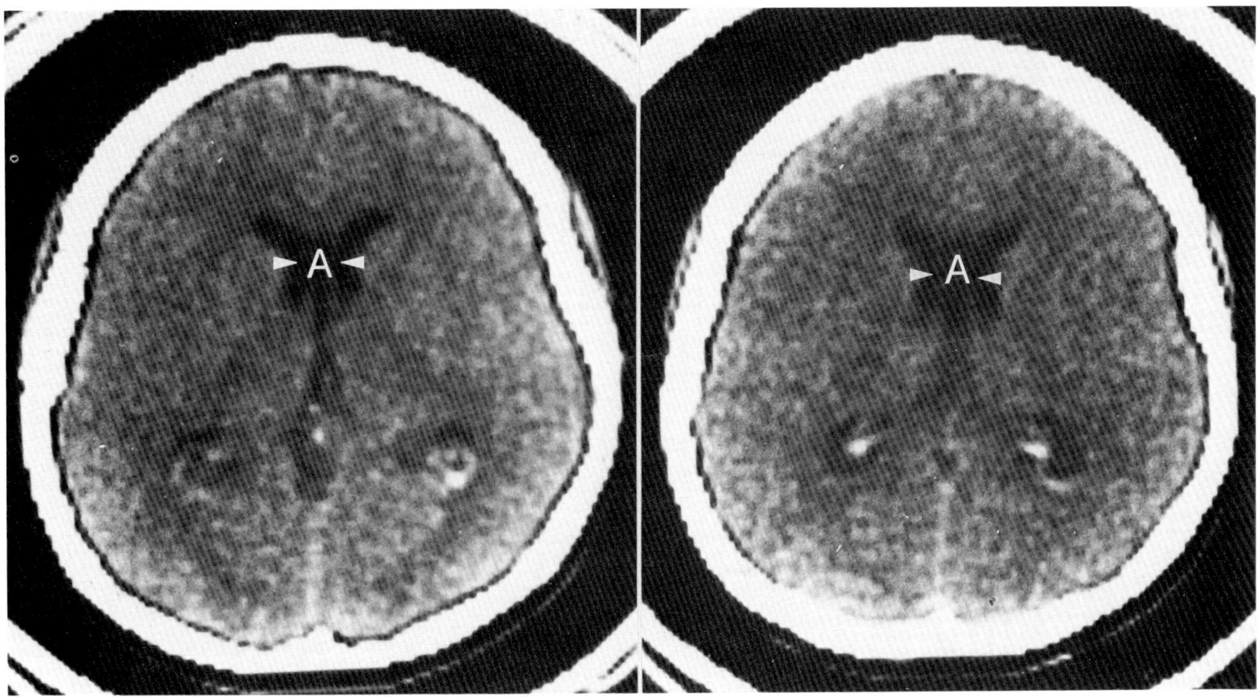

Figure 3-3-2. **Cavum Septi Pellucidi, Computed Tomography.** A cavum septi pellucidi(A), a normal variant, is identified between the anterior lateral ventricles. The lateral extent of the cavum is outlined by arrowheads. Pathological cysts of the septum pellucidum may produce obstructive hydrocephalus of the lateral ventricles, thus distinguishing the pathologic from the normal cavum.

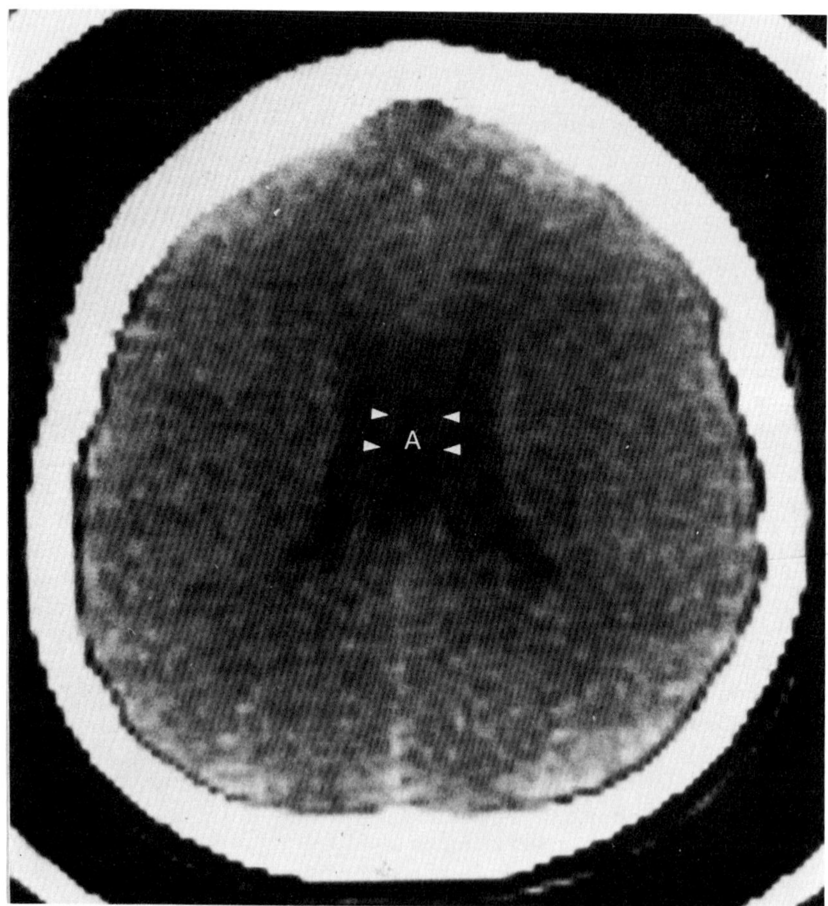

Figure 3-3-3. **Cavum Vergae, Computed Tomography.** A cavum septi pellucidi which extends posteriorly to the level of the interventricular foramina is defined as a cavum vergae (A, with the lateral extent outlined by arrowheads), and is a normal variant.

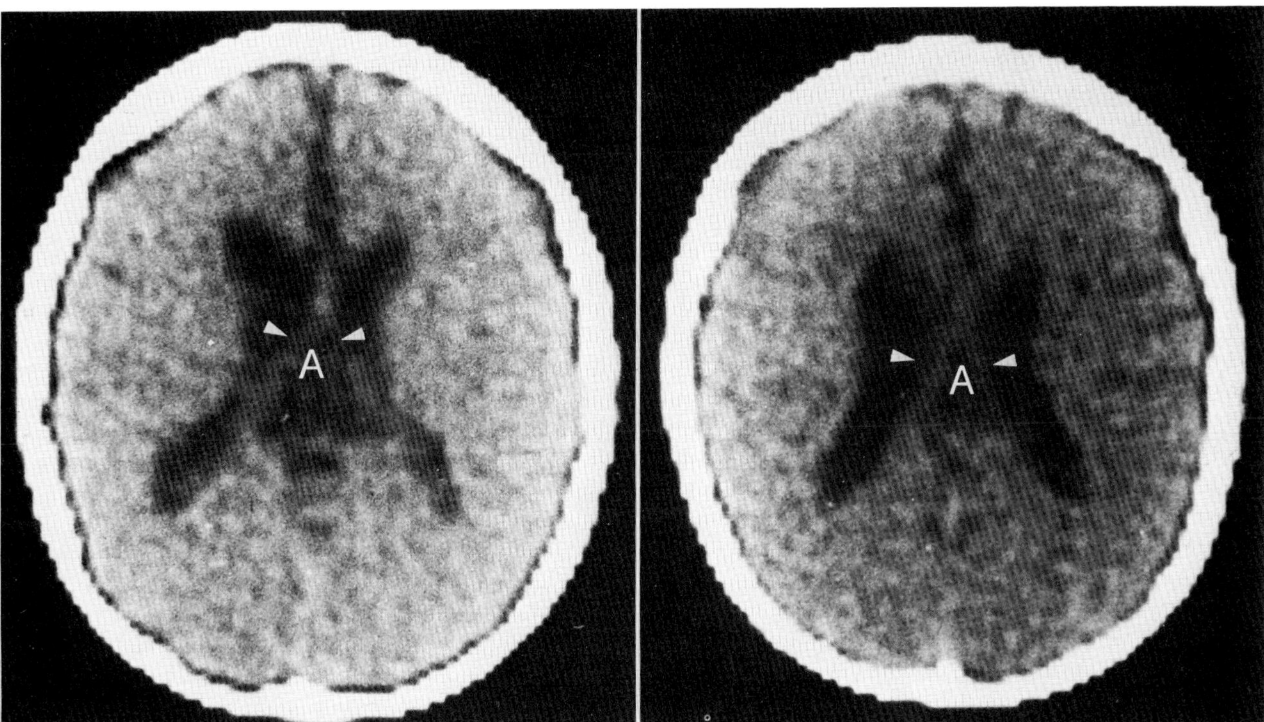

Figure 3-3-4. **Cavum Veli Interpositi, Computed Tomography.** Two sections through the superior portion of the third ventricle demonstrate a triangular-shaped CSF structure which represents the cavum veli interpositi (A), with its lateral extent identified by arrowheads. This cavum or cistern is formed between the pial covering of the roof of the third ventricle, and a second pial layer on the under surface of the corpus callosum. This cavum communicates posteriorly with the superior cerebellar cistern and the cisterns about the pineal gland and great cerebral vein, and is a normal variant.

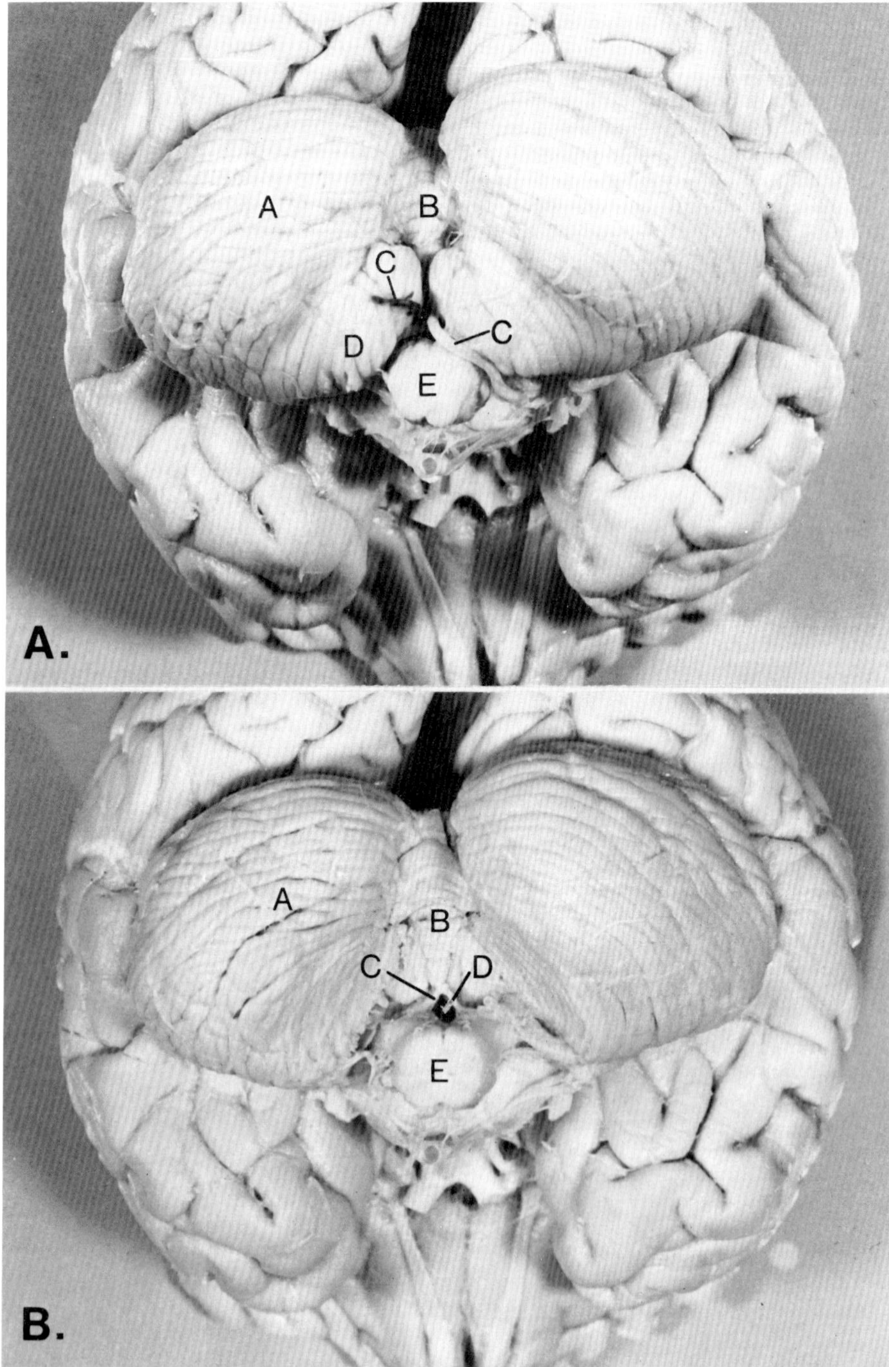

Figure 3-4-1. **Posteroinferior View of Cerebellum and Medulla.**
A. A. Cerebellar hemisphere.
  B. Vermis.
  C. Posterior inferior cerebellar arteries (left, containing blood).
  D. Tonsil (slight coning).
  E. Medulla.
B. Tissue removed to show foramen of Magendie.
  A. Cerebellar hemisphere.
  B. Vermis.
  C. Posterior medullary velum.
  D. Foramen of Magendie.
  E. Medulla.

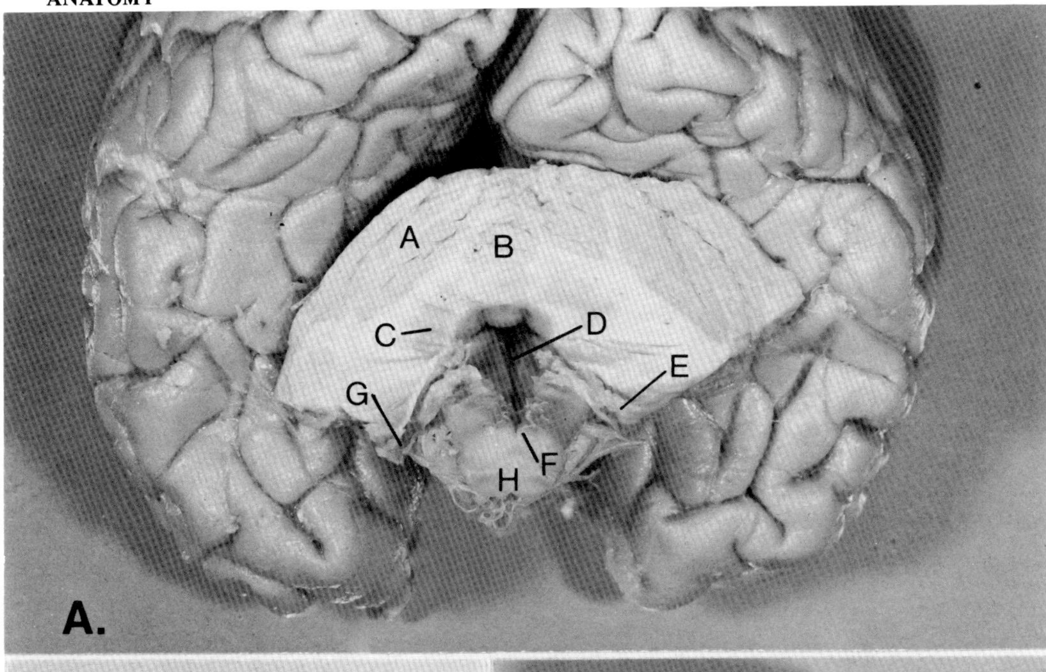

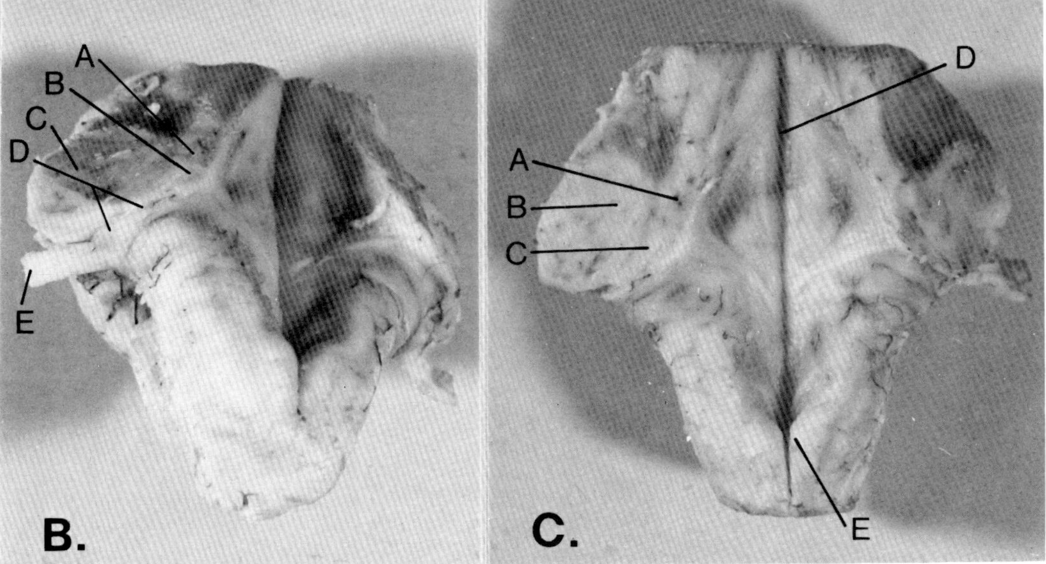

Figure 3-4-2. **Fourth Ventricle.**
A. Continuation of Figure 3-4-1. Added tissue is removed to show the fourth ventricle.
   A. Cerebellar hemisphere.
   B. Vermis.
   C. Dentate nucleus.
   D. Midline, floor of fourth ventricle.
   E. Lateral recess of fourth ventricle, containing choroid plexus.
   F. Obex.
   G. Foramen of Luschka.
   H. Medulla.
B. Oblique view of pontomedullary junction. (With **C,** from a case other than that of **A.**)
   A. Superior cerebellar peduncle.
   B. Inferior cerebellar peduncle.
   C. Middle cerebellar peduncle.
   D. Cochlear nuclei, overlying inferior cerebellar peduncle.
   E. Auditory nerve.
C. A. Superior cerebellar peduncle.
   B. Middle cerebellar peduncle.
   C. Inferior cerebellar peduncle.
   D. Midline, floor of fourth ventricle.
   E. Obex.

$\longrightarrow$

Figure 3-5-1 **Basal Ganglia and Some Surrounding Structures—15° Axial
Sections,** progressing inferiorly.
A. A. Head of caudate nucleus.
   B. Beginning of tail of caudate nucleus.
B. A. Head of caudate nucleus.
   B. Choroid plexus.
   C. Tail of caudate nucleus.
   D. Beginning of posterior horn of lateral ventricle, from atrium.
C. A. Anterior cerebral arteries in longitudinal fissure.
   B. Corpus callosum.
   C. Anterior horn of lateral ventricle.
   D. Head of caudate nucleus.
   E. Body of lateral ventricle.
   F. Internal capsule.
   G. Frontal operculum.
   H. Insula.
   I. Anterior commissure.
   J. Thalamostriate vein.
   K. Putamen.
   L. Thalamus.
   M. Globus pallidus.
   N. Third ventricle.
   O. Middle cerebral artery branch in lateral cerebral sulcus.
   P. Tail of caudate nucleus.
   Q. Lateral geniculate body.
   R. Medial geniculate body.
   S. Choroidal fissure.
   T. Hippocampus.
   U. Choroid plexus in inferior horn of lateral ventricle.
   V. Cerebral aqueduct.
D. A. Corpus callosum.
   B. Anterior horn of lateral ventricle.
   C. Head of caudate nucleus.
   D. Internal capsule.
   E. Thalamostriate vein.
   F. Body of fornix. The septum pellucidum, just above, extends up to the corpus
      callosum.
   G. Putamen.
   H. Globus pallidus.
   I. Thalamus.
   J. Medial geniculate body.
   K. Lateral geniculate body.
   L. Insula.
   M. Middle cerebral artery branch in suprainsular sulcus.
   N. Tail of caudate nucleus.
   O. Choroidal fissure.
   P. Hippocampus.
   Q. Third ventricle.
   R. Cerebral aqueduct.

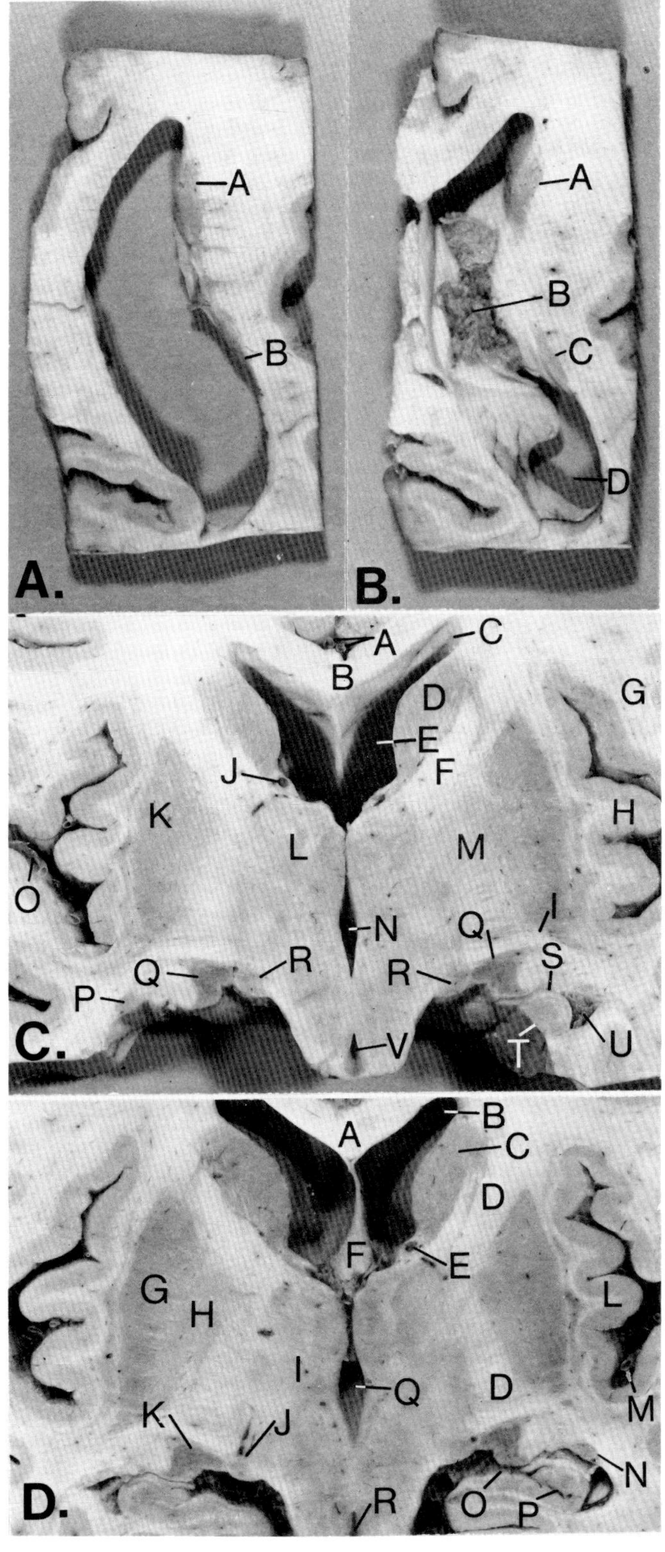

$\rightarrow$

Figure 3-5-2. **Basal Ganglia—15° Axial Sections,** continued.
A. A. Corpus callosum.
    B. Anterior horn of lateral ventricle.
    C. Frontal operculum.
    D. Head of caudate nucleus.
    E. Subcallosal gyrus (paraolfactory area).
    F. Anterior commissure.
    G. Third ventricle.
    H. Mammillothalamic tract.
    I. Mammillary body.
    J. Cerebral peduncle.
    K. Interpeduncular fossa.
    L. Internal capsule.
    M. Putamen.
    N. Globus pallidus.
    O. Claustrum.
    P. Insula.
    Q. Middle cerebral artery branch in suprainsular sulcus.
    R. Lateral sulcus.
    S. Anterior oblique temporal gyrus (see Fig. 2-5).
    T. Tail of caudate nucleus.
    U. Hippocampus.
    V. Posterior cerebral artery.
    W. Superior cerebellar artery.
B. A. Amygdala.
    B. Tail of caudate nucleus.
    C. Ependymal adherence of inferior horn of lateral ventricle (developmental variant).
    D. Inferior horn of lateral ventricle.

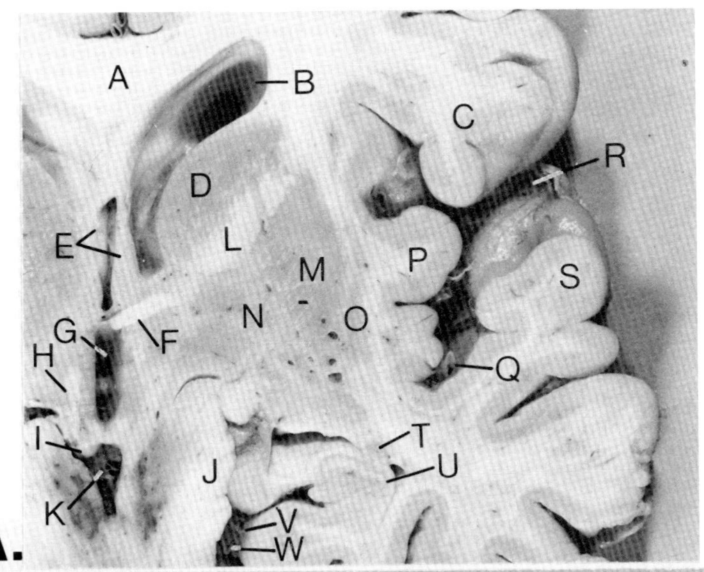
A
B
C
D
E
L
M
P
R
N
O
S
F
G
H
Q
I
K
J
T
U
V
W
A.

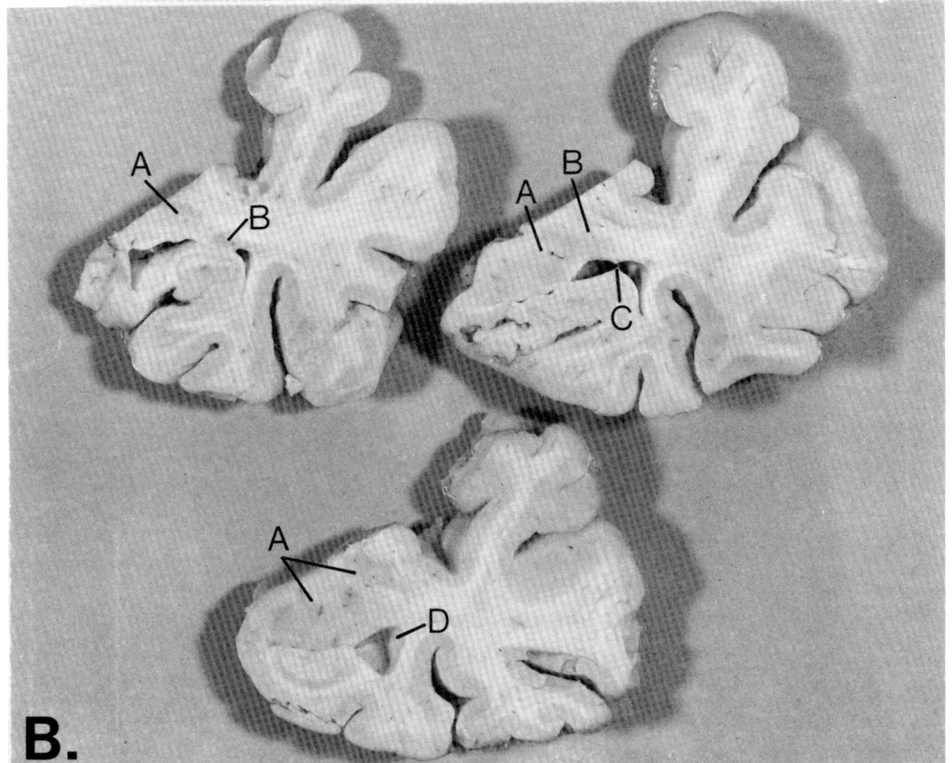
A
B
A
B
C
A
D
B.

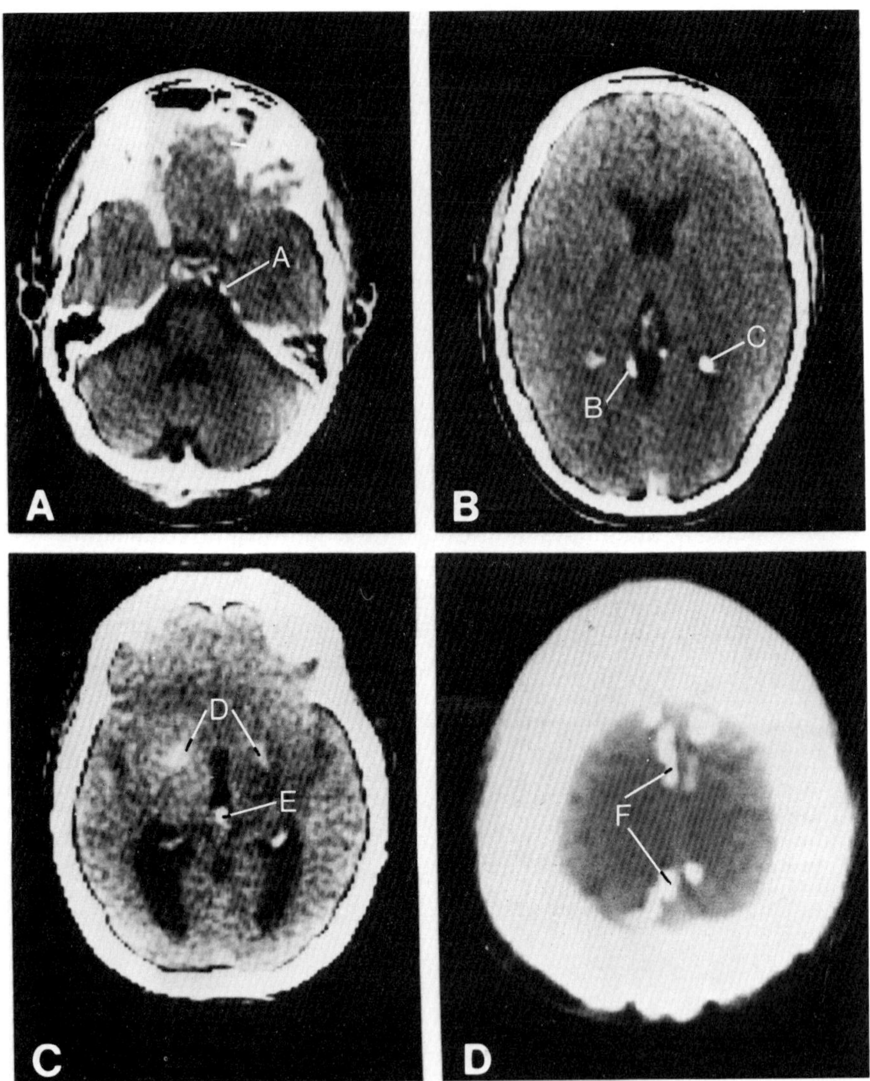

Figure 3-6. **Normal Intracranial Calcification.** Various CT levels (*A-D*) from different patients illustrate normal physiological calcifications. Letters in italics refer to larger letters denoting subdivisions of the illustration. Nonitalicised letters refer to smaller letters that indicate individual structures in the illustration.

A. B. C. D.   A. Petroclinoid.
B. High tentorial hiatus.
C. Choroid (glomus).
D. Globus pallidus.
E. Pineal.
F. Parasagittal dural.

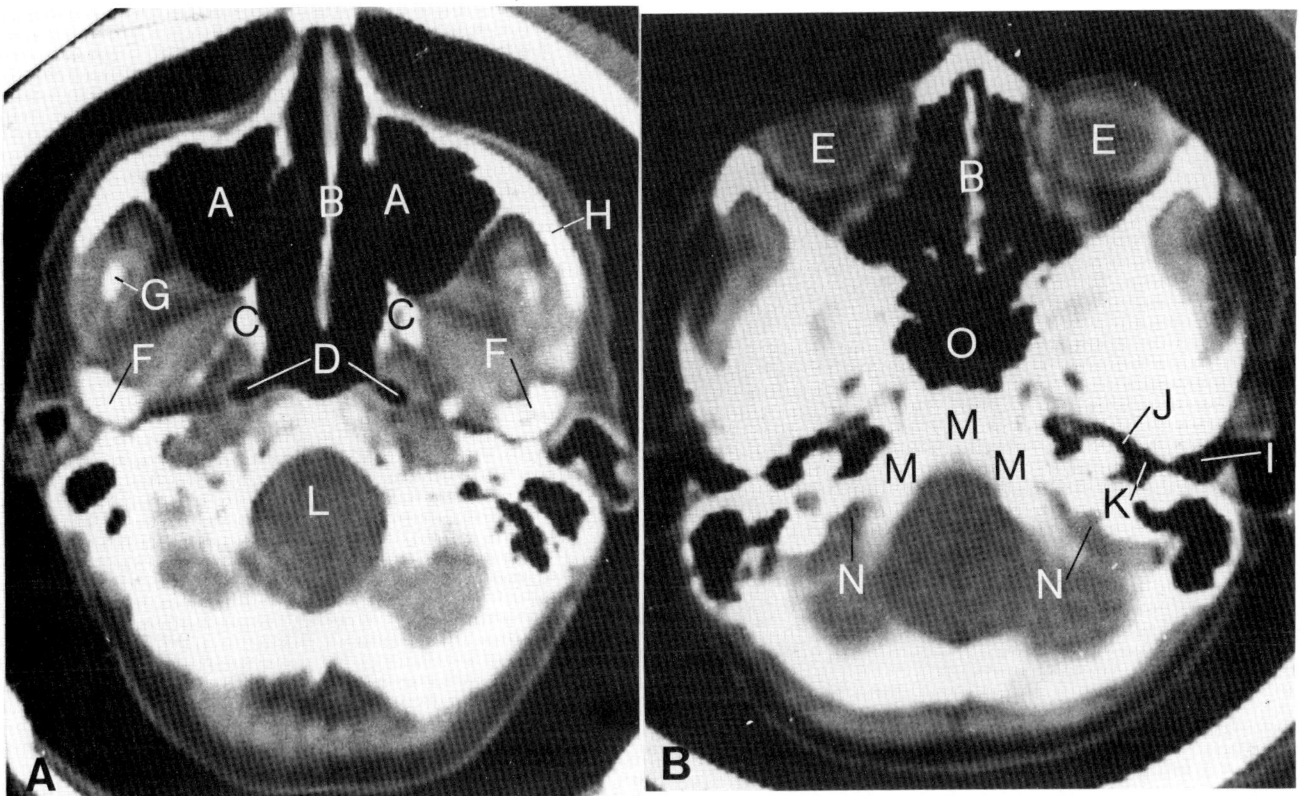

Figure 4-1. **Base of Skull and Upper Nasopharynx, Normal.** Two views (*A, B*) which are caudal and cephalic respectively, demonstrate the following:
A. Maxillary sinus.
B. Nasal septum.
C. Pterygoid plates.
D. Fossa of Rosenmüller.
E. Optic globes.
F. Mandibular condyles.
G. Coronoid process of the mandible.
H. Anterior zygomatic arch.
I. External auditory canal.
J. Eustachian canal.
K. Middle ear.
L. Medulla at level of foramen magnum.
M. Clivus.
N. Upper jugular foramina.
O. Lower sphenoid sinus.

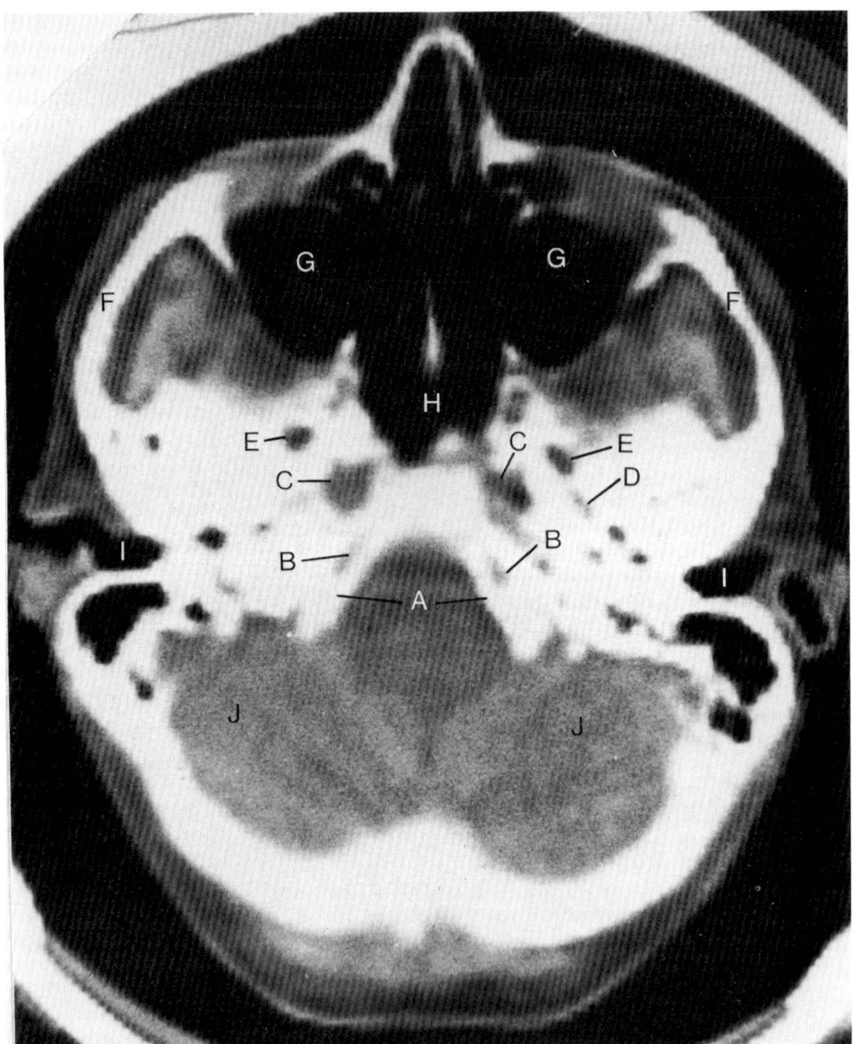

Figure 4-2. **Base of Skull and Upper Nasopharynx, Normal.**
A. Clivus.
B. Hypoglossal canal foramina.
C. Foramen lacerum.
D. Foramen spinosum.
E. Foramen ovale.
F. Zygomatic arches.
G. Maxillary sinuses.
H. Sphenoid sinus.
I. External auditory canals.
J. Cerebellum.

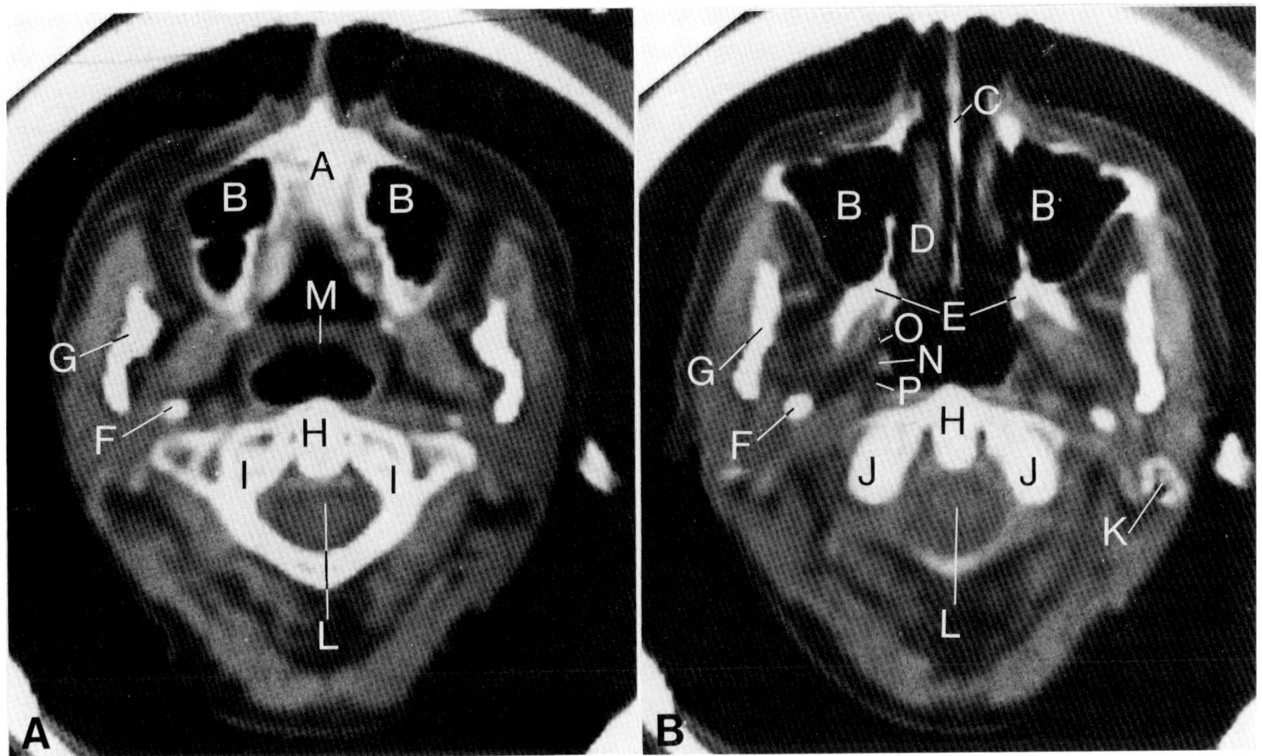

Figure 4-3. **Normal Nasopharynx and Base Views of the Skull.**

A. Maxilla.
B. Maxillary sinuses.
C. Nasal septum.
D. Nasal turbinate.
E. Pterygoid plates.
F. Styloid process.
G. Mandible.
H. Odontoid (dens).
I. C-1 vertebral body.
J. Atlanto-occipital articulation.
K. Mastoid tip.
L. Combination of cervical spinal cord and CSF.
M. Soft palate.
N. Torus tubarus.
O. Eustachian tube orifice.
P. Fossa of Rosenmüller.

CISTERNS—CSF FLOW

→

Figure 5-1. **Cisterns, as seen in Sagittal View.**
A. Cerebellomedullary cistern (cisterna magna).
B. Arachnoid over the cistern.
C. Quadrigeminal cistern.
D. Pineal cistern.
E. Cistern of great cerebral vein.
F. Superior cerebellar cistern.
G. Cistern of corpus callosum.
H. Cistern of lamina terminalis.
I. Chiasmatic cistern.
J. Interpeduncular cistern.
K. Pontine cistern.
L. Superior frontal gyrus.
M. Callosomarginal artery. (Atypical course is illustrated.)
N. Cingulate gyrus.
O. Superior superficial cerebral vein, opening into superior sagittal sinus, at P.
Q. Occipitoparietal sulcus and artery.
R. Calcarine sulcus and artery.
S. Choroid plexus in interventricular foramen.
T. Internal cerebral vein (open).
U. Frontal pole.
V. Occipital pole.
W. Temporal pole.
X. Approximate position of central sulcus—point of demarcation between frontal and parietal lobes.
Y. Point of demarcation between parietal and occipital lobes (in addition to Q, and with reference to lateral surface.
Z. Corpus callosum.

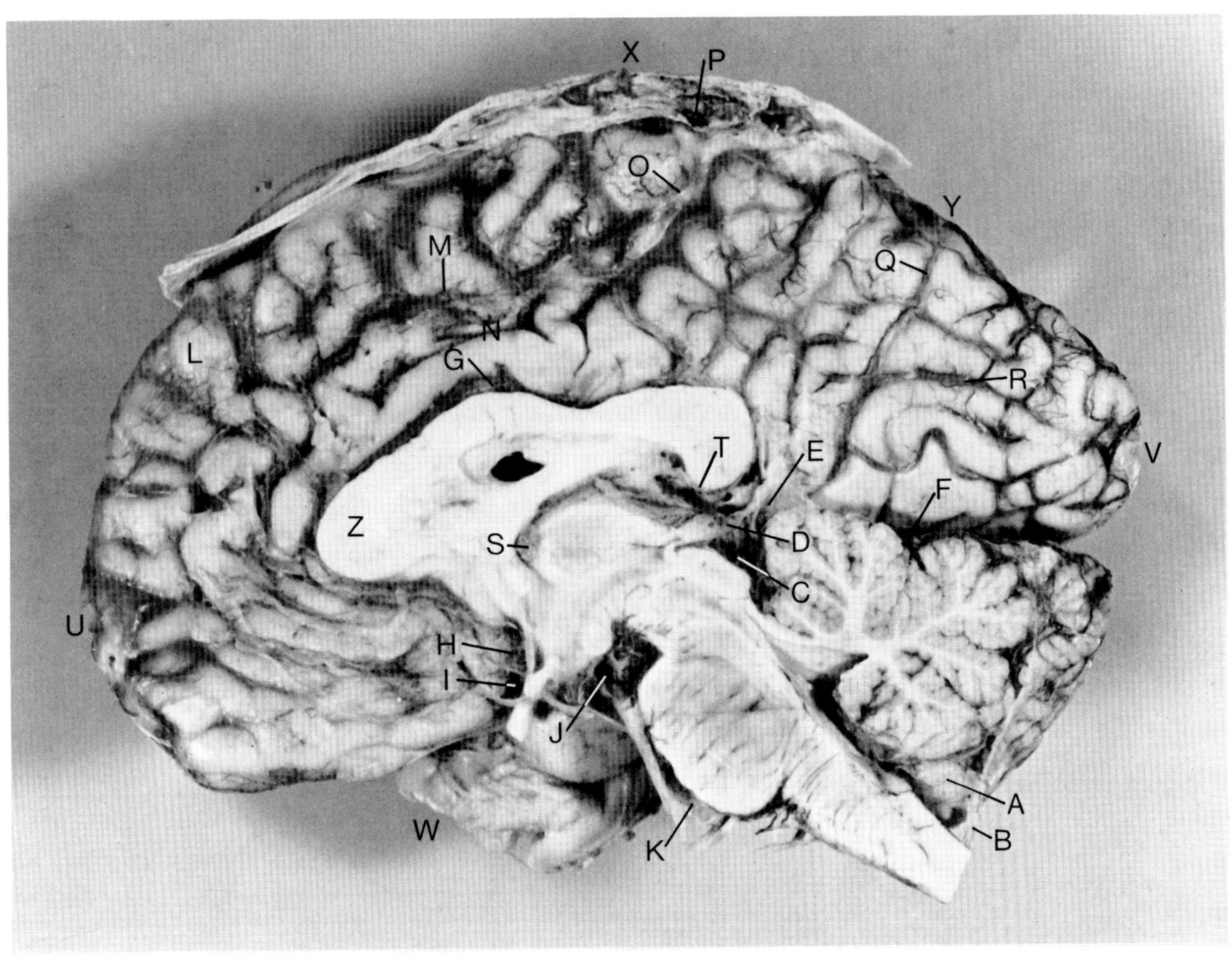
X
P
O
M
Y
N
Q
L
G
R
T
E
V
Z
D
S
F
C
U
H
I
J
A
W
K
B

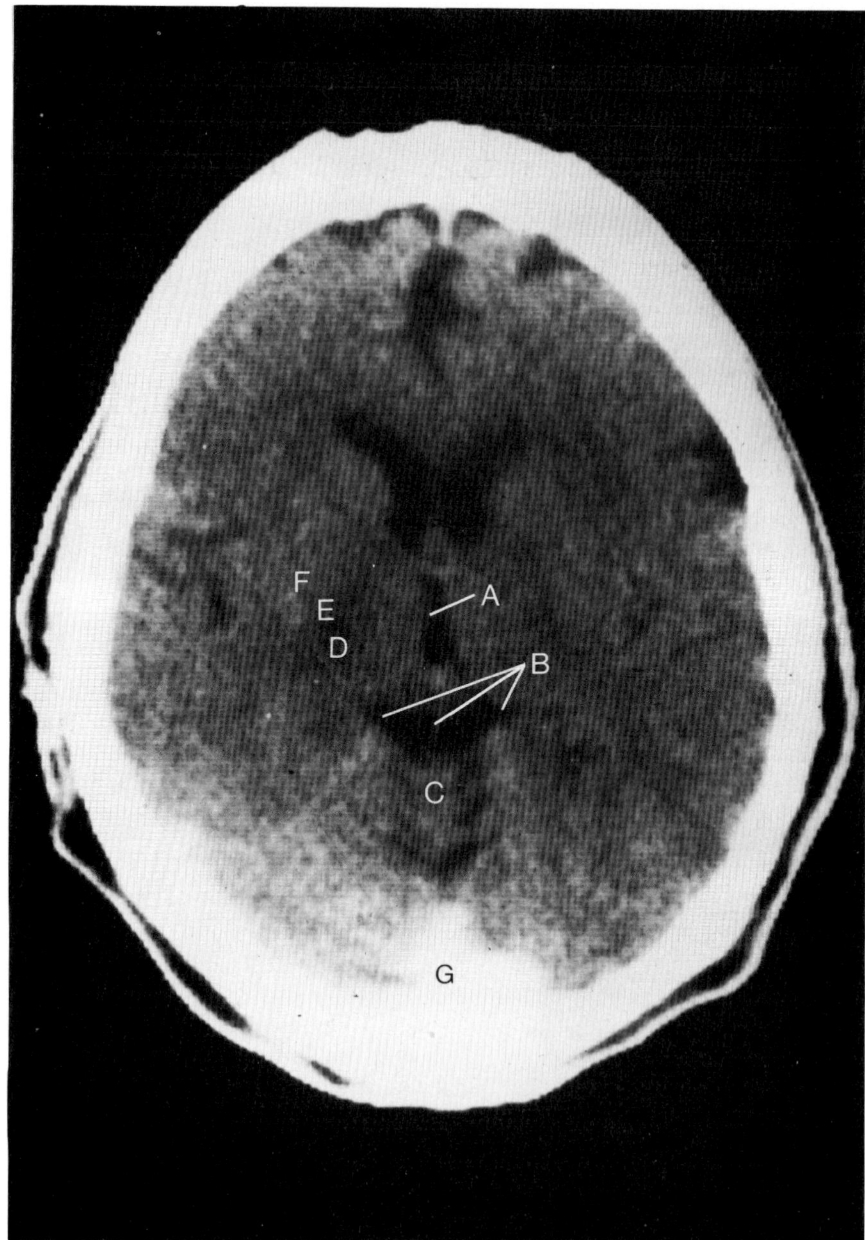

Figure 5-2. **Normal Cerebrospinal Fluid Anatomy, "The Dagger Sign."** A post contrast axial section demonstrates a dagger-like configuration made up of several CSF structures.

- A. Third ventricle (the handle).
- B. Lateral aspects, retropulvinar cisterns. Midline aspects, great cerebal vein and pineal cisterns (the hilt).
- C. Cerebellar vermis in the superior cerebellar cistern (the blade).
- D. Thalamus.
- E. Posterior internal capsule.
- F. Lenticular nucleus.
- G. Torcular Herophili.

Enlargement of the blade coincides with cerebellar atrophy. A large handle is often associated with hydrocephalus. Obliteration of the hilt suggests, among other things, mass effects in the thalami, lateral ventricles, cerebellum (i.e., upward herniation through the tentorial hiatus), collicular plate or tegmentum, and pineal gland.

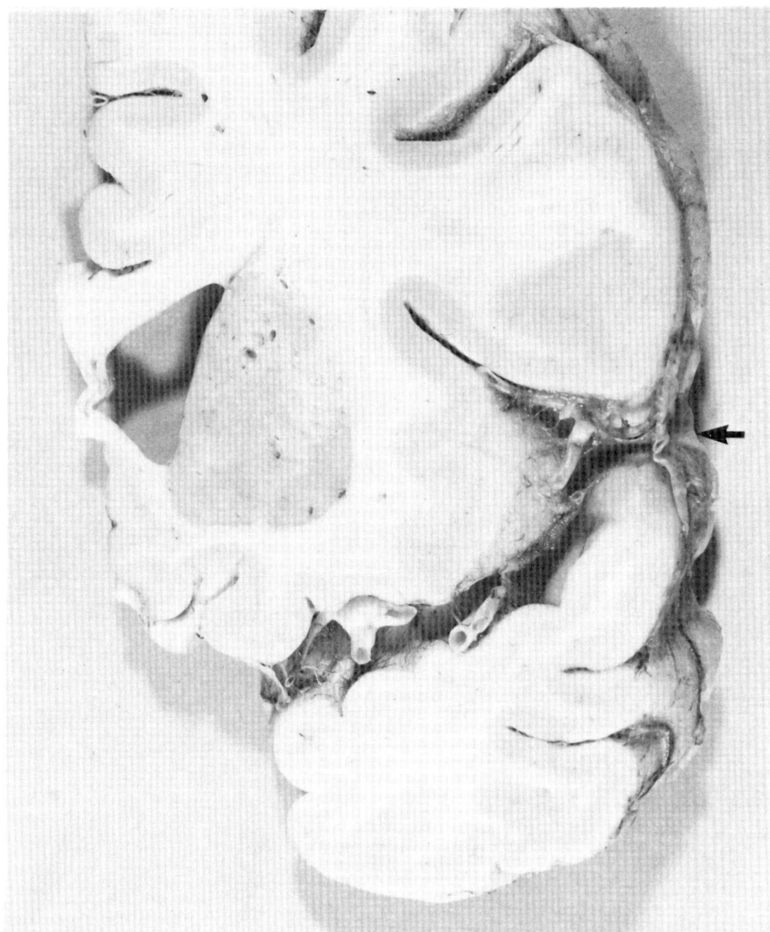

Figure 5-3. **Cistern of Lateral Sulcus.** The cistern contains branches of the middle cerebral artery. It is covered by arachnoid (*arrow*).

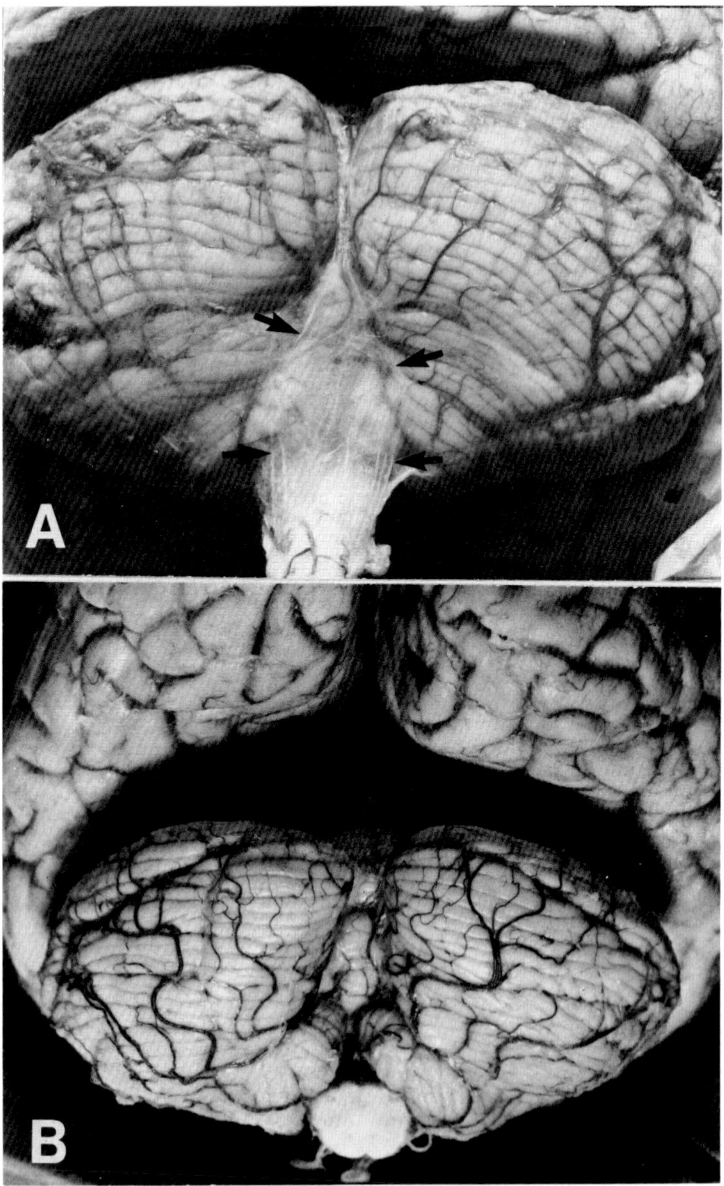

Figure 5-4. **Cerebellomedullary Cistern (Cistern Magna).**
A. With arachnoid in place. Arrows indicate lateral margins of the cistern.
B. With arachnoid removed.

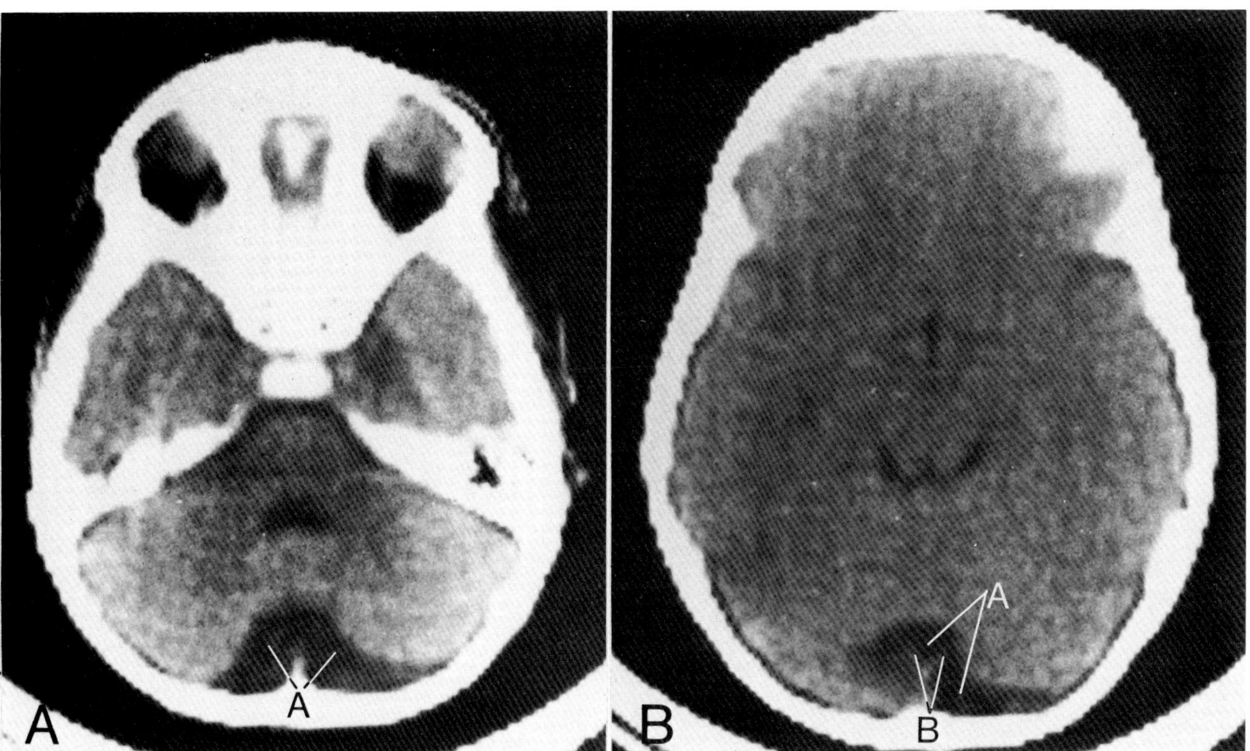

Figure 5-5. **Normal Cerebellomedullary Cistern.** Two CT levels **A-B** caudal to
cephalad), demonstrate a large cisterna magna (A) with some superior extension
through the tentorium (B), a normal variant.

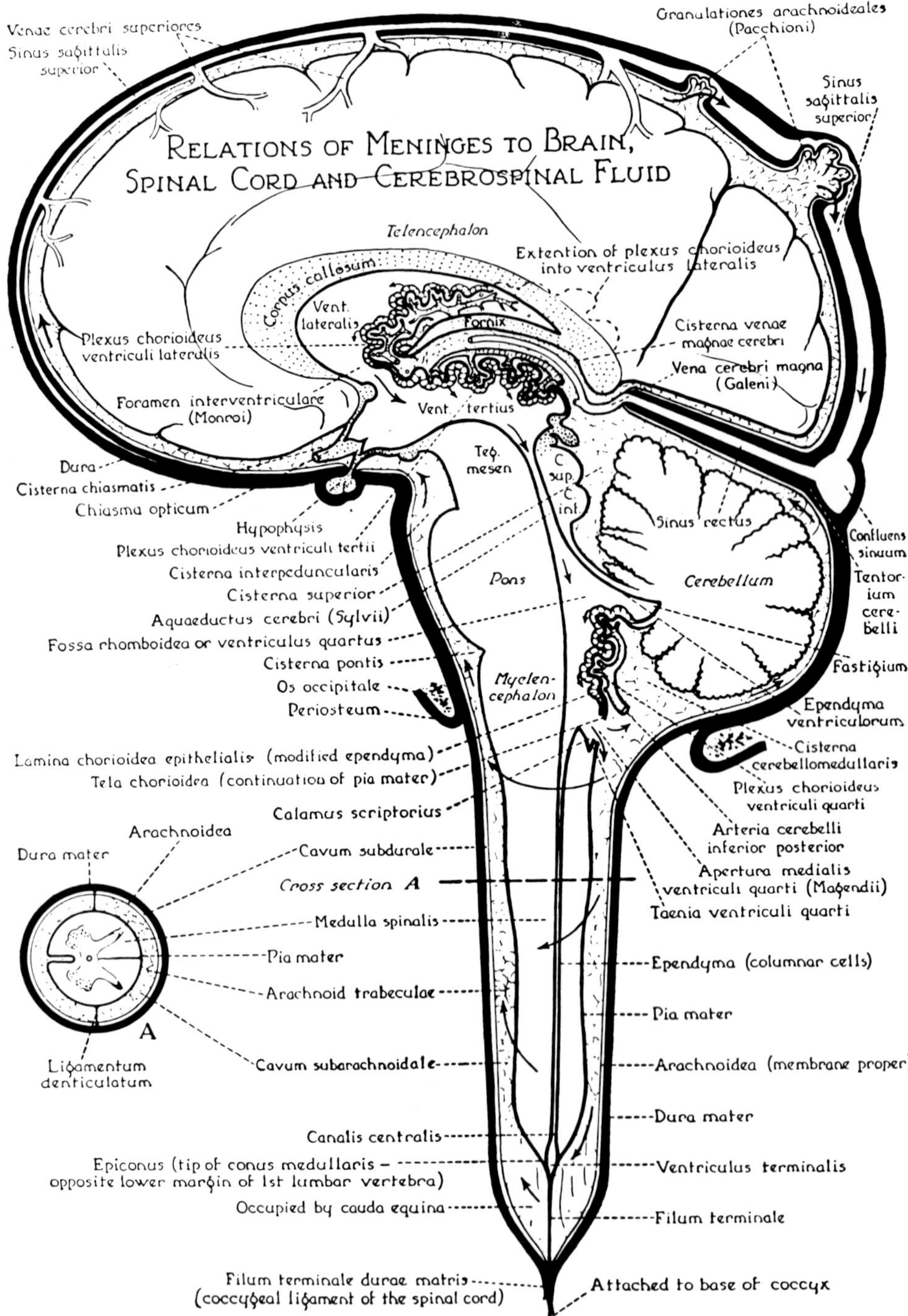

Figure 5-6. **The Relations of the Meninges to the Brain, Spinal Cord, and Cerebrospinal Fluid.** After Gray, H.: *Anatomy of the Human Body,* Ed., XXVIII, Goss, C. M., Ed., 1966, Lea and Febiger, Philadelphia; from Rasmussen, A. T.: *The Principal Nervous Pathways,* the Macmillan Company.

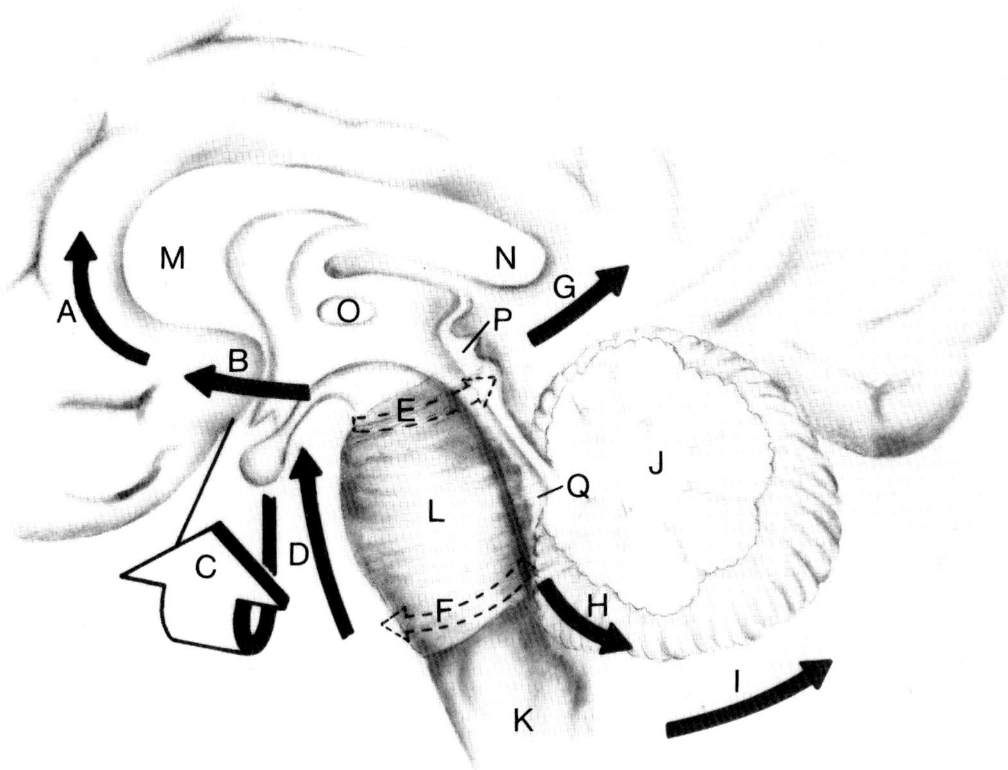

Figure 5-7. **Schematic Representation of Midline and Basal Cisterns.** A schematic drawing through a sagittal view of the brain demonstrates the following major cisterns as represented by lettered figures adjacent to arrows, the latter of which represent directional flow; included are also major anatomic structures.

A. Anterior longitudinal fissure/pericallosal cistern.

B. Suprasellar (chiasmatic) cistern running forward into the cistern of the lamina terminalis (located just in front of the anterior inferior third ventricle).

C. Cistern of the middle cerebral artery extending into the proximal suprainsular cistern.

D. Prepontine cistern, extending superiorly into the interpeduncular cistern.

E. Perimesencephalic cistern.

F. Peripontine cistern.

G. Quadrigeminal cistern extending superiorly into the great cerebral vein and pineal cisterns.

H. CSF in the vallecula medial to the cerebellar tonsils.

I. Cerebellomedullary cistern.

J. Cerebellum.

K. Medulla.

L. Pons.

M. Genu of the corpus callosum.

N. Splenium of the corpus callosum.

O. Third ventricle.

P. Quadrigeminal plate.

Q. Fourth ventricle.

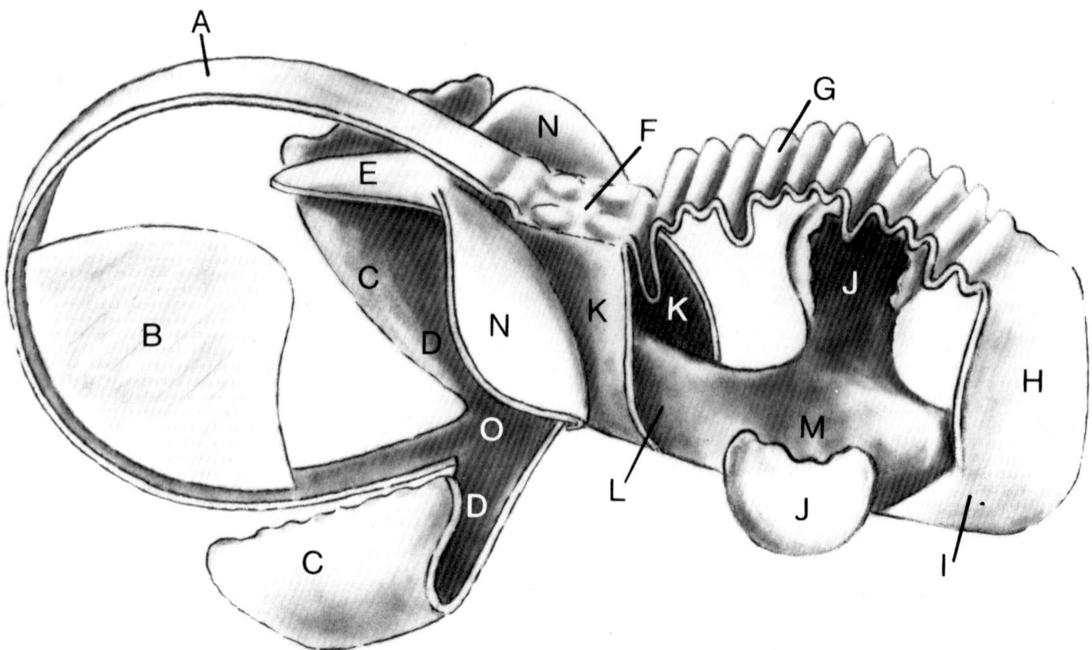

Figure 5-8. **Major Cerebrospinal Fluid Cisterns.** A highly schematic composite drawing of the major cerebrospinal cisterns is seen from the left and slightly above.

A. Pericallosal cistern.
B. Cavum septi pellucidi.
C. Suprainsular cistern.
D. Cistern of the middle cerebral artery.
E. Cavum veli interpositi.
F. Collicular cistern (shown very diagramatically, folded over the collicular plate).
G. Superior cerebellar cistern
H. Cerebellomedullary cistern.
I. Lateral medullary cistern.
J. Cistern of acoustic recess.
K. Perimesencephalic or circum-mesencephalic (ambient) cistern.
L. Prepeduncular cistern (crural cistern).
M. Prepontine cistern.
N. Retropulvinar (wing of ambient) cistern.
O. Suprasellar (chiasmatic) cistern.

Modified, after Hodges, F. J., III: Anatomy of the Ventricles and Subarachnoid Space, in: *Seminars in Roentgenology,* vol. 5, 1970, Grune and Stratton, New York.

CRANIAL NERVES

with

Visual Pathway

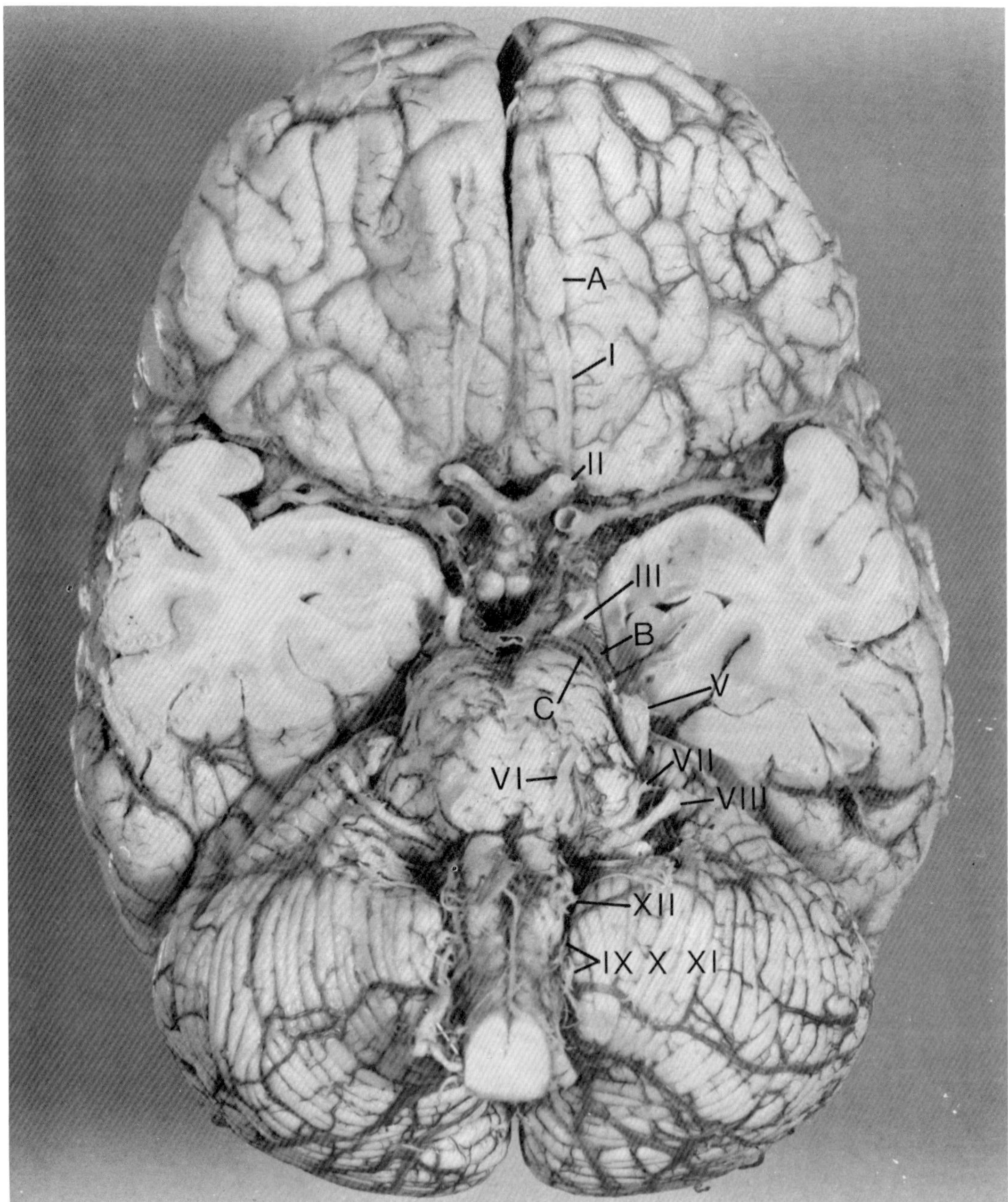

Figure 6-1. **Cranial Nerves, as seen in View of Base of Brain.**
     I. Olfactory tract (A, olfactory bulb).
    II. Optic nerve.
   III. Oculomotor nerve. It passes between the posterior cerebral (B) and superior cerebellar (C) arteries.
   IV. The trochlear nerve is shown in a special preparation (see Fig. 6-5).
    V. Trigeminal nerve.
   VI. Abducens nerve.
  VII. Facial nerve.
 VIII. Auditory nerve.
IX, X, XI. The glossopharyngeal, vagus and accessory nerve rootlets emerge from the medulla just dorsal to the ventral olivary nucleus.
  XII. The hypoglossal nerve rootlets emerge between the olive and the pyramid.

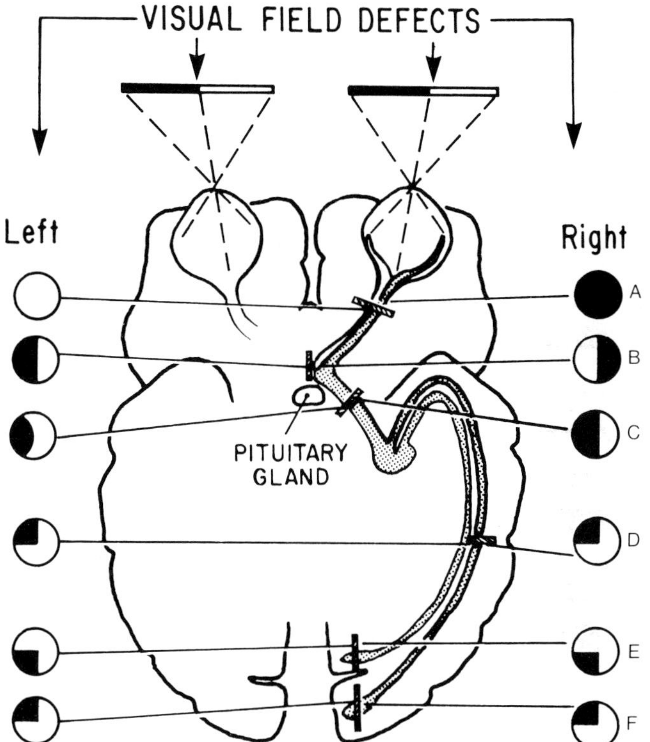

Figure 6-2. **Schematic Diagram of Visual Pathway with Illustrative Pathologic Defects.** An axial section through the orbits and brain demonstrates the normal visual pathway with appropriate visual field defects. A small circle with darkened areas represents the field defects as the patient sees the field testing objects.

A. Optic nerve defect, right field blindness.

B. Optic chiasm defect (typical pituitary tumor), bitemporal hemianopia.

C. Optic tract defect, incongruous homonomous hemianopia.

D. Partial optic radiation defect, homonomous quadrantanopia.

E. and F. Calcarine defects, inferior or superior homonomous quadrantanopia, depending upon the defect.

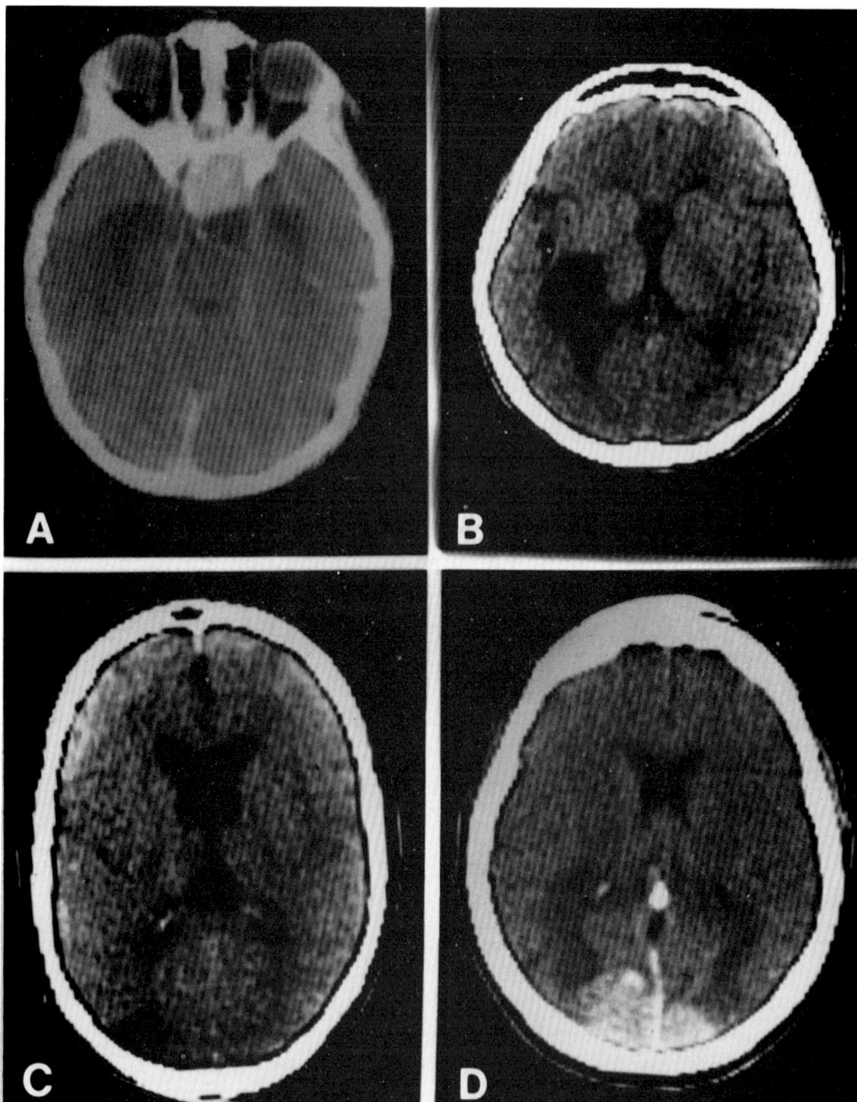

Figure 6-3. **Examples of Lesions Along the Visual Pathway.** (For application to anatomy.) **A.** An ovoid enhancing lesion is seen superimposed within the chiasmatic cistern with some destruction of the anterior clinoids. This represents an optic chiasmatic glioma which resulted in severe bilateral field defects, with predominance of bitemporal hemianopia. **B.** An area of porencephaly adjacent to the atrium of the left lateral ventricle resulted in a right homonomous hemianopia. The etiology of the lesion is unclear, but was thought to be congenital. **C.** A wedge-shaped area representing an infarct is seen in the left occipital lobe resulting in a disassociated visual optic defect, and a right quadrant homonomous hemianopia. **D.** Bilateral enhancing lesions are seen in each occipital pole, representing metastases from the breast. The patient had severe central macular defects as well as bilateral homonomous incongruous field defects.

Figure 6-4-1. **Normal Orbital Views, Coronal and Axial** *(A-H).* (See pages 56 and 57.)

Figure 6-4-1. **Normal Orbital Views, Coronal and Axial** (*A-H*). The following letters A-N refer to small capitals denoting individual structures in the illustrations.

A. Lens.
B. Superior oblique muscle.
C. Optic globe.
D. Medial rectus muscle.
E. Levator palpebrae muscle.
F. Superior rectus muscle.
G. Lacrimal gland.
H. Inferior oblique and inferior rectus muscle group.
I. Superior ophthalmic vein.
J. Optic nerve.
K. Maxillary sinus.
L. Lateral rectus muscle.
M. Superior orbital fissure.
N. Inferior orbital fissure.

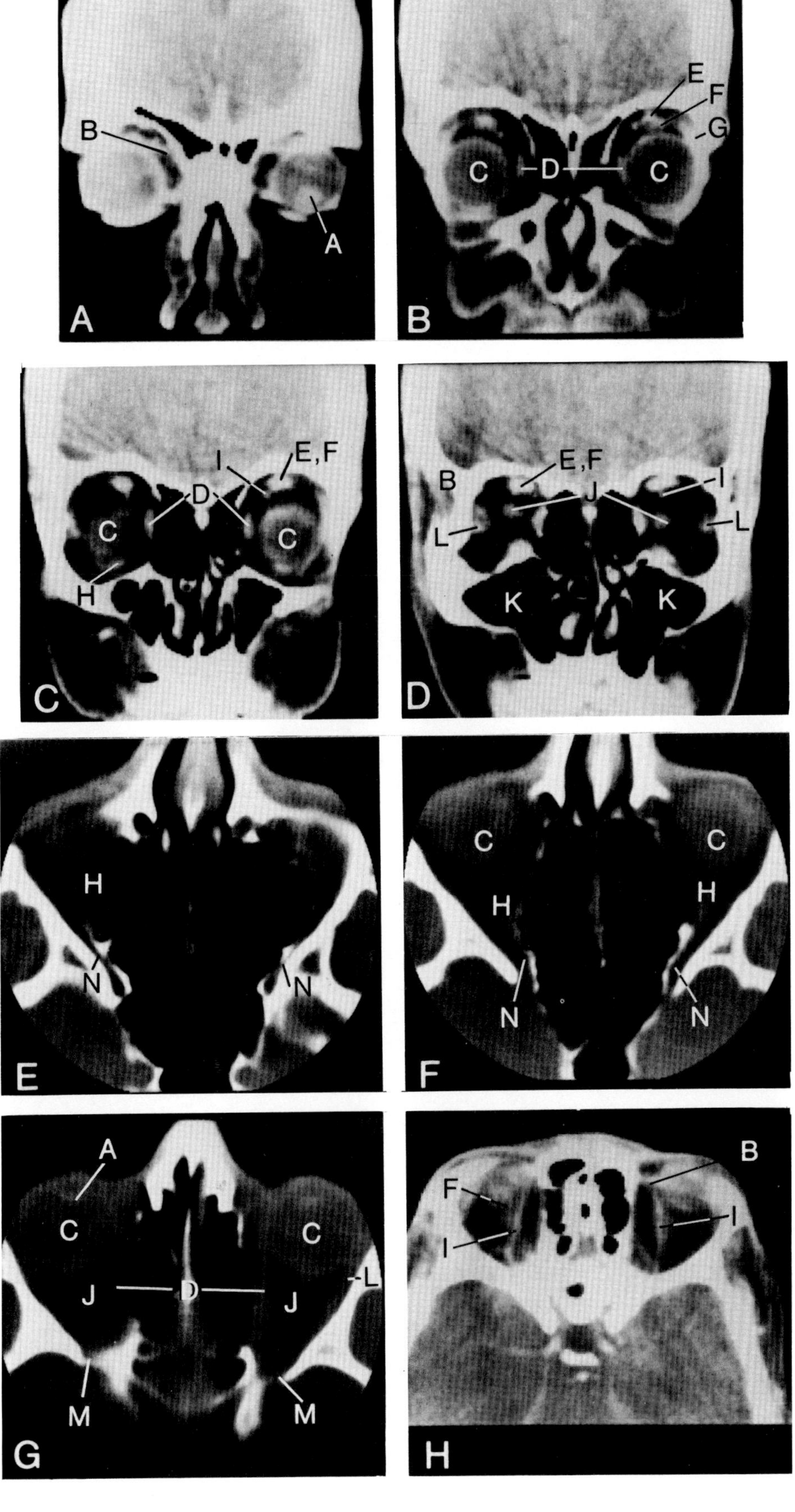

$\longrightarrow$

Figure 6-4-2. **Coronal Views of Orbits, Predental Positioning.**
A. Palpebral fissure.
B. Optic globe.
C. Superior oblique muscle.
D. Levator palpebrae muscle.
E. Superior rectus muscle.
F. Medial rectus muscle.
G. Lateral rectus muscle.
H. Nasal septum.
I. Inferior rectus muscle group.
J. Maxillary sinus.
K. Superior oblique muscle.
L. Optic nerve.
M. Inferior orbital fissure.
N. Inferior turbinate.
O. Portion of superior orbital fissure.
P. Middle turbinate.
Q. Anterior clinoids.
R. Zygoma.
S. Dorsum sella/clivus.
T. Temporal lobe.

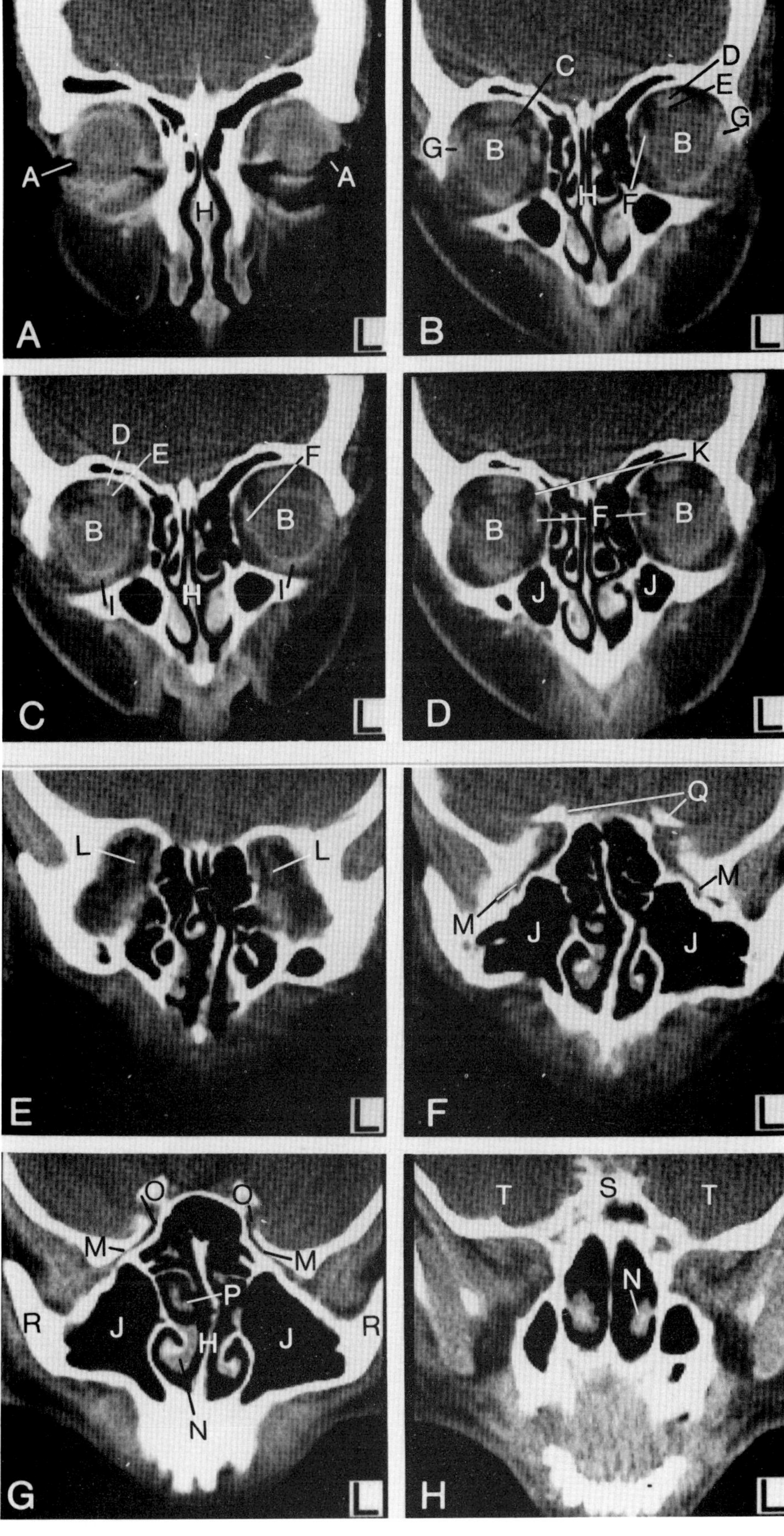

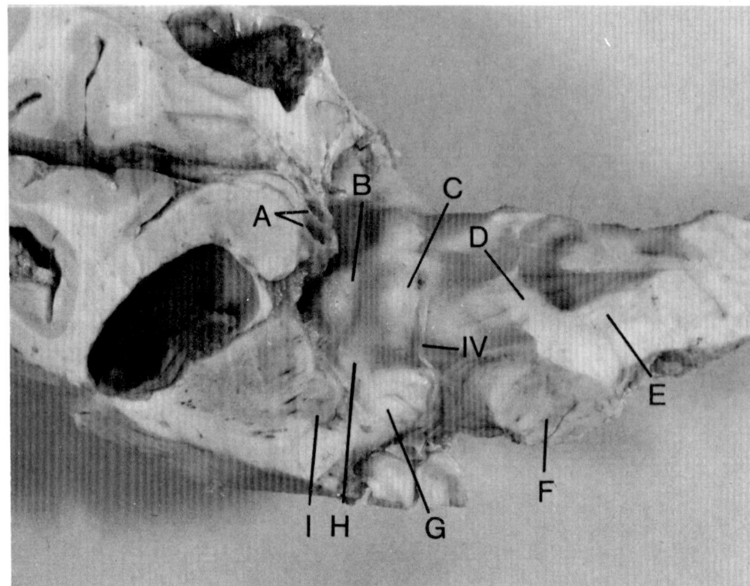

Figure 6-5. **Midbrain, with Nerve IV.** Following decussation in the superior medullary velum, the fourth cranial verve (trochlear) emerges from the dorsal aspect of the midbrain just caudal to the inferior colliculus. It winds around the lateral aspect of the cerebral peduncle and passes forward along with nerves II and VI.

IV. Trochlear nerve.

A. Internal cerebral veins just before joining to form the great cerebral vein.

B. Superior colliculus.

C. Inferior colliculus.

D. Superior cerebellar peduncle.

E. Inferior cerebellar peduncle.

F. Middle cerebellar peduncle.

G. Cerebral peduncle.

H. Brachium of the inferior colliculus, extending from the inferior colliculus to the medial geniculate body.

I. Medial geniculate body, in cross section.

ARTERIES

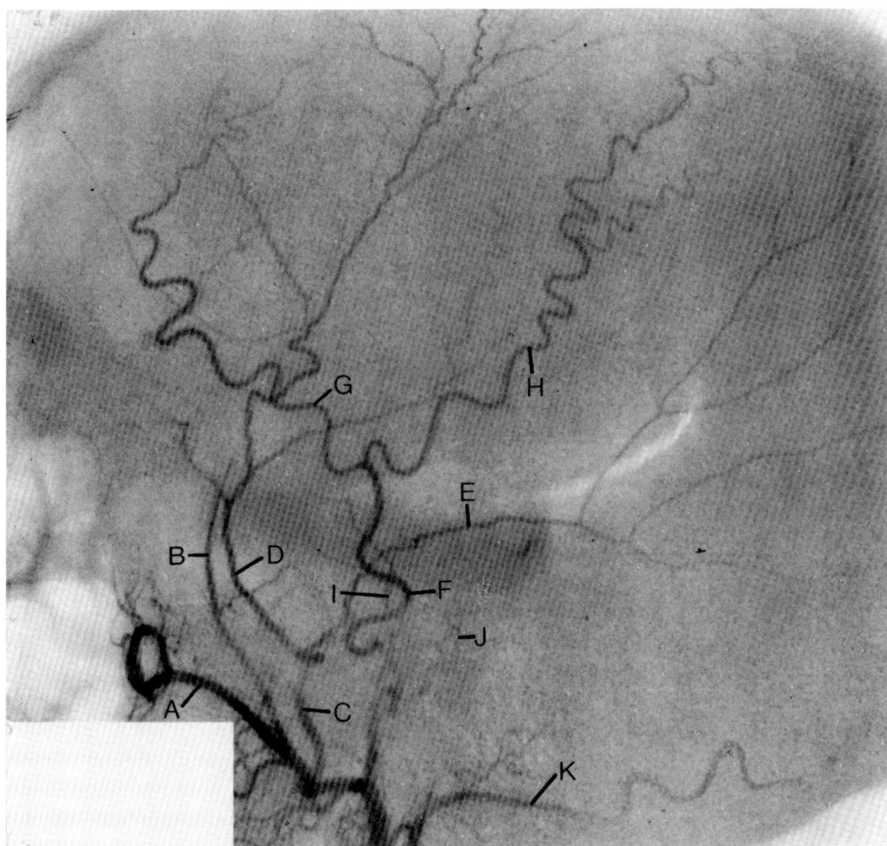

Figure 7-1. **Angiogram: Normal Lateral of External Carotid Artery.**
A. Internal maxillary artery.
B. Deep temporal artery.
C. Middle meningeal artery, main trunk.
D. Middle meningeal artery, anterior trunk.
E. Middle meningeal artery, posterior trunk.
F. Superficial temporal artery, main trunk.
G. Superficial temporal artery, anterior branch.
H. Superficial temporal artery, posterior branch.
I. Ascending pharyngeal artery.
J. Posterior auricular atery.
K. Occipital artery.

Figure 7-2. **Major Arteries of Brain as seen in View of Base of Brain.** Some portions
of frontal and temporal lobes have been removed.

Arteries:
A. Internal carotid.
B. Middle cerebral.
C. Anterior cerebral.
D. Anterior communicating.
E. Posterior communicating.
F. Posterior cerebral.
The foregoing arteries form the circle of Willis.
G. Superior cerebellar.
H. Basilar.
I. Anterior inferior cerebellar.
J. Vertebral.
K. Posterior inferior cerebellar.
L. Anterior spinal.

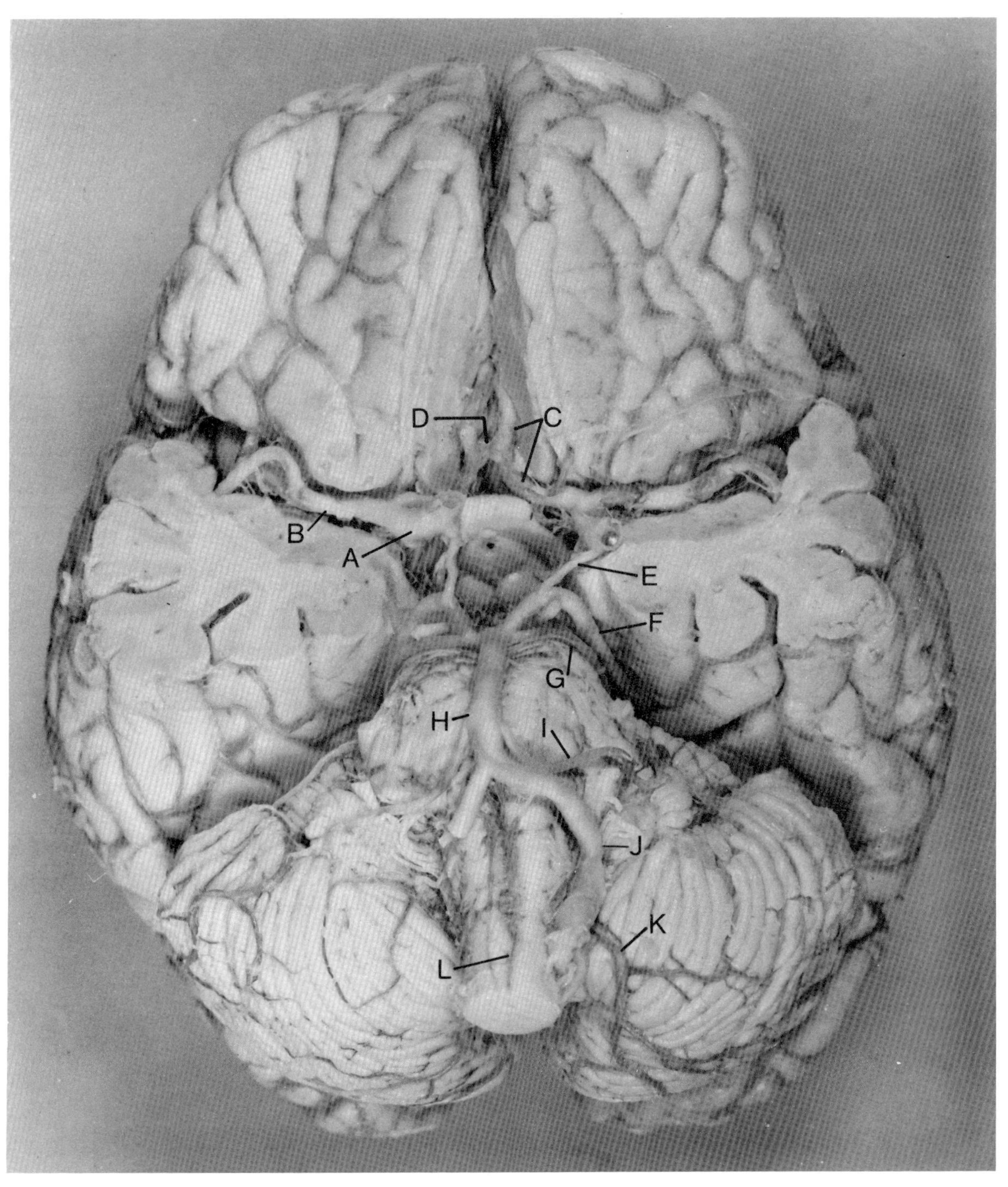

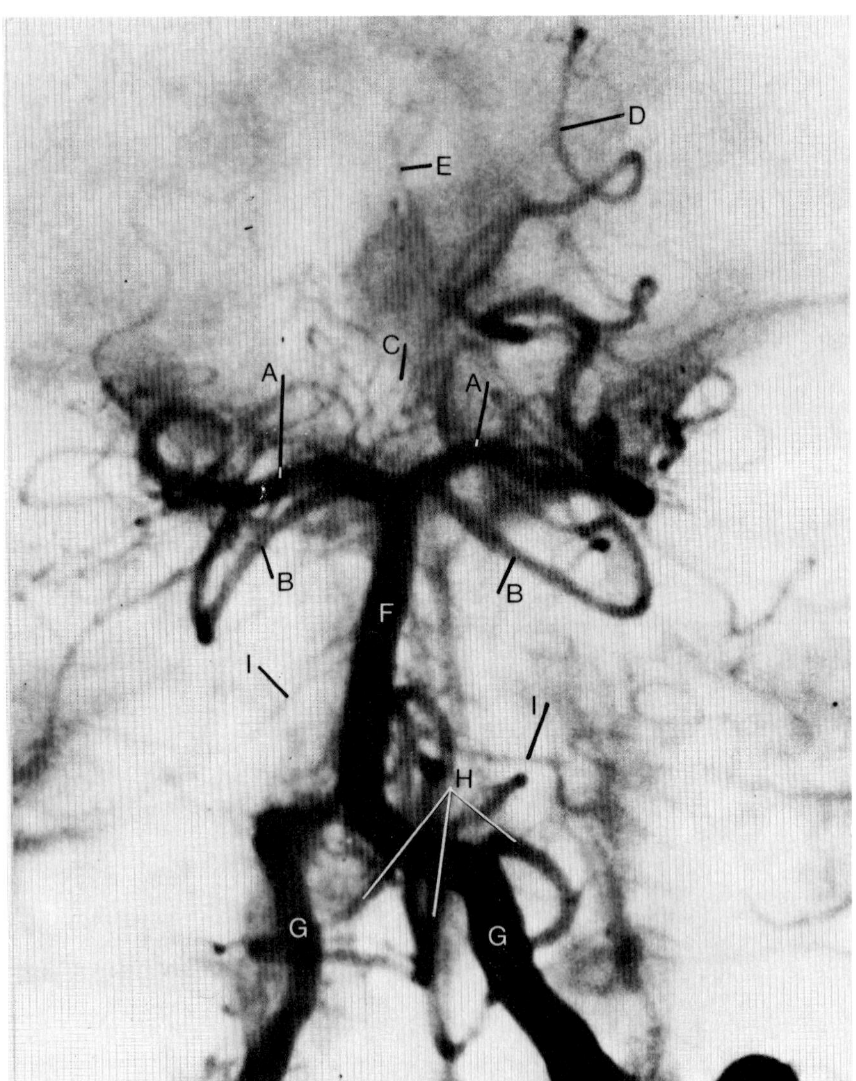

Figure 7-3. **Vertebral Arteriogram, AP Transfacial Arterial Phase.**
A. Posterior cerebral arteries, main trunk.
B. Superior cerebellar arteries, main trunk.
C. Thalamo-perforate arteries.
D. Posterior cerebral artery, parieto-occipital branch.
E. Posterior cerebral artery, calcarine branch.
F. Basilar artery.
G. Vertebral arteries.
H. Posterior inferior cerebellar arteries (PICAs).
I. Anterior inferior cerebellar arteries (AICAs).

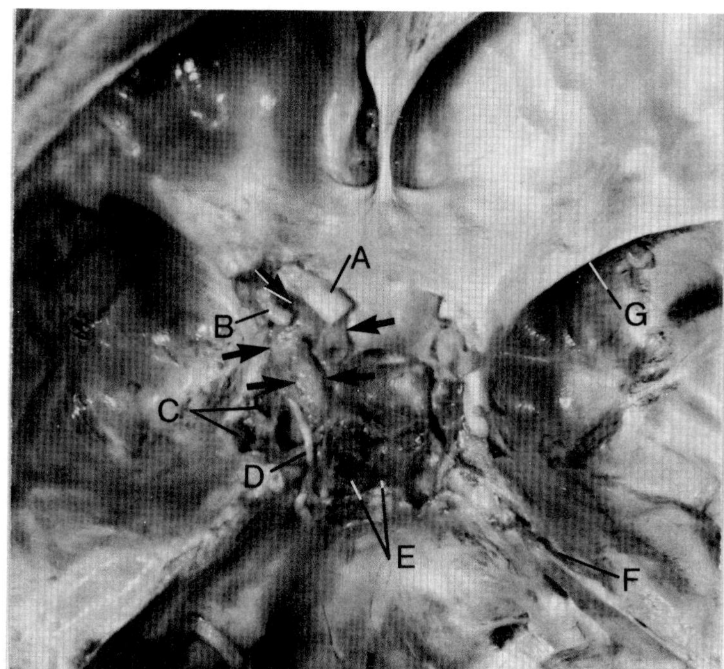

Figure 7-4. **Internal Carotid Artery—Intracranial (Intracavernous and Supraclinoid) Portion.** The left posterior clinoid, pituitary, and portions of dura covering cavernous and posterior intercavernous sinuses have been removed. The artery is indicated with arrows. Its essentially sigmoid course is shown.

A. Optic nerve.
B. Oculomotor nerve.
C. Locules of the cavernous sinus.
D. Abducens nerve.
E. Locules of the posterior intercavernous sinus.
F. Superior petrosal sinus.
G. Lesser wing of sphenoid bone. The sphenoparietal sinus is within the marginal portion of the dura.

Figure 7-5. **Internal Carotid Arteriogram, AP** (*A*) **and Lateral** (*B*), **Views** →
Arterial Phase.

A. Internal carotid artery, supraclinoid segment
B. Internal carotid artery, cavernous segment
C. Internal carotid artery, petrous segment
D. Horizontal (M-1) segment of middle cerebral artery
E. Horizontal (A-1) segment of the anterior cerebral artery
F. Lenticulostriate arteries
G. Sylvian point. In the AP projection, this point lies at the midpoint, or within one centimeter below the midpoint, of a perpendicular line drawn from the orbital roof or apex of the petrous pyramid (whichever is lower), to a tangent drawn along the inner table of the skull at the vertex. In the lateral projection, G lies within a centimeter of the midportion of a line drawn from the bregma to the internal occipital protuberance.
H. Angular artery
I. Posterior temporal artery
J. Posterior parietal artery
K. Central artery
L. Precentral artery
M. Ascending frontal artery
N. Pericallosal artery
O. Callosomarginal artery
P. Frontopolar artery
Q. Ophthalmic artery
R. Anterior internal frontal artery
S. Middle internal frontal artery
T. Posterior internal frontal artery
U. Superior internal parietal artery
V. Inferior internal parietal artery
W. Anterior choroidal artery
X. Anterior temporal artery
Y. Orbitofrontal artery
1. Measurement of the middle cerebral artery (insular curve). This distance, measured from the inner table of the skull to the most medial branch of the middle cerebral artery should be between 20 to 30 mm.
2. Relationship of the middle cerebral arteries to the lenticulostriate arteries. The distance between the most lateral lenticulostriate artery and the closest branch of the middle cerebral artery should be between 11 to 14 mm.

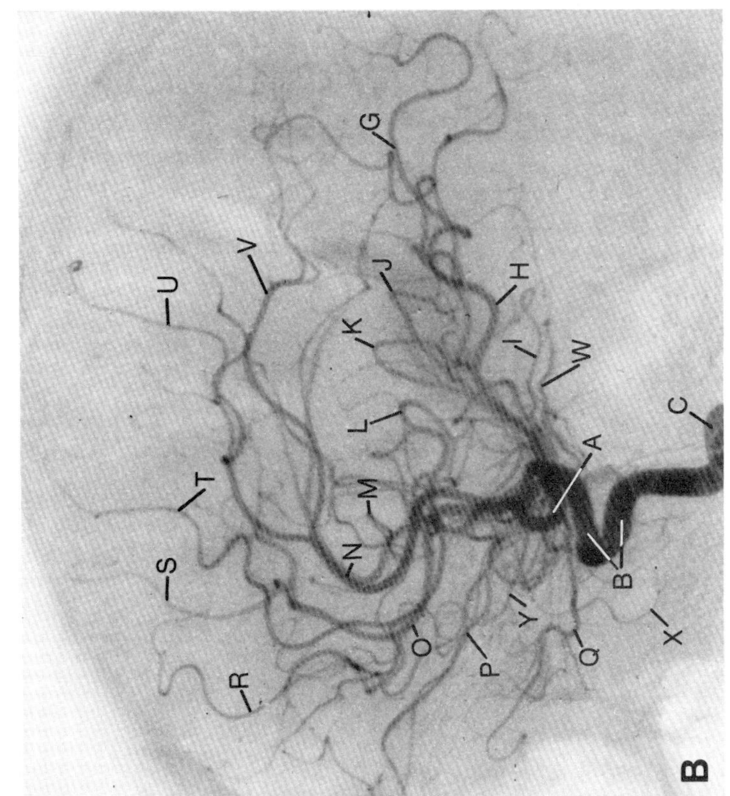

B
G
V
U
J
H
K
I
W
L
A
C
T
M
S
N
B
Y
X
O
Q
P
R

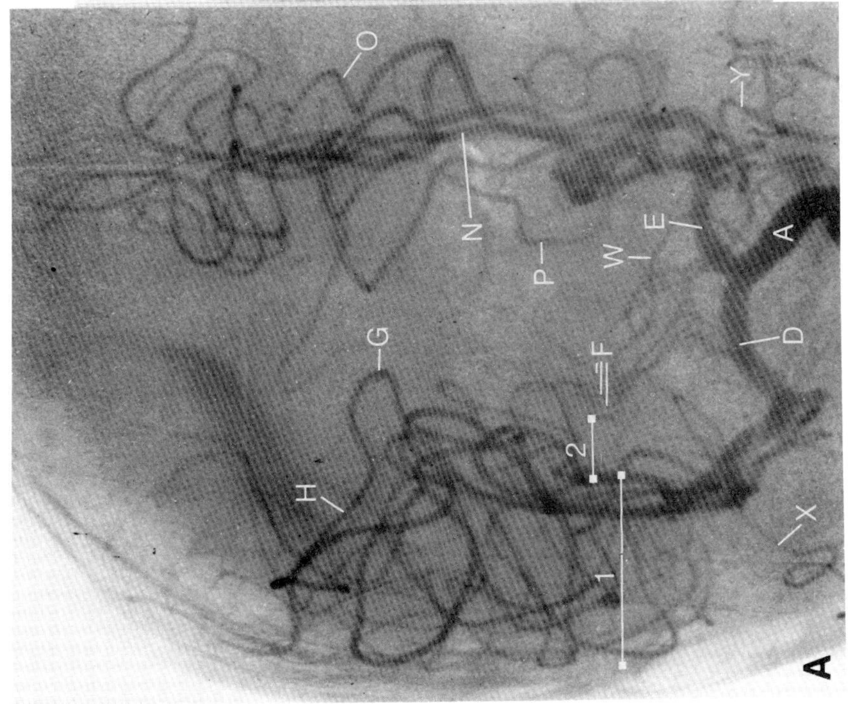

O
Y
N
P
E
W
I
A
G
F
D
2
H
1
X
A

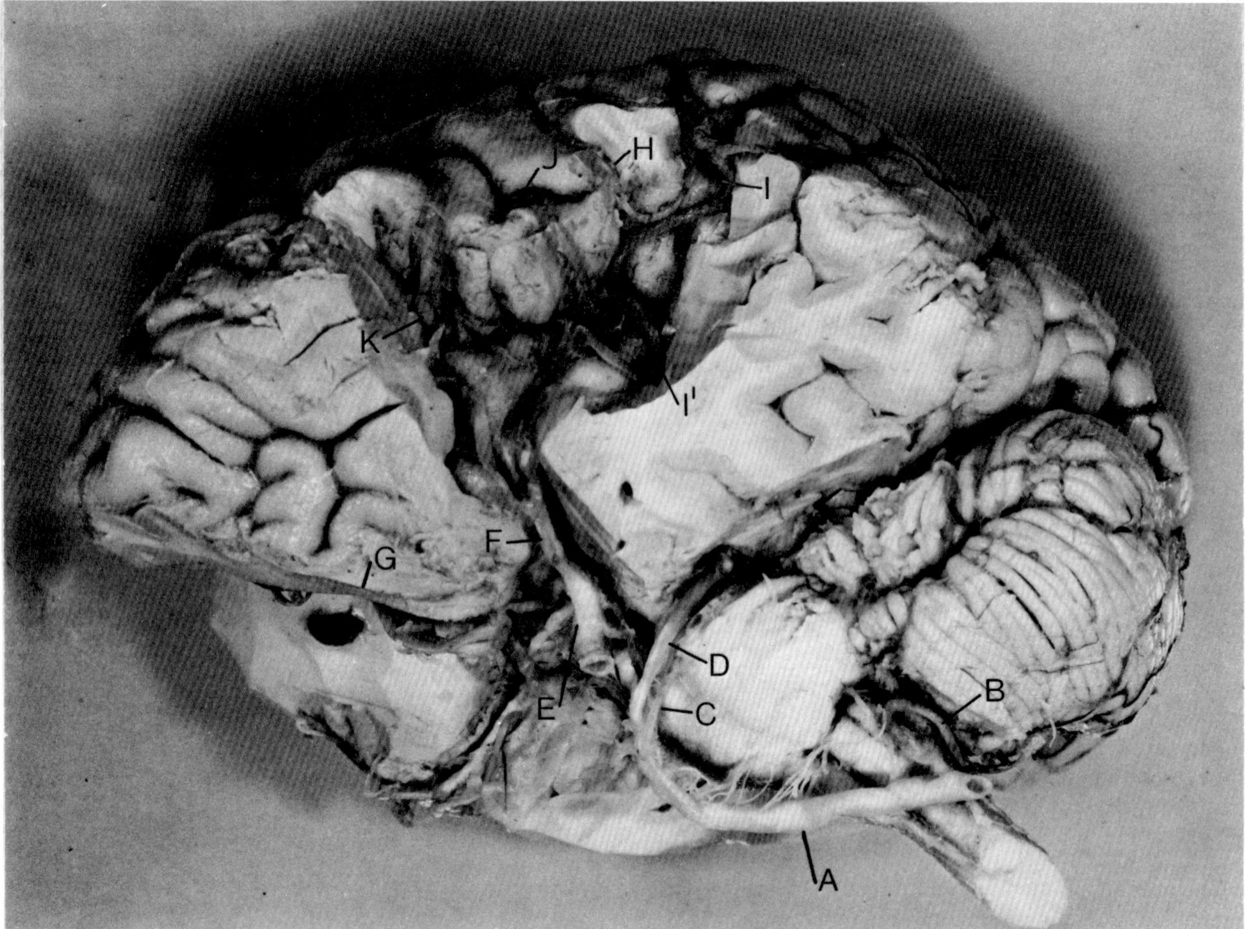

Figure 7-6-1. **Arteries seen in lateral aspect of brain.** Oblique view of a dissection. Portions of frontal, parietal and temporal lobes have been removed to enhance visibility of the vessels.

Arteries:

A. Basilar.

B. Posterior inferior cerebellar. The characteristic loop is seen.

C. Superior cerebellar (residual portion).

D. Posterior cerebral (residual portion).

E. Internal carotid.

F. Middle cerebral. An arcade of branches is formed; the branches ramify in the suprainsular sulcus, and in due course, pass up over the surrounding opercular convolutions. The pattern of arrangement of the branches is variable. Applicability of the standard nomenclature categories to the arteries as they appear in a given case may vary accordingly.

G. Anterior cerebral.

H. Central.

I. Postcentral (anterior parietal). Superior to the point indicated, two branches extend posteriorly to constitute the equivalent of a posterior parietal artery.

I'. The postcentral artery illustrates the variability of course of the arteries, in forming a prominent loop, part of a figure S described by the artery as it passes to the postcentral sulcus.

J. Precentral.

K. Orbitofrontal (a more fitting term, at least in the present case, might be anterior frontal).

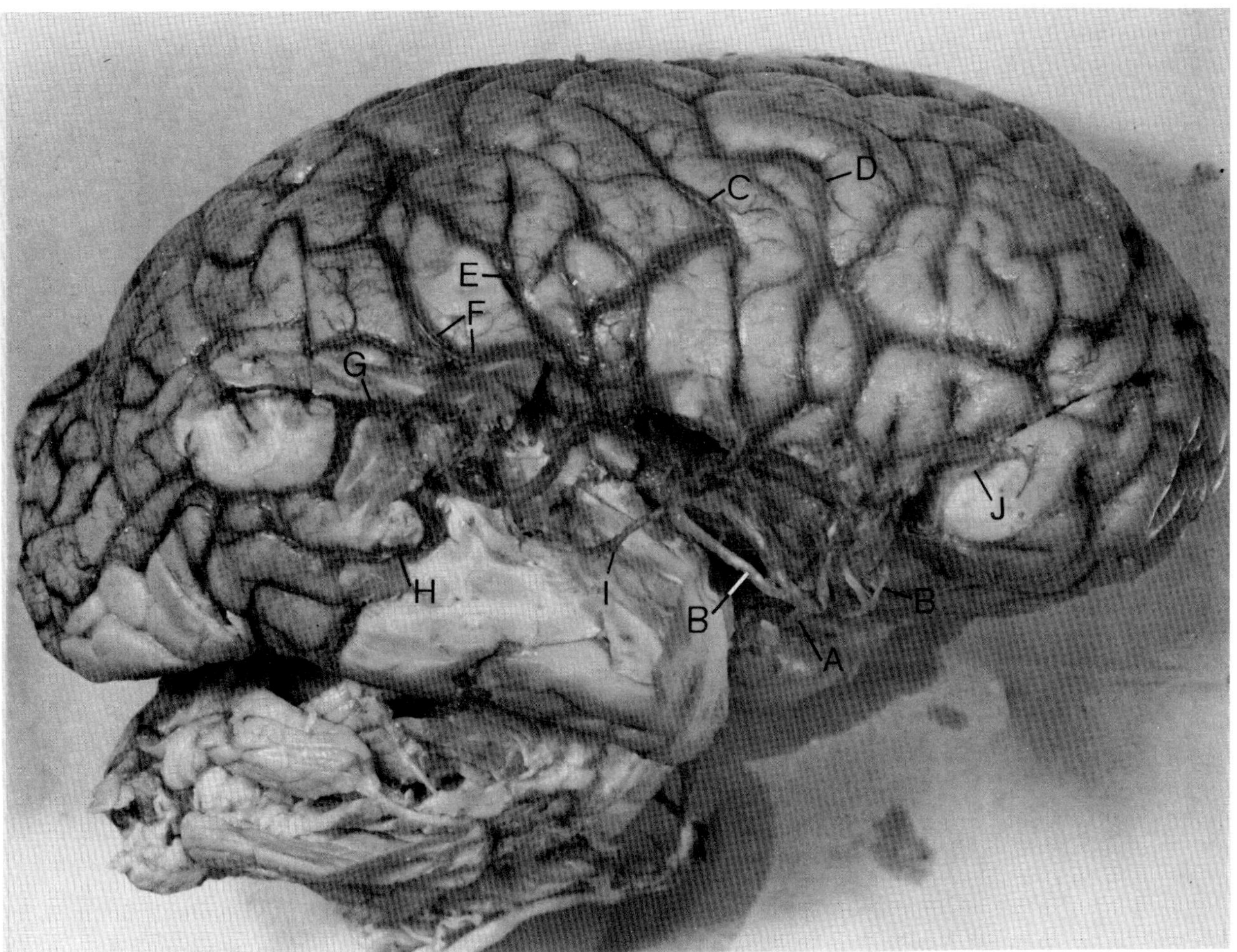

Figure 7-6-2. **Middle cerebral artery distribution.** A portion of the temporal lobe has
been removed to enhance visibility of the arteries.

Arteries:

A. Middle cerebral
B. Middle cerebral forms a triangular branching arcade.
C. Central. The artery traverses the postcentral gyrus and part of another (illustrating
   variability of pattern).
D. Precentral.
E. Postcentral (anterior parietal)
F. Posterior parietal
G. Angular
H. Posterior temporal
I. Anterior temporal
J. Orbitofrontal

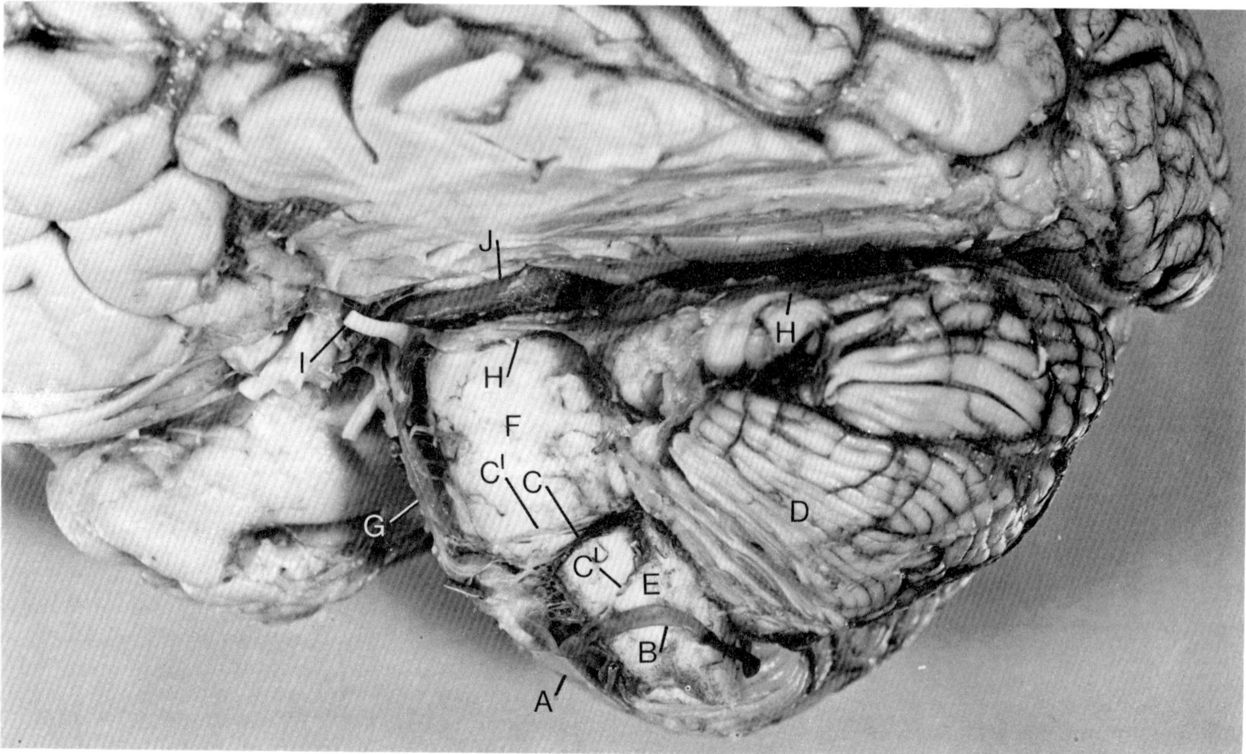

Figure 7-7. **Arteries. Lateral View Especially of Cerebellar.**

A. Vertebral artery.

B. Posterior inferior cerebellar a.

C. Anterior inferior cerebellar a. The variability of formation of the surface arteries is shown with the appearance of added small arteries (C^1), one of them appearing to anastomose between the two inferior cerebellar arteries.

    (Note: The terms anterior inferior and posterior inferior cerebellar arteries are not meaningful; the two arteries bear more of a superior-inferior relation. In due course, it may be hoped that the cerebellar arteries will be named properly: superior, middle, and inferior, reflecting the three cerebellar penduncles.)

D. Cerebellar hemisphere.

E. Medulla.

F. Pons.

G. Basilar a. An arcade of penetrating branches is seen on the deep side of the basilar artery.

H. Superior cerebellar a.

I. Oculomotor nerve.

J. Posterior cerebral a.

Figure 7-8. **Lateral Vertebral Angiography, Arterial Phase.** (See pages 72 and 73.)

→

Figure 7-8. **Lateral Vertebral Angiography, Arterial Phase. A** and **B** show routine and autotomographic views of the lateral vertebral arterial circulation.

A. Posterior inferior cerebellar artery (PICA), anterior medullary segment.
B. PICA, lateral medullary segment.
C. PICA, retromedullary segment.
D. PICA, choroidal point.
E. PICA, retrotonsillar branch.
F. PICA, inferior vermian branch.
G. PICA, hemispheric branch.
H. Basilar artery.
I. Thalamoperforate arteries.
J. Medial posterior choroidal artery.
K. Lateral posterior choroidal artery.
L. Posterior cerebral artery, major trunk.
M. Superior cerebral artery, major trunk.
N. Tonsillohemispheric branch from PICA.
O. Superior cerebellar artery, vermis branch passing over the culmen of the cerebellar vermis.
P. Posterior cerebral artery, parieto-occipital branch.
Q. Posterior cerebral artery, calcarine branch.
R. Anterior inferior cerebellar artery (AICA) near internal auditory canal orifice.

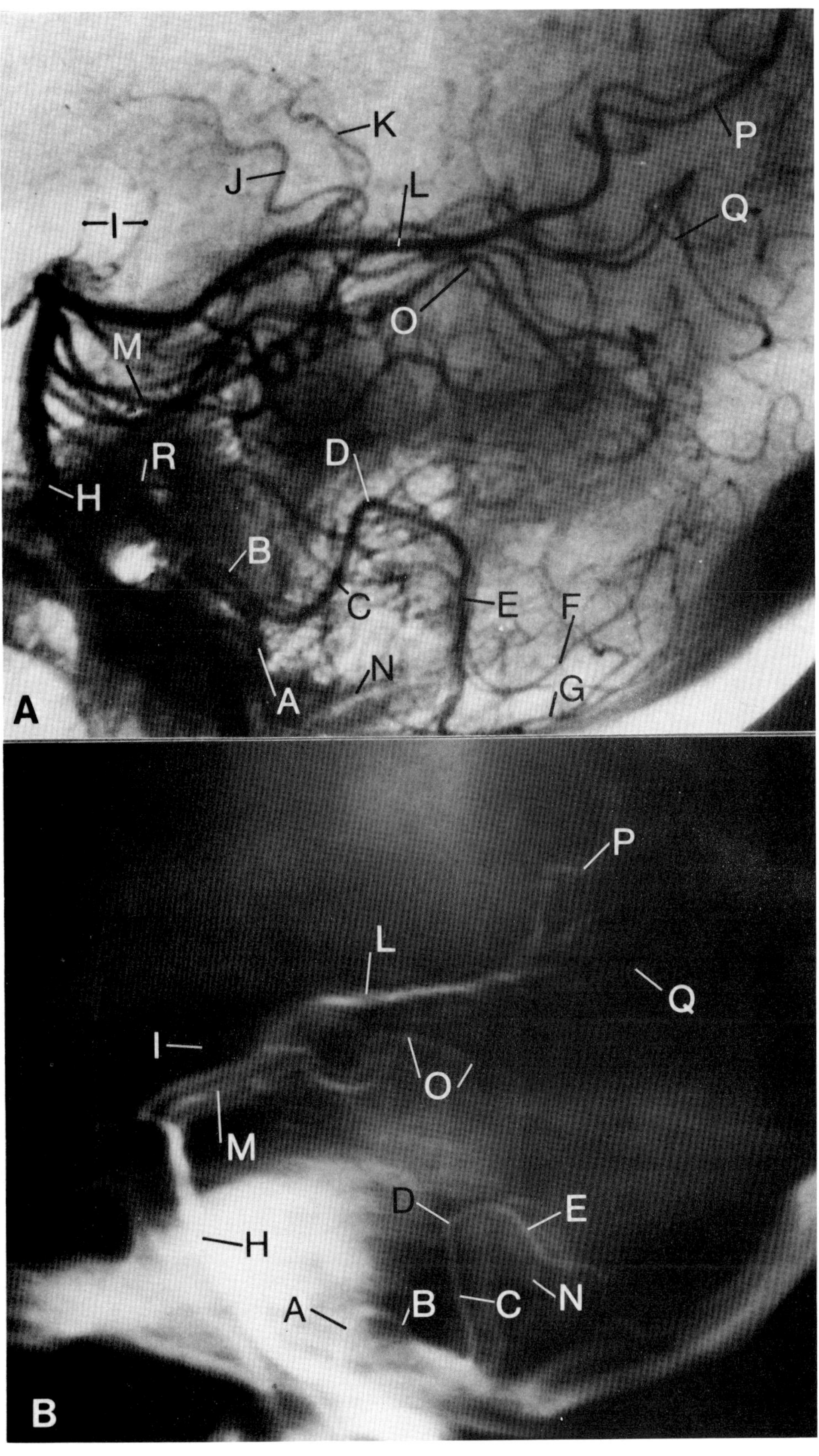
A
K
J
I
L
P
Q
M
O
R
D
H
B
C
E
F
G
A
N
B
P
L
Q
I
O
M
D
E
H
A
B
C
N

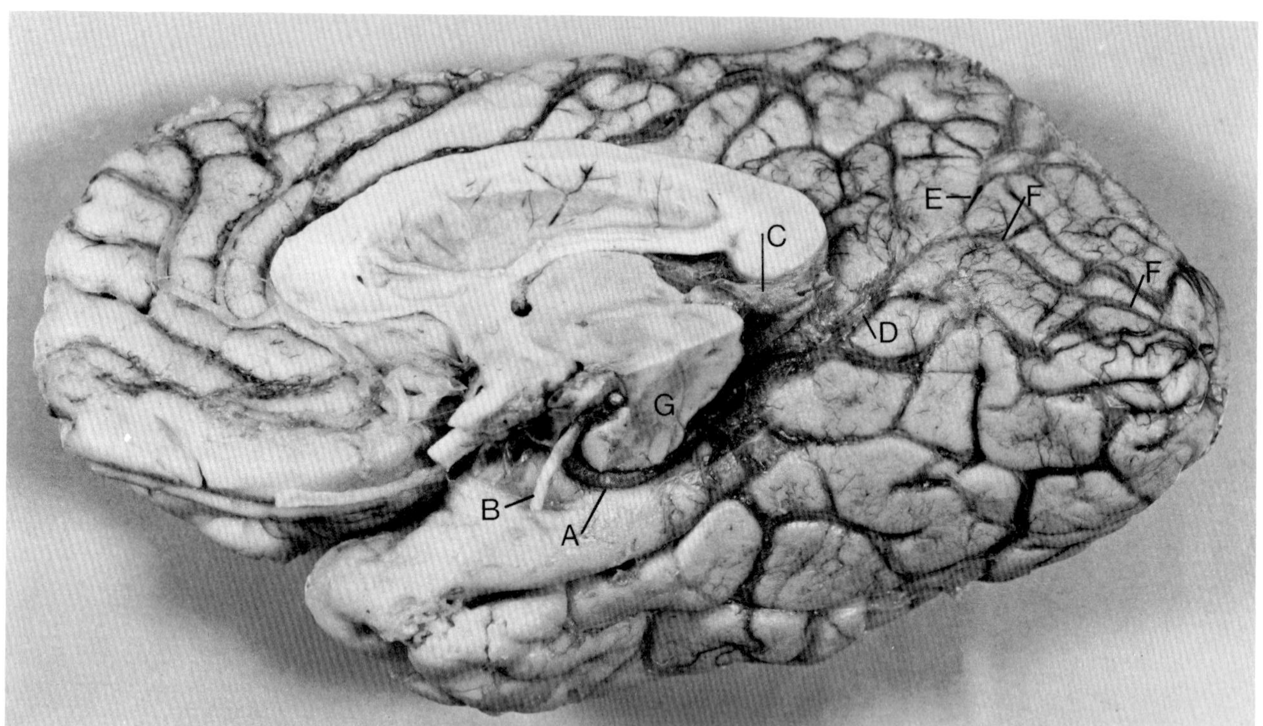

Figure 7-9. **Posterior Cerebral Artery.**

A. Posterior cerebral artery.

B. Oculomotor nerve.

C. Great cerebral vein.

D. Internal occipital artery. Before the origin of this artery, some sizeable branches extend down and to reader's right. This illustrates the variability of pattern of distribution of the surface arteries.

E. Occipital sulcus and artery.

F. Calcarine sulcus and artery. Compare with Figure 7-14.

Figure 7-10 A, B and C. **Arteries.** (See pages 76 and 77.)

$\rightarrow$

Figure 7-10. **Arteries.**
A. Anterior choroidal artery. This vessel usually arises from the internal carotid artery, as in the case illustrated. It courses back over the optic tract and enters the choroidal fissure.

    A. Internal carotid artery.
    B. Anterior choroidal a.
    B′. Point of entrance into the choroidal fissure.
    C. Optic tract.

B. Medial striate artery. This vessel arises from the anterior cerebral artery. It may not be found regularly to stand out individually. It supplies the anteromedial extremity of the head of the caudate nucleus; this latter tissue tends to survive major middle cerebral (distribution) infarction. (See **D.**)

    A. Anterior cerebral artery.
    B. Medial striate a.

C. Ganglionic arterial groups. Small deeply-penetrating branches arise from the under surfaces of the major arteries at the base of the brain. Some of these are scarcely more than arterioles. Particular clusters arise from the parts of the circle of Willis.

    A. Internal carotid artery.
    B. Middle cerebral a.
    C. Anterior cerebral a.
    D. Lateral striate group.
    E. Anteromedial group.
    F. Posteromedial group. (The posterolateral group is covered by the posterior cerebral artery (G′.)
    G. Posterior cerebral a.
    G′.Portion of posterior cerebral artery giving rise to the posterolateral group (covered by the artery).

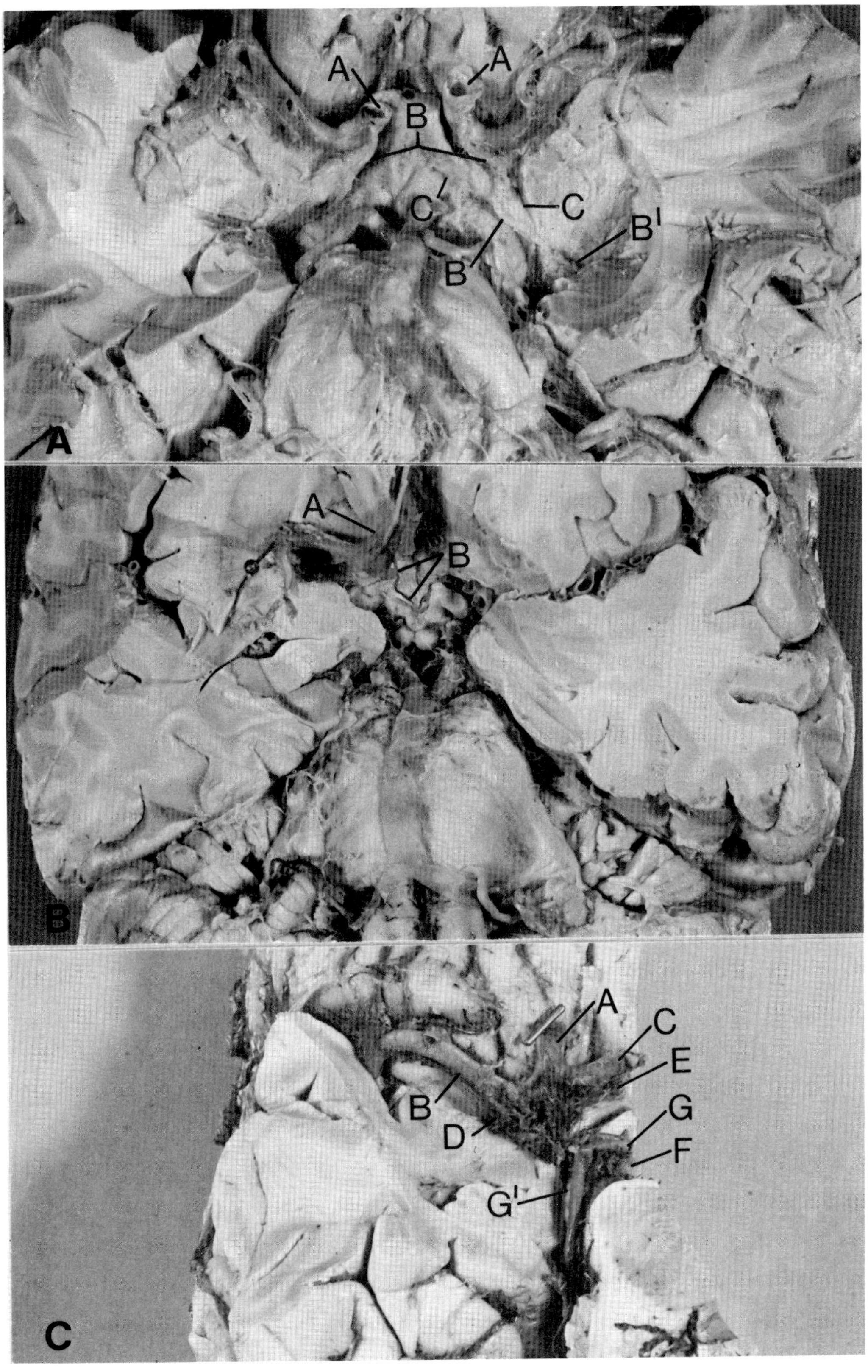
A
A
B
C'
C
B
B'
A
B
A
C
E
B
G
D
F
G'

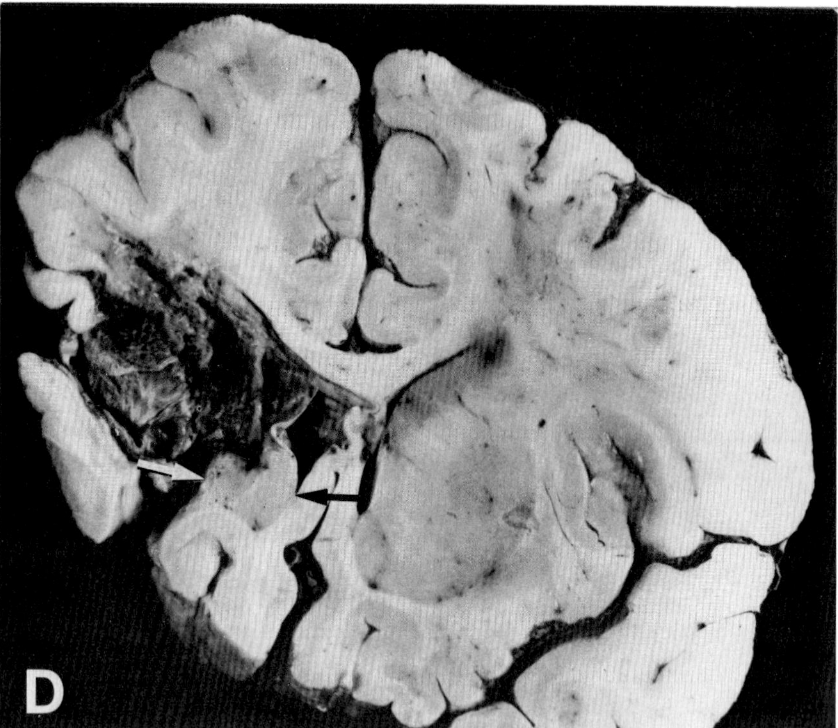

Figure 7-10. **Arteries.**
D. Old infarct in rheumatic vascular disease, for anatomy. Middle cerebral region of supply has been destroyed. Anteromedial extremity of head of caudate nucleus (*arrows*) escaped, being supplied by medial striate artery, branch of anterior cerebral (see **B**). From Dublin, W.B.: *Fundamentals of Neuropathology.* Ed. II, 1967, Charles C. Thomas, Springfield, Illinois.

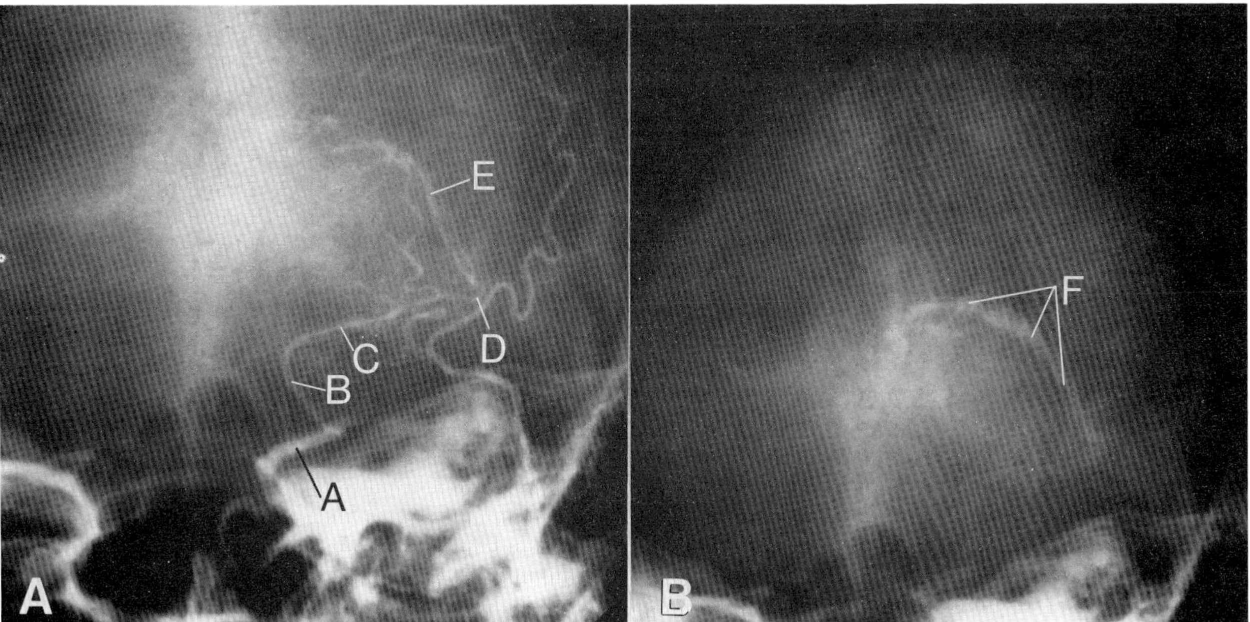

Figure 7-11-1. **Angiogram: Anterior Choroidal Artery. A.** Anterior-posterior view, arterial phase. **B.** Anterior-posterior view, capillary phase. The anatomy of the anterior choroidal artery is demonstrated in an individual with internal carotid occlusion both above and below the origin of the main artery from the internal carotid vessel.

A. Internal carotid artery.

B. Anterior choroidal artery, prepeduncular portion.

C. Anterior choroidal artery, prepeduncular or perimesencephalic (ambient) segment.

D. Plexal point. Point at which the anterior choroidal enters the temporal horn.

E. Anterior choroidal artery within the inferior horn.

F. Inferior horn choroid vascular blush.

$\longrightarrow$

Figure 7-11-2. **Angiogram: Anterior Choroidal Artery, Lateral Projection.** Arterial (**A**), and capillary late venous phase (**B**) views of the same patient as Figure 7-11-1, demonstrate the following:

A. Internal carotid artery.
B. Anterior choroidal artery, prepeduncular segment.
C. Anterior choroidal artery, peripeduncular or perimesencephalic segment.
D. Plexal point.
E. Anterior choroidal artery, inferior horn segment.
F. Choroid, temporal horn.
G. Choroid, posterior body lateral ventricle.

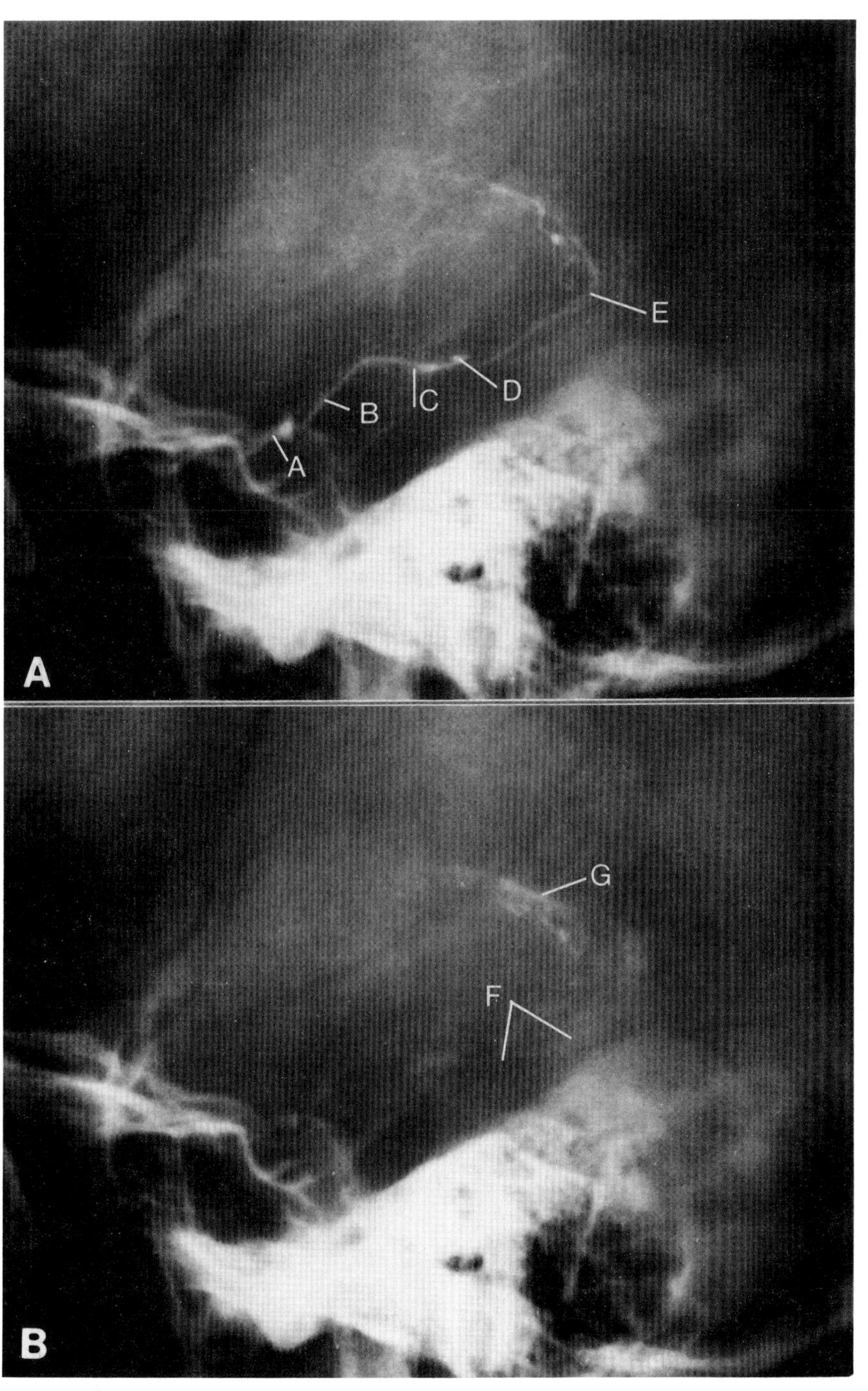

$\longrightarrow$

Figure 7-12. **Posterior inferior cerebellar artery.**

A. The posterior inferior cerebellar artery (P.I.C.A.) (*larger arrows*) describes an S-shaped loop beneath the vermis. A portion of the medulla has been removed, and the remainder is pinned aside (downward). This aids clarity of the choroid plexus (*smaller arrows*), with which P.I.C.A. comes in contact (the artery has separated, as artifact, from the inferiormost portion of the plexus) and which it supplies through small branches. After giving off vermian branches, P.I.C.A. continues (toward reader's right) as a tonsillohemispheric artery.

B. P.I.C.A. (*larger arrows*) describes, in this case, a figure-eight loop. Proximation with the choroid plexus (*smaller arrows*) is shown. The artery gives off a vermian branch (*arrowhead*); the latter anastomoses with the main branch of the anterior inferior cerebellar artery, the first part of which has been removed along with cerebellar tissue, for clarity. P.I.C.A. continues, toward reader's left, as a tonsillohemispheric branch.

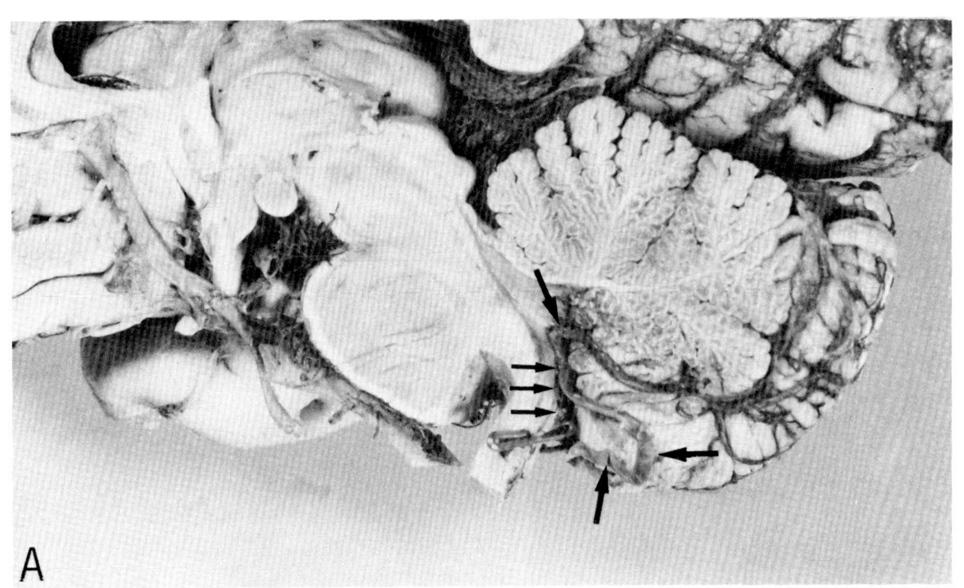

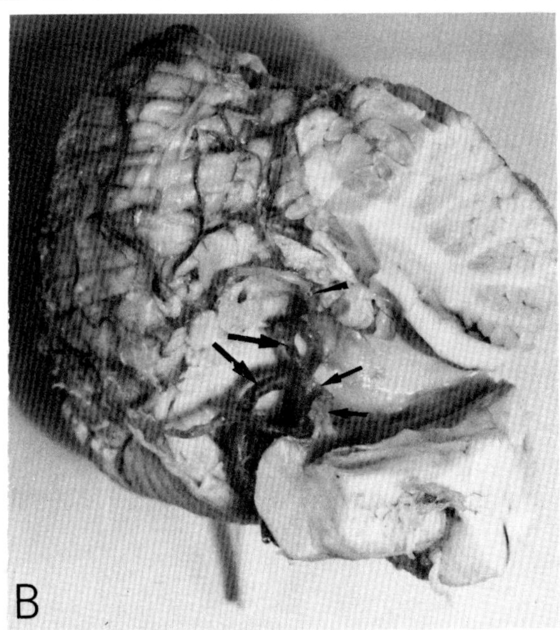

Figure 7-13. **Angiogram: Posterior Inferior Cerebellar Artery (PICA). A** and **B** (lateral and anterior-posterior arterial views, respectively) demonstrate a small vertebral artery ending essentially in PICA. The following anatomic points are:
A. Vertebral Artery.
Posterior Inferior Cerebellar Artery (PICA):
B. Anterior medullary segment.
C. Lateral medullary segment.
D. Retromedullary segment.
E. Choroidal point.
F. Retrotonsilar segment.
G. Tonsilohemispheric branch.
H. Inferior vermian branch.

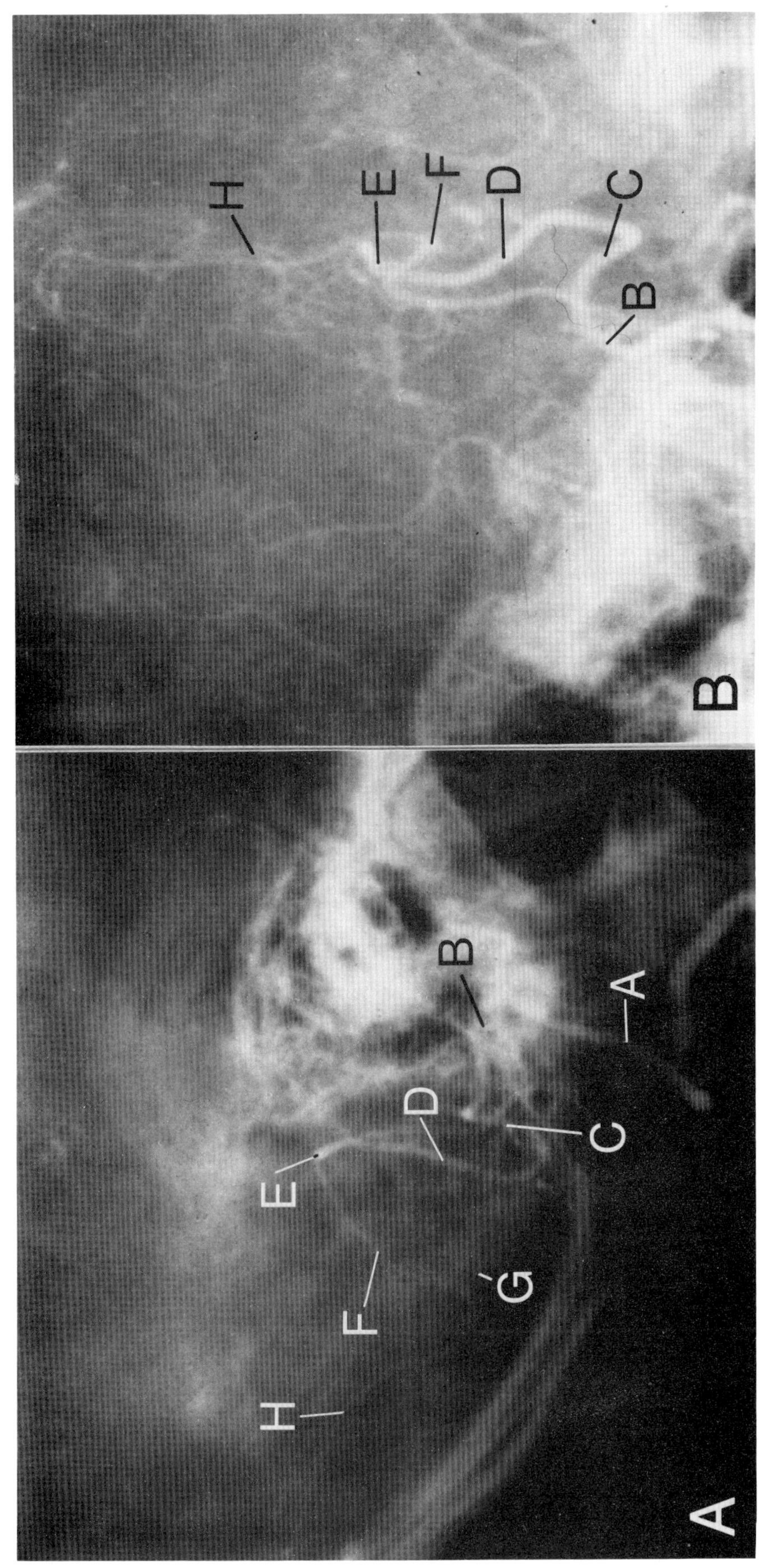
A
B
C
D
E
F
G
H

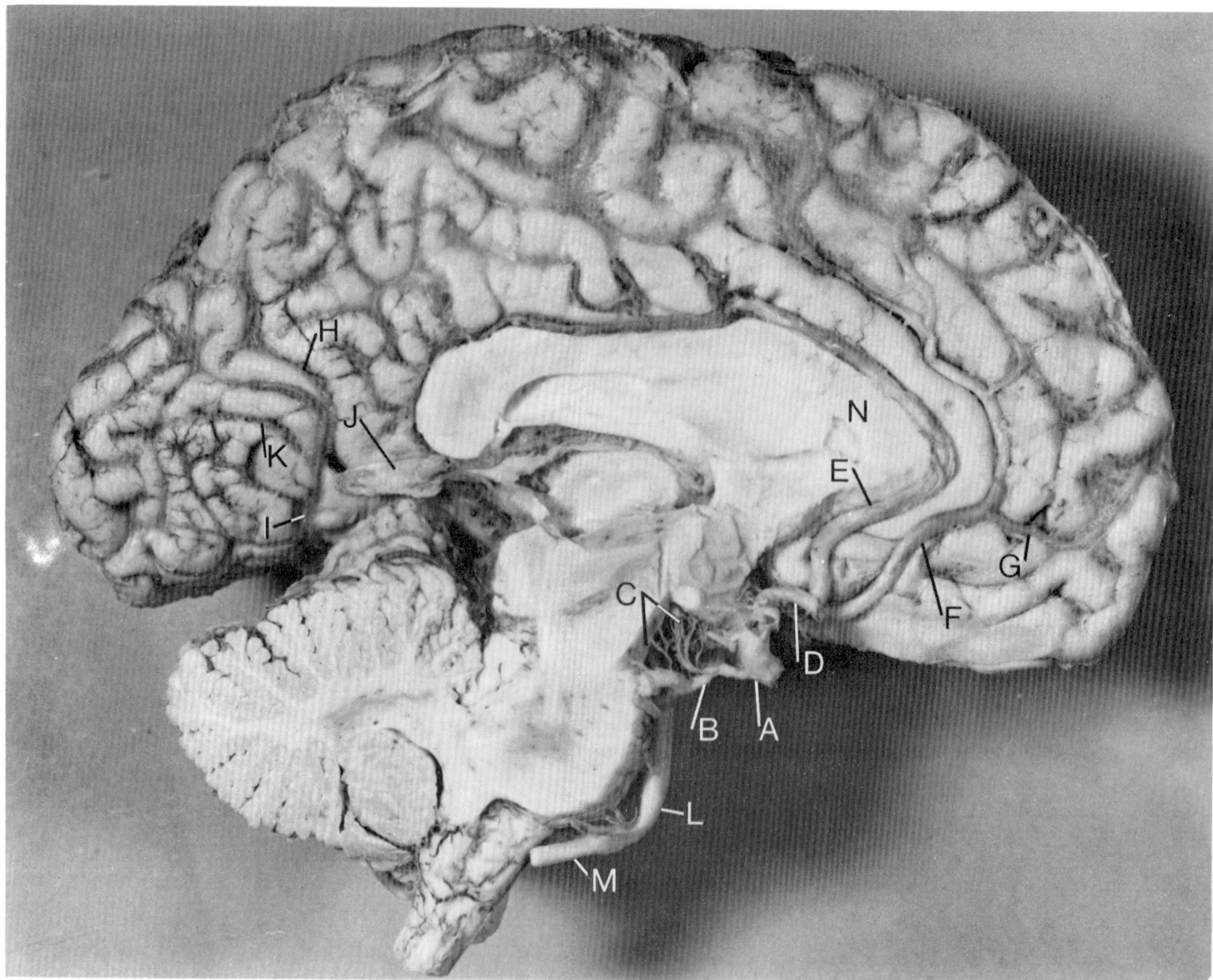

Figure 7-14. **Arteries, as seen in Sagittal View of Brain.** See also Figure 8-13.

A. Internal carotid artery.

B. Posterior communicating a.

C. Arcade of posterior striate arteries.

D. Anterior cerebral a.

E. Pericallosal a.

F. Callosomarginal a. It is derived early in the source of the anterior cerebral artery, in this case. At point of origin of the callosomarginal artery, the lumen of the transected anterior communicating artery is seen.

G. Frontopolar a.

H. Occipitoparietal sulcus and a.

I. Internal occipital a.

J. Great cerebral vein.

K. Calcarine sulcus and a. The variability of formation of gyri and sulci, and of the vascular arrangement, is illustrated; the posterior portion of the calcarine sulcus and artery appears displaced, with formation of an irregular cluster of small gyri. See also Figure 11-1-1.

L. Basilar a. Penetrating pontine branches appear on the deep side of the artery.

M. Vertebral a.

N. Corpus callosum.

SINUSES AND VEINS

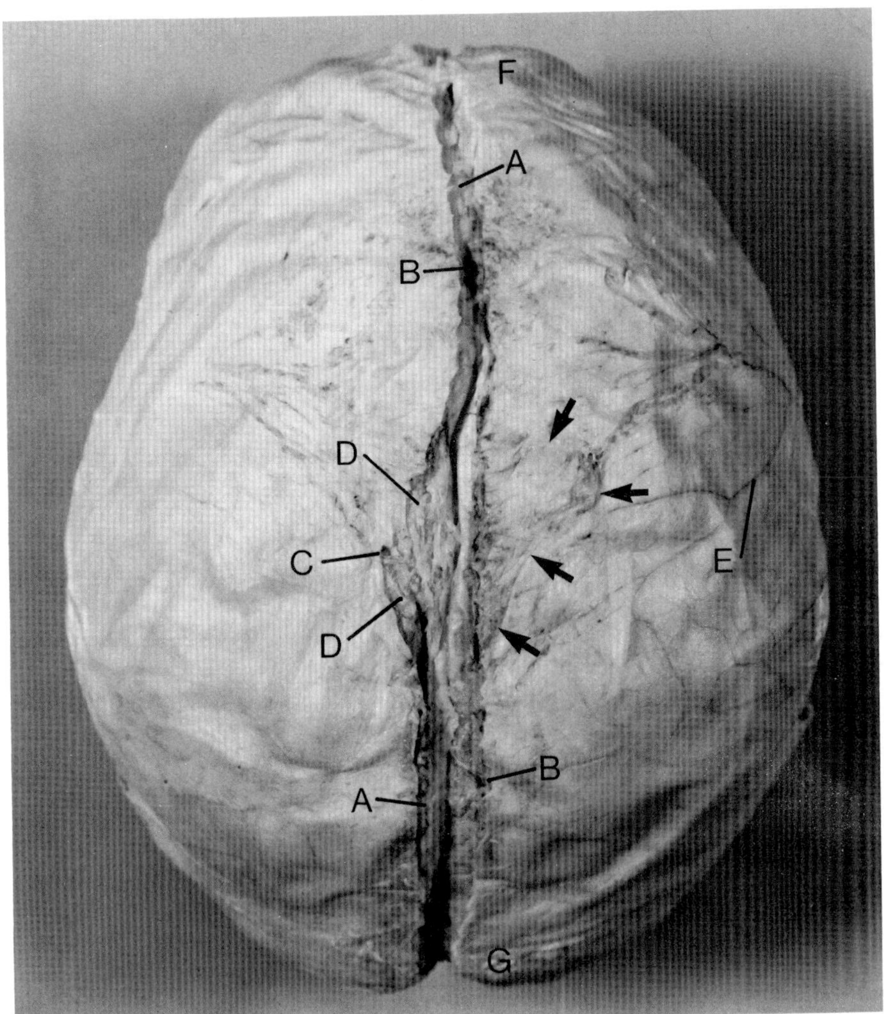

Figure 8-1. **Superior Sagittal Sinus, with Dura.**

A. Open superior sagittal sinus.
B. Opening of vein into the sinus.
C. Opening of vein into a lacuna.
D. Lacuna. A larger one is outlined with arrows, on the right.
E. Middle meningeal artery, branch.
F. Frontal pole.
G. Occipital pole.

$\longrightarrow$

Figure 8-2. **Superior Sagittal Sinus, and portions of Superior Cerebral Veins.**
A. Frontal pole.
B. Longitudinal fissure.
C. Occipital pole.
D. Remnant of dura, most of which has been removed.
E. Large superior cerebral veins. The one of the left drains into a lacuna (F) of the
   superior sagittal sinus.
F. Lacuna of the superior sagittal sinus.
G. Superior sagittal sinus.
H. Openings of veins into the sinus.
I. (Added) large superior cerebral veins. The one on the left opens into a lacuna (J),
   that is smaller than the one at F.
J. Lacuna of superior sagittal sinus.

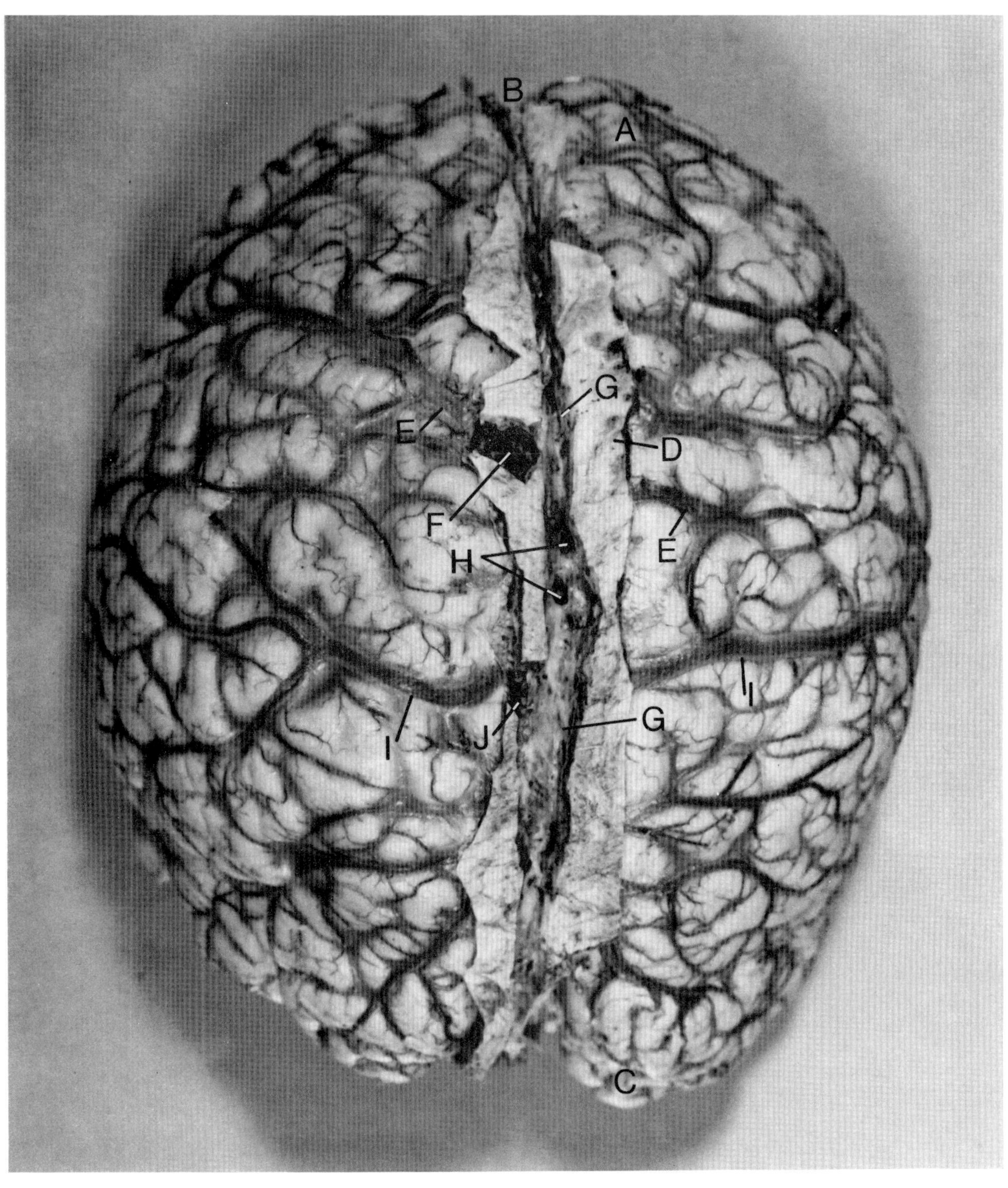

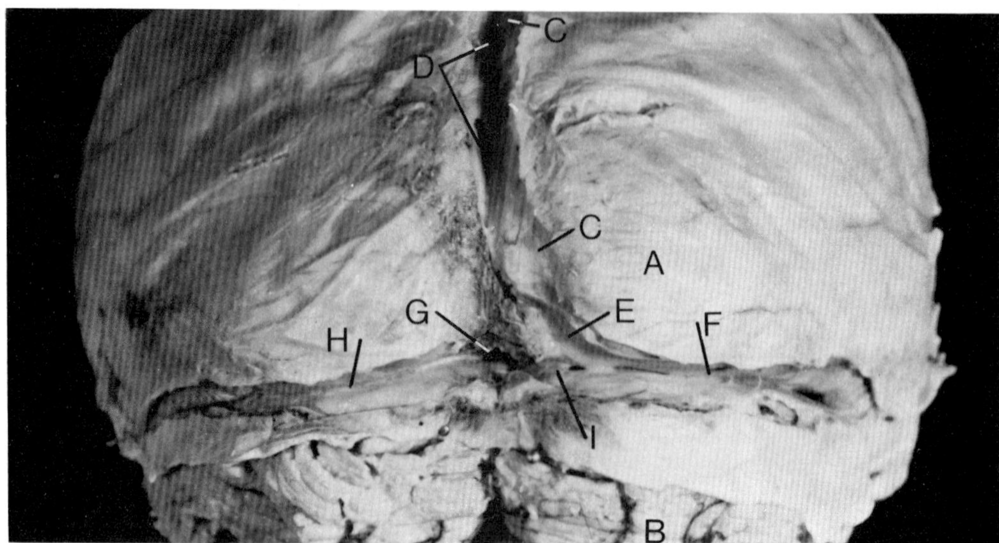

Figure 8-3. **Dural Sinuses as seen in Posterior View.**

A. Dura covering occipital pole.

B. Cerebellar hemisphere.

C. Lumen of superior sagittal sinus.

D. Openings of veins into the sinus.

E. The superior sagittal sinus turns to the right to connect with the transverse sinus.

F. Right transverse sinus.

G. Opening of the straight sinus, connecting with the left transverse sinus.

H. Left transverse sinus.

I. Channel of communication between the two transverse sinuses, with formation of the confluens sinuum.

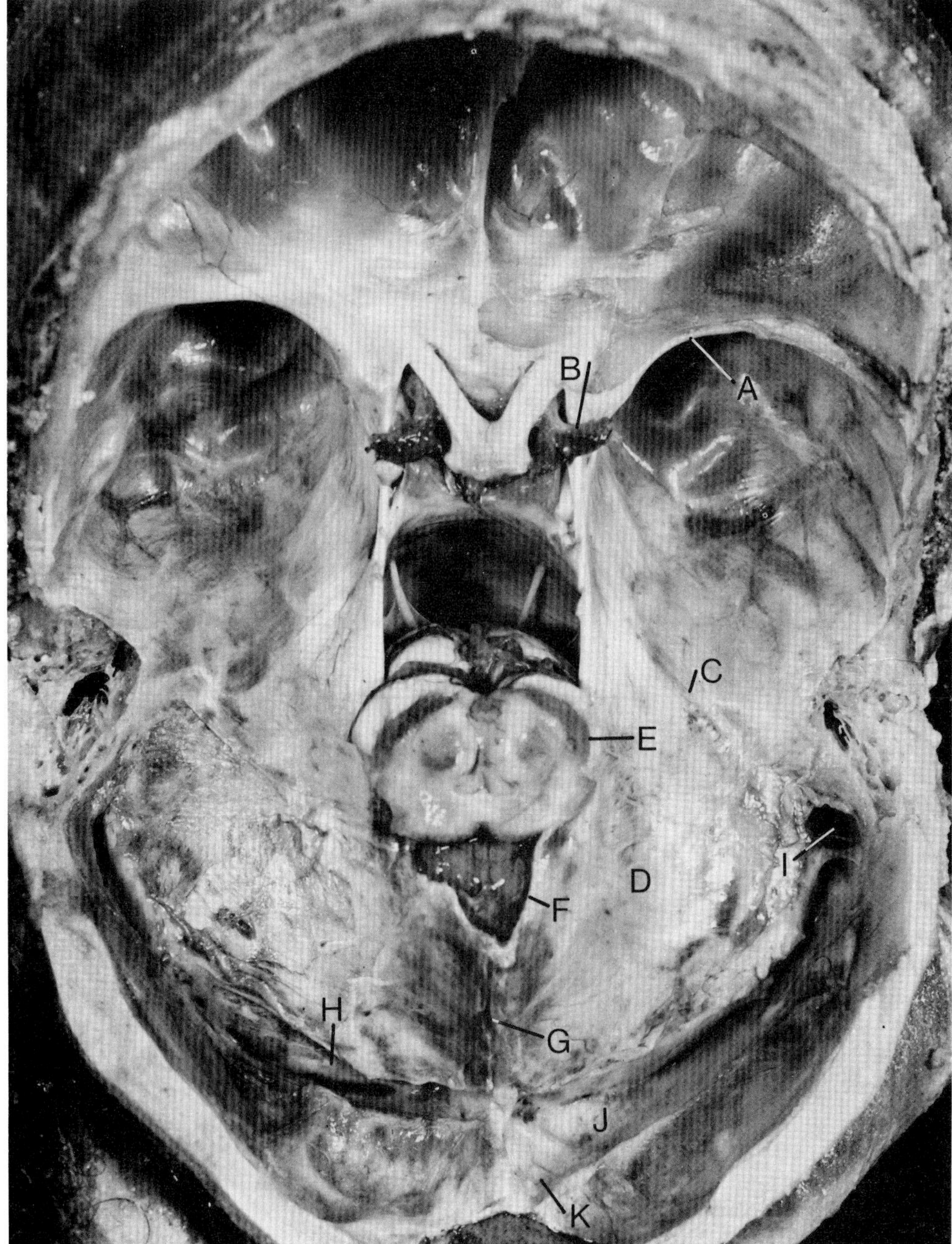

Figure 8-4. **Dural Sinuses as seen with Cerebrum Removed.**

A. Sphenoparietal sinus runs in the margin of the dura bordering the lesser wing of the sphenoid.

B. Internal carotid artery.

C. The superior petrosal sinus within the junction of tentorium with that portion of the dura covering the upper margin of the petrous bone.

D. Tentorium.

E. The edge of the tentorium extends across the cerebral peduncle on each side; if swelling occurs, there may be grooving of the peduncle.

F. Continuation of incisural margin of tentorium.

G. Straight sinus (open) lies in the triangle formed by the junction of tentorium with falx cerebri (removed).

H. Left lateral sinus; it receives mainly the straight sinus.

I. Point of turning downward of right lateral sinus to continue as sigmoid sinus.

J. Right lateral sinus.

K. Point of turning of the superior sagittal sinus to the right to continue as the lateral sinus.

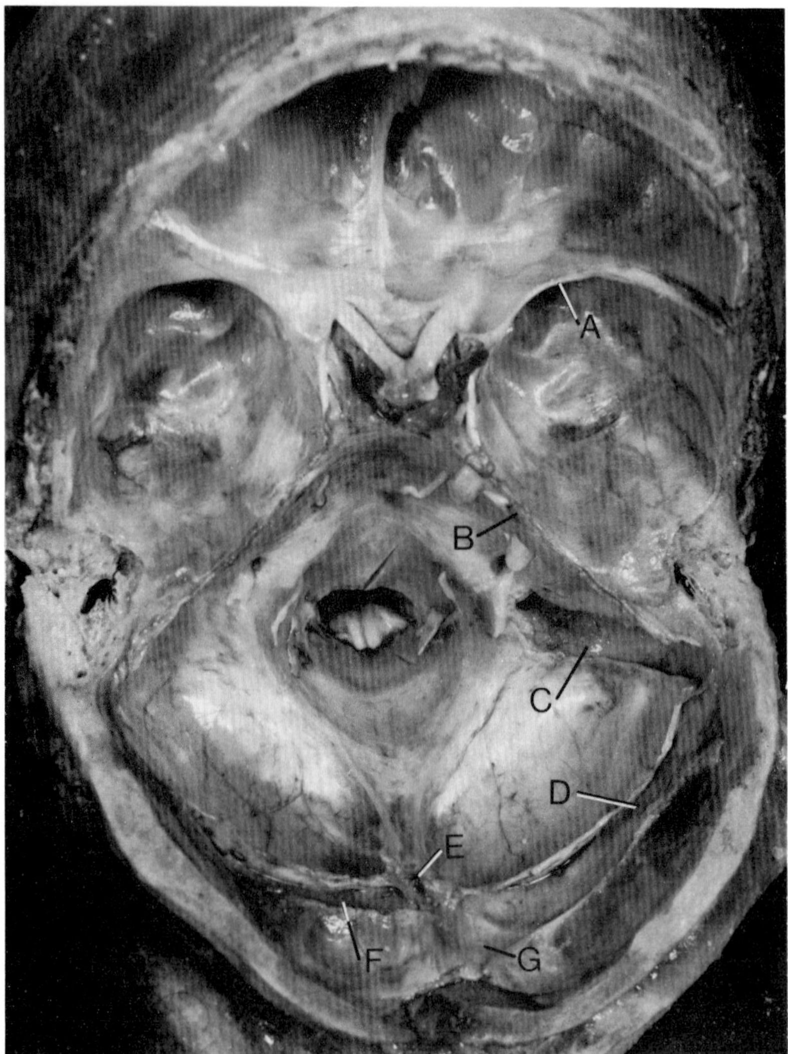

Figure 8-5. **Dural Sinuses.** continuation from 8-4. with removal of tentorium, cerebellum, and brain stem.

A. Sphenoparietal sinus runs within the border of the dura covering the margin of the lesser wing of the sphenoid.

B. Superior petrosal sinus lies within the point of junction of tentorium and the dura covering the upper margin of the petrous bone. The tentorium has been removed, resulting in opening the sinus.

C. Sigmoid sinus.

D. Transverse sinus.

E. Point of junction of occipital sinus with straight sinus.

F. Left lateral sinus. It appears smaller than the right.

G. Point of turning to the right of the superior sagittal sinus to continue as the right lateral sinus.

Figure 8-6. **Jugular Venogram.** (See pages 94 and 95.)

Figure 8-6. **Jugular Venogram.** Lateral (**A**) and Anterior-Posterior (**B**) Views. →
A. Transverse sinus.
B. Sigmoid sinus.
C. Jugular bulb.
D. Internal jugular vein.
E. Collateral veins of the neck.
F. Torcular Herophili.

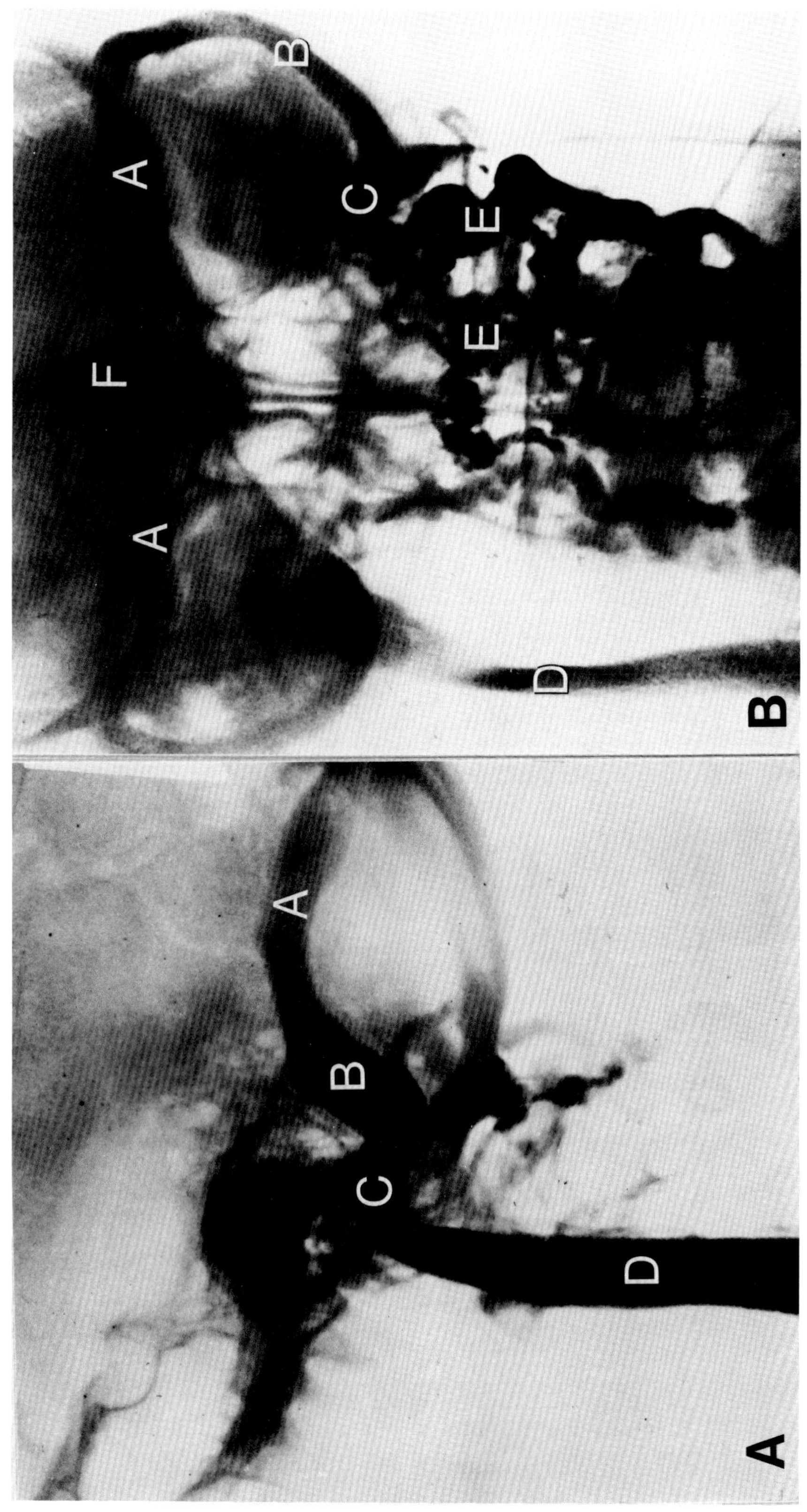

Figure 8-7. **Lateral Vertebral Angiogram, Capillary (A) and Venous (B) Views, Normal Anatomy.**

A. Capillary stain of the thalamus and choroid plexus of the third ventricle.
B. Capillary stain of the occipital lobes.
C. Capillary stain of the cerebellum.
D. Internal cerebral vein.
E. Great cerebral vein (Galen).
F. Precentral cerebellar vein.
G. Superior vermian vein.
H. Lateral mesencephalic vein.
I. Posterior mesencephalic vein.
J. Anterior pontomesencephalic vein.
K. Superior petrosal vein.
L. Straight sinus.
M. Inferior vermian vein,copular point.
N. Internal occipital vein.

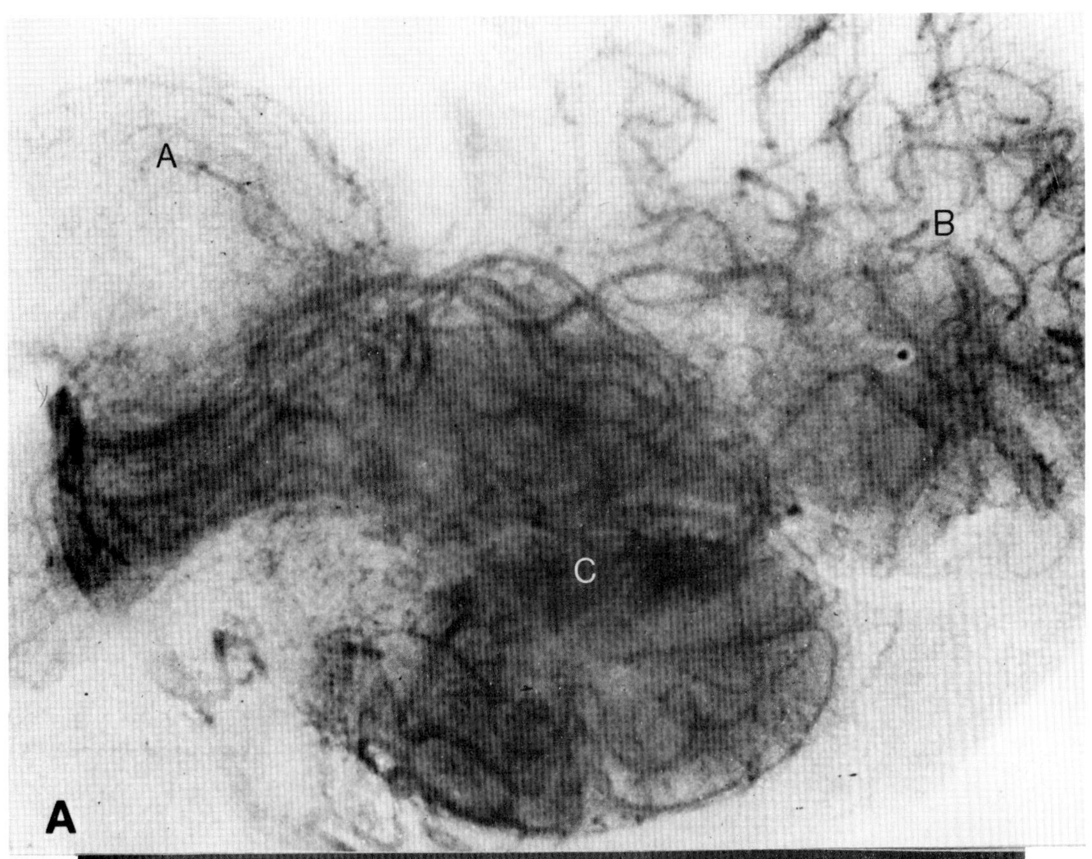
A
B
C
A

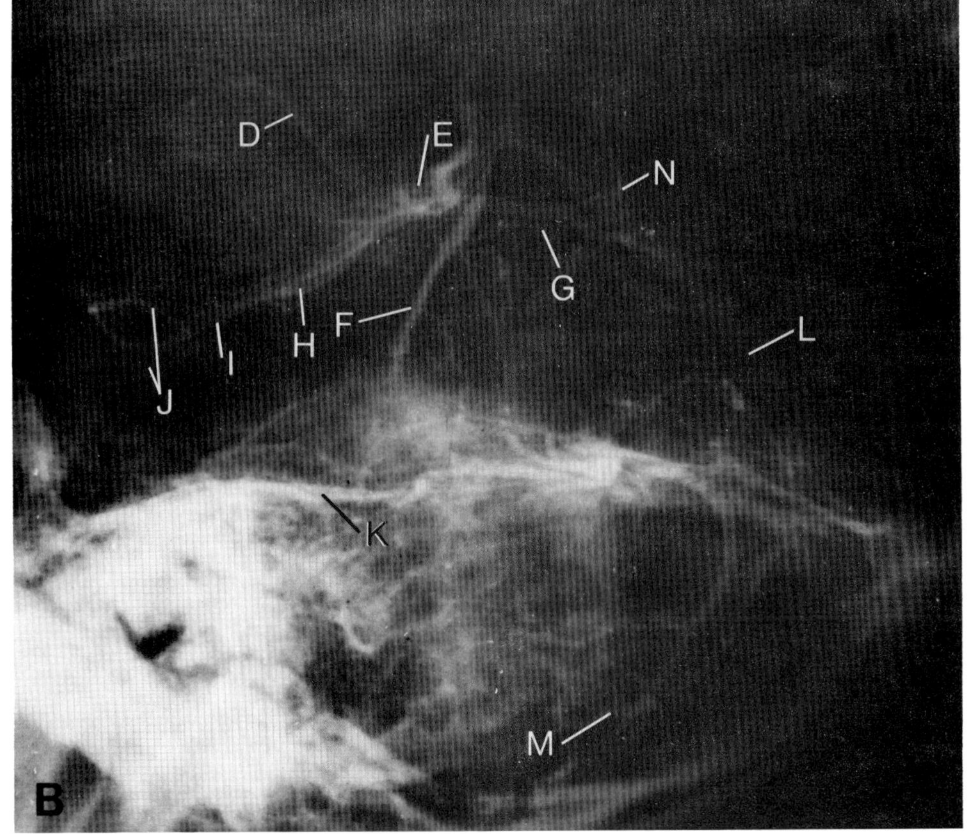
D
E
N
G
F
H
I
J
L
K
M
B

Figure 8-8. **AP Vertebral Posterior Fossa, Normal Venous Anatomy. A and B** →
demonstrate various aspects of venous anatomy from two different patients.
A. Transverse sinus.
B. Torcular Herophili.
C. Superior sagittal sinus.
D. Inferior vermian vein, main trunk.
E. Inferior vermian vein, inferior retrotonsillar branch.
F. Inferior vermian vein, superior retrotonsillar branch.
G. Petrosal vein.
H. Superior petrosal sinus.
I. Peduncular veins.
J. Lateral mesencephalic vein.
K. Transverse pontine vein.
L. Precentral cerebellar vein.
M. Brachial vein.
N. Inferior hemispheric vein.

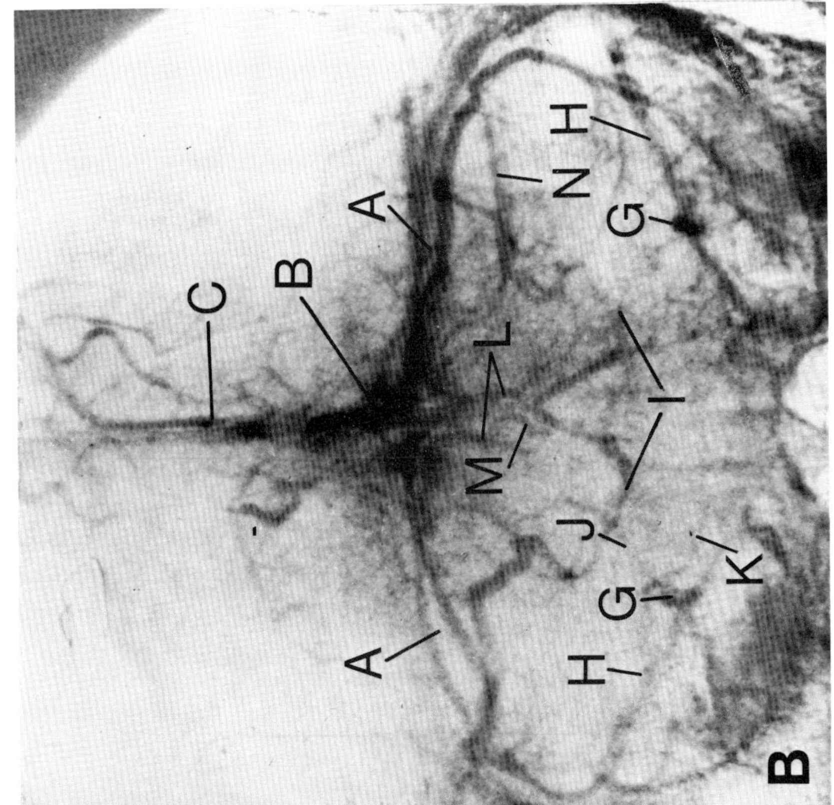

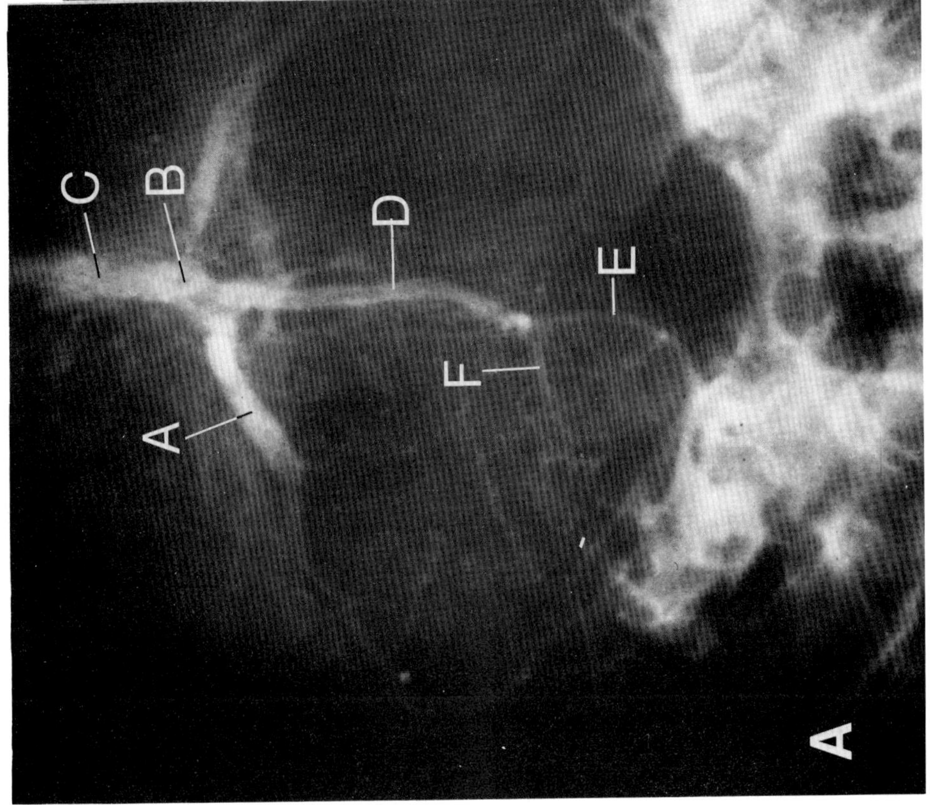

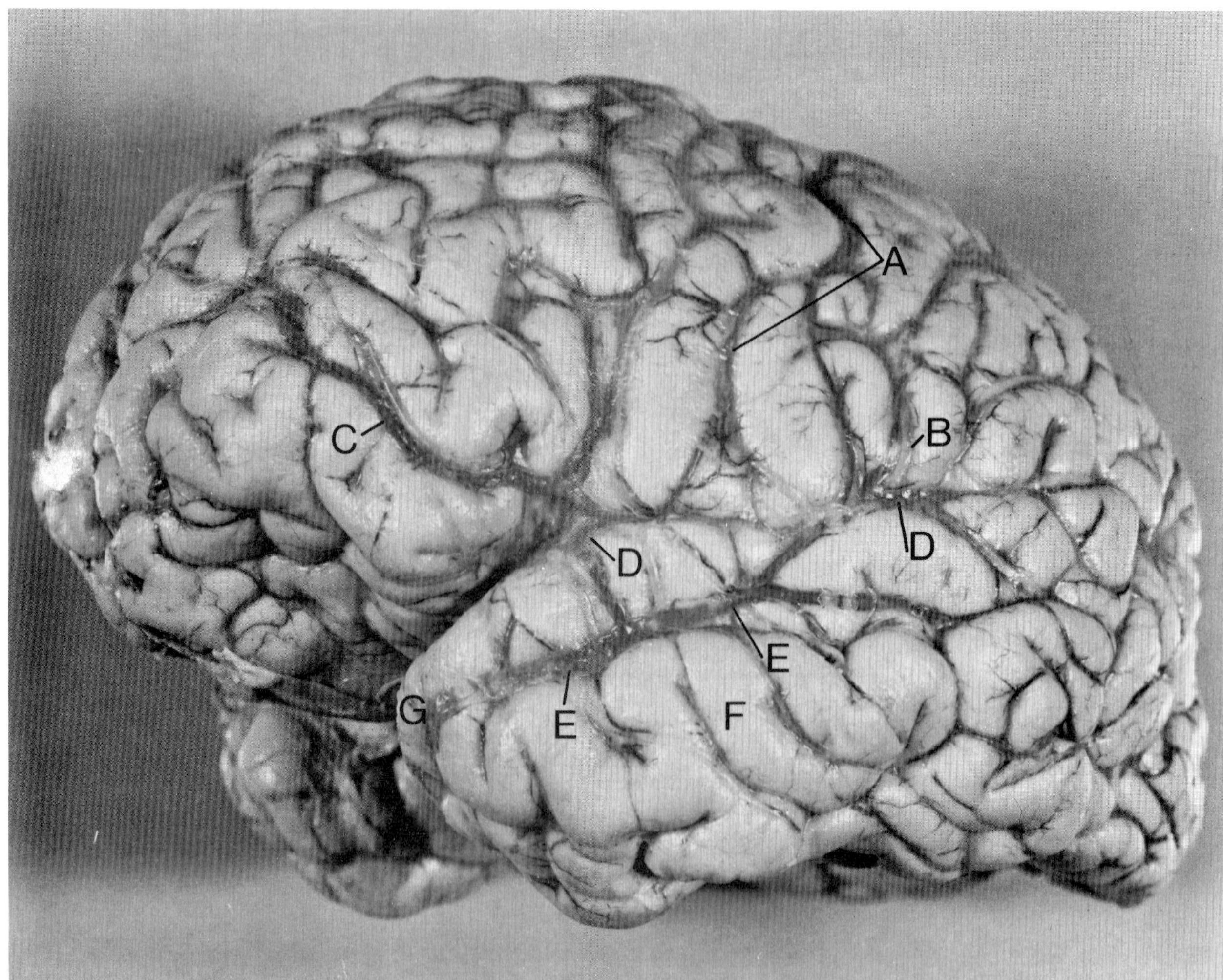

Figure 8-9. **Superficial Cerebral Veins, as seen in Lateral View of Brain.** The variability of pattern of vessels and convolutions is illustrated in this case. The precentral gyrus, anterior to the central sulcus, the latter marked A, is somewhat serpiginous near the vertex. The arachnoid is in place over the cerebral surface, and a plentiful network of veins is apparent. Two of them, marked A and C, appear to extend from the vertex to the lateral sulcus, and are of large size, and qualify as superior anastomotic veins. An added, branched venous segment extending along a sulcus marked B appears to fit into the same functional category. The middle cerebral vein (D) appears to extend along the lateral sulcus in the usual way. A still larger vein, however, appears to qualify as a middle cerebral vein; extending along the superior temporal sulcus (E), it ends at the temporal pole (G). In situ, it joined the sphenoparietal sinus. The middle temporal gyrus (F) appears somewhat broader (vertical dimension) than usual.

A. Central sulcus.
A, B, C. Superior cerebral veins, appearing to qualify as anastomotic.
D. Middle cerebral vein.
E. Vein appearing to serve similarly as middle cerebral.
F. Middle temporal gyrus.
G. Temporal pole; end of the vein designated E.

Figure 8-10. **Deep Veins.** (See pages 102 and 103.)

$\longrightarrow$

Figure 8-10. **Deep Veins.**
A. Dural sinuses and deep venous tributaries. Viewed from side and above obliquely, with portions of right cerebral hemisphere removed.
  A. Falx cerebri.
  B. Superior sagittal sinus.
  C. Tentorium.
  D. Inferior sagittal sinus.
  E. Straight sinus.
  F. Point of junction of great cerebral vein with straight sinus.
  G. Great cerebral vein.
  H. Left internal cerebral vein.
  I. Right internal cerebral vein.
  J. Basal vein.
B. Horizontal view of deep veins as viewed from above. (Compare with Fig. **A.**)
  A. Great cerebral vein.
  B. Internal cerebral vein.
  C. Basal vein.
  D. Thalamostriate vein.
  E. Choroidal vein with choroid plexus.

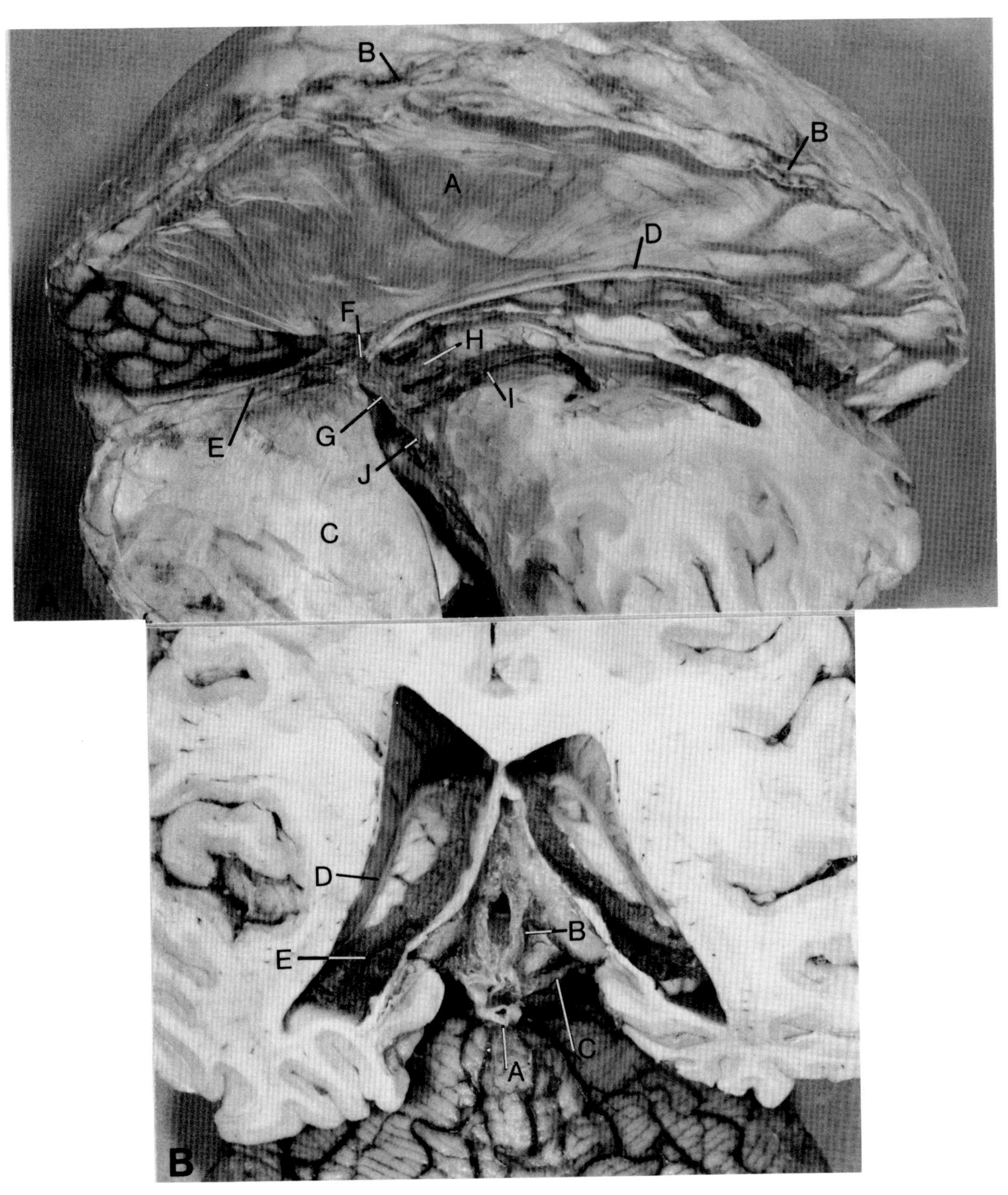

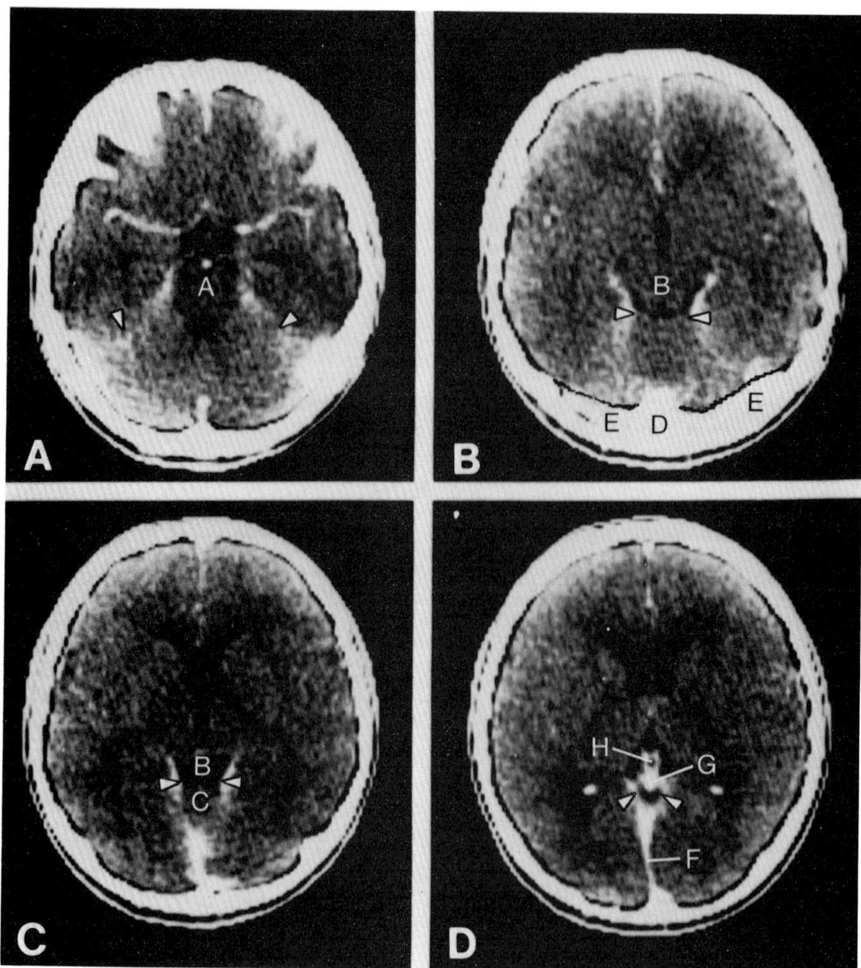

Figure 8-11. **Normal Tentorium in Axial CT Projection.** Four contrast enhanced levels, progressing cephalad (**A-D**) demonstrate the tentorial edge (*Arrowheads*) with a "Y" or "tuning fork" appearance which progressively narrows cephalad. Related structures include: (A) brain stem, (B) collicular plate (tectum), (C) superior cerebellar cistern with vermis, (D) torcular Herophili, (E) transverse sinus, (F) straight sinus, (G) great cerebral vein, and (H) internal cerebral veins.

Figure 8-12. **Deep Cerebral Veins: Thalamostriate, Choroidal, Internal Cerebral, Great Cerebral.** (See pages 106 and 107.)

Figure 8-12. **Deep Cerebral Veins: Thalamostriate, Choroidal, Internal Cerebral, Great Cerebral.** Portions of brain have been removed.

A. Medial view of right lateral ventricle and superior third ventricle with portions of cerebrum removed.

    A. Head of caudate nucleus.

    B. Thalamostriate vein. The collection of subependymal veins into the thalamostriate is shown.

    C. Thalamus.

    D. Choroid plexus.

    E. Choroidal vein.

    F. Internal cerebral vein.

    G. Corpus callosum. The course of venous channels tranverse to the ependymal surface of the ventricle is shown, together with the tangential surface course when the veins reach the ventricular surface.

B. Same general view in another case. Compare with **A.**

    A. Head of caudate nucleus.

    B. Thalamus.

    C. Thalamostriate vein. It is higher in the ventricular wall than usual. This configuration could produce artifactual widening of the venous angle, in lateral view angiographic studies. The variability of pattern of vessels is again illustrated.

    D. An aberrant subependymal vein of substantial size.

    E. Choroidal vein.

    F. Internal cerebral vein.

    G. Point of junction of the internal cerebral veins to form the great cerebral vein.

    H. Quadrigeminal cistern.

    I. Pons in sagittal section, showing the deep transverse course of the small penetrating vessels.

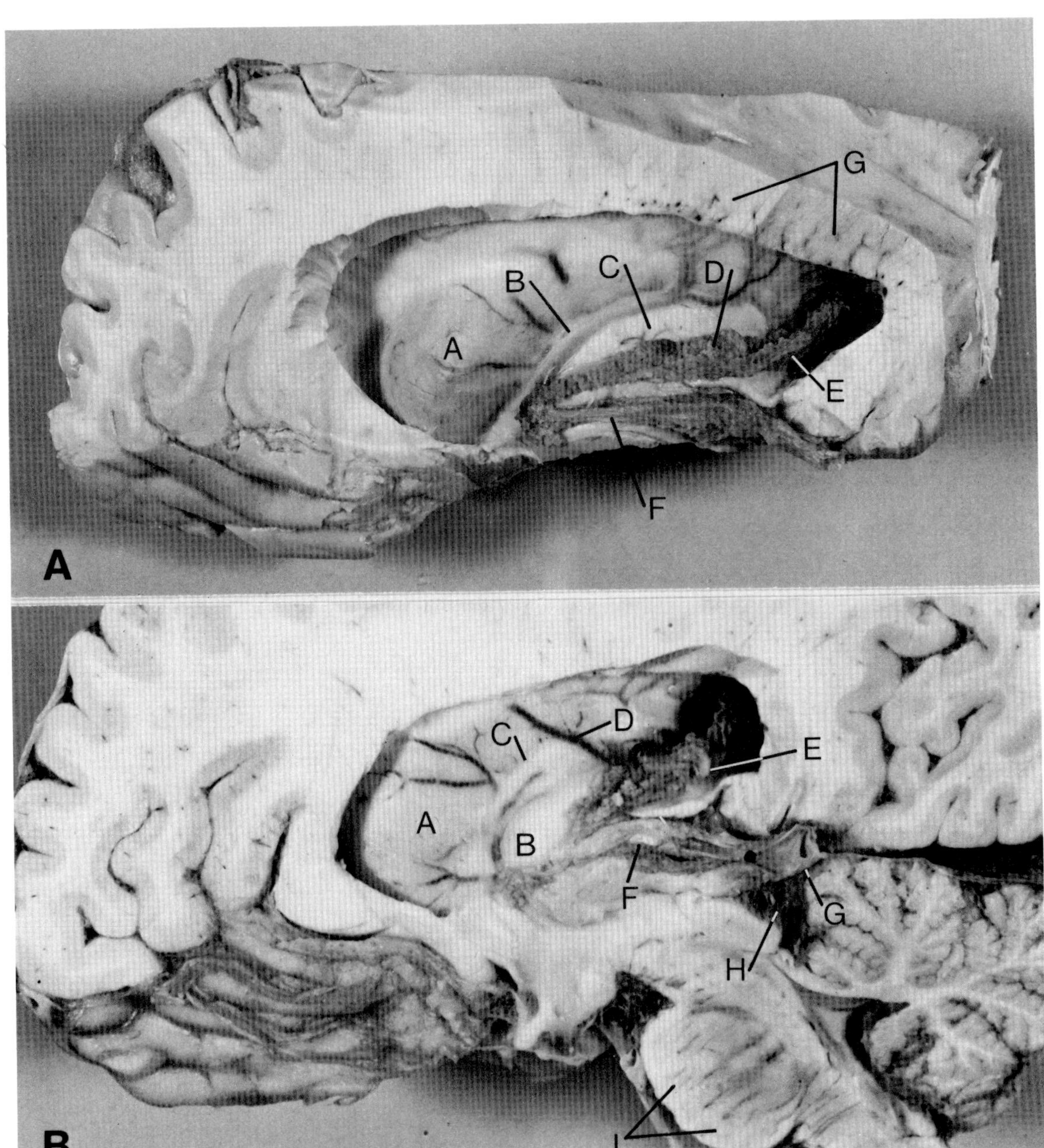
G
B
C
D
A
E
F
A
D
C
E
A
B
F
G
H
I
B

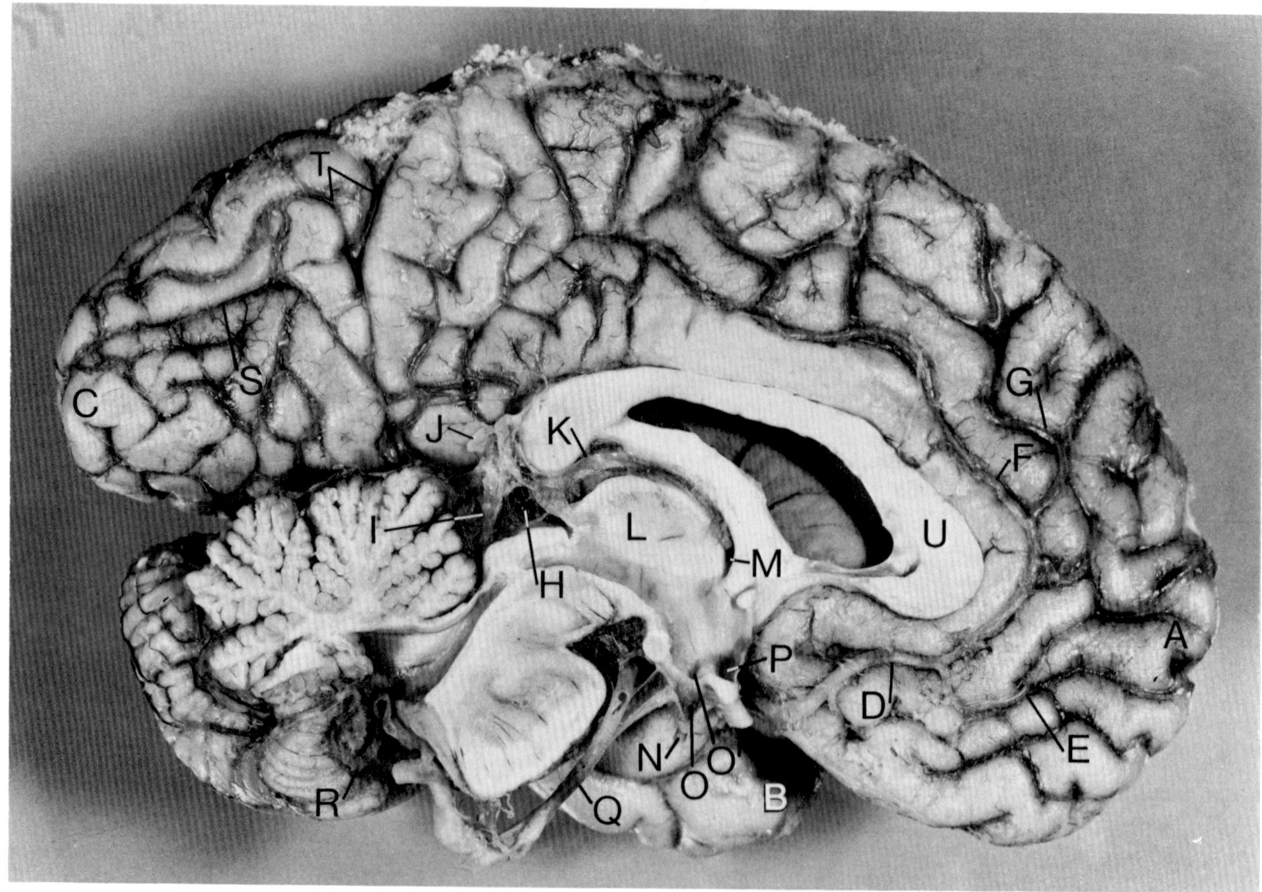

Figure 8-13. **Precentral Cerebellar Vein and Various Other Structures seen in Sagittal Section.** Compare with Figure 11-1.

A. Frontal pole.
B. Temporal pole.
C. Occipital pole.
D. Anterior cerebral artery. It is situated farther than usual from the corpus callosum, and so also is its continuation as the pericallosal artery (F), and the same applies to the callosomarginal artery (G).
E. Frontopolar artery.
F. Pericallosal a.
G. Callosomarginal a.
H. Quadrigeminal cistern.
I. Precentral cerebellar vein.
J. Great cerebral vein.
K. Internal cerebral vein.
L. Interthalamic connection ("massa intermedia"), involving almost the full extent of the medial aspect of the thalamus. (In some cases, there is none or almost none; this again illustrates the variability of structural formation of the brain.)
M. Interventricular foramen.
N. Stalk of pituitary.
O. Infundibulum; it presents a recess (O').
P. Optic recess.
Q. Basilar artery.
R. Posterior inferior cerebellar artery. It exhibits a double loop.
S. Calcarine artery and sulcus. The artery appears higher than usual. This demonstrates, again, the variability of formation of convolutions and vessels; compare with Figure 7-14. The occipitotemporal artery (T) is especially atypical in arrangement.
T. Occipitotemporal artery.
U. Corpus callosum genu.

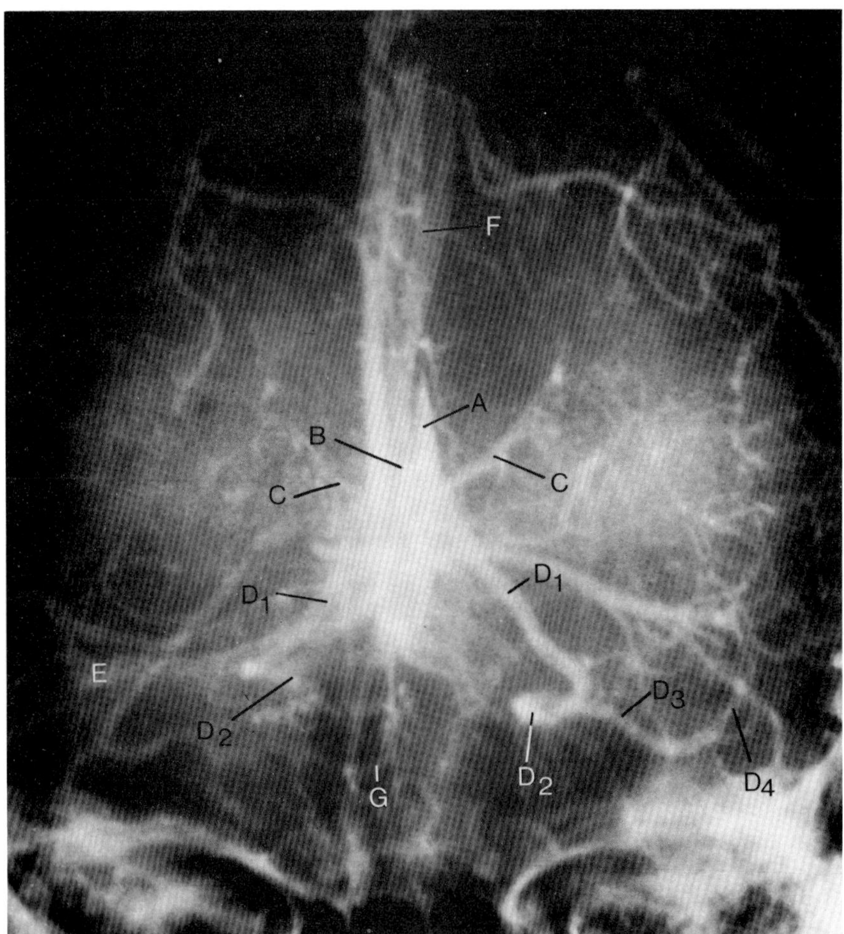

Figure 8-14. **AP Carotid Injection, Venous Phase.**
A. Great cerebral vein (Galen).
B. Internal cerebral vein.
C. Thalamostriate vein.
D.-1. Basal vein, lateral mesencephalic portion.
D.-2. Basal vein, prepeduncular portion.
D.-3. Deep middle cerebral vein, draining into basal vein.
D.-4. Insular vein, draining into deep middle cerebral vein.
E. Transverse sinus.
F. Superior sagittal sinus.
G. Septal vein.

Figure 8-15. **Internal Carotid Injection, AP (A) and Lateral (B) Venous Phase.**
A. Superior sagittal sinus.
B. Torcular Herophili.
C. Transverse sinus.
D. Sigmoid sinus.
E. Jugular bulb.
F. Internal jugular vein.
G. Straight sinus.
H. Superior anastomotic vein (Trolard).
I. Inferior anastomotic veins (Labbé).
J. Basal vein (Rosenthal).
K. Internal cerebral vein.
L. Septal vein.
M. Thalamostriate vein.
N. Anterior caudate vein.
O. Venous angle at interventricular foramen.
P. Prepeduncular veins draining into basal vein.
Q. Inferior petrosal sinus.
R. Great cerebral vein (Galen).

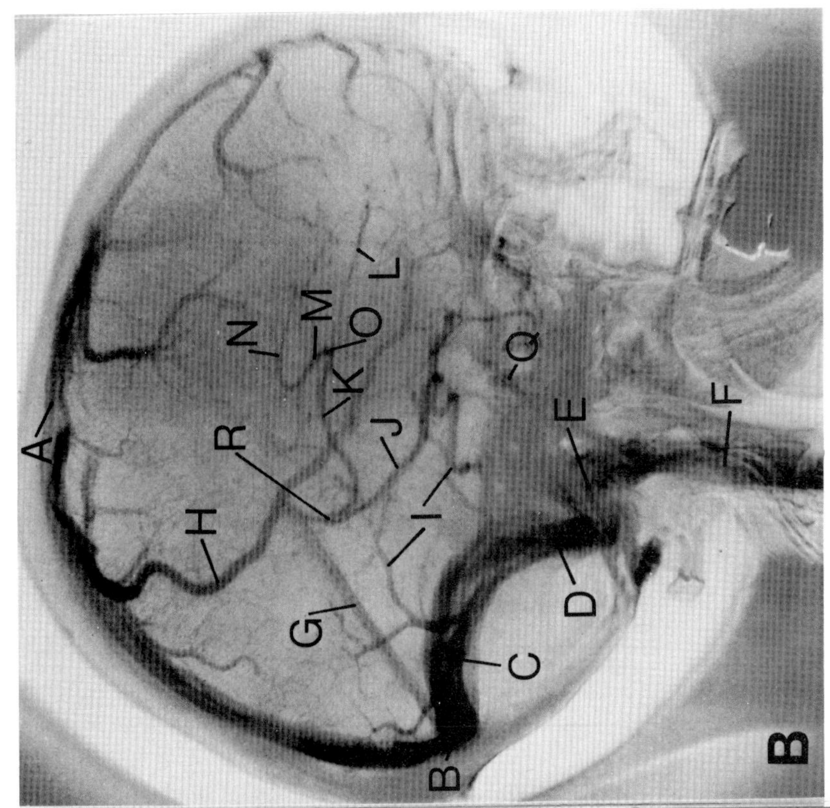
A
H
M
J
O
K
C
P
A

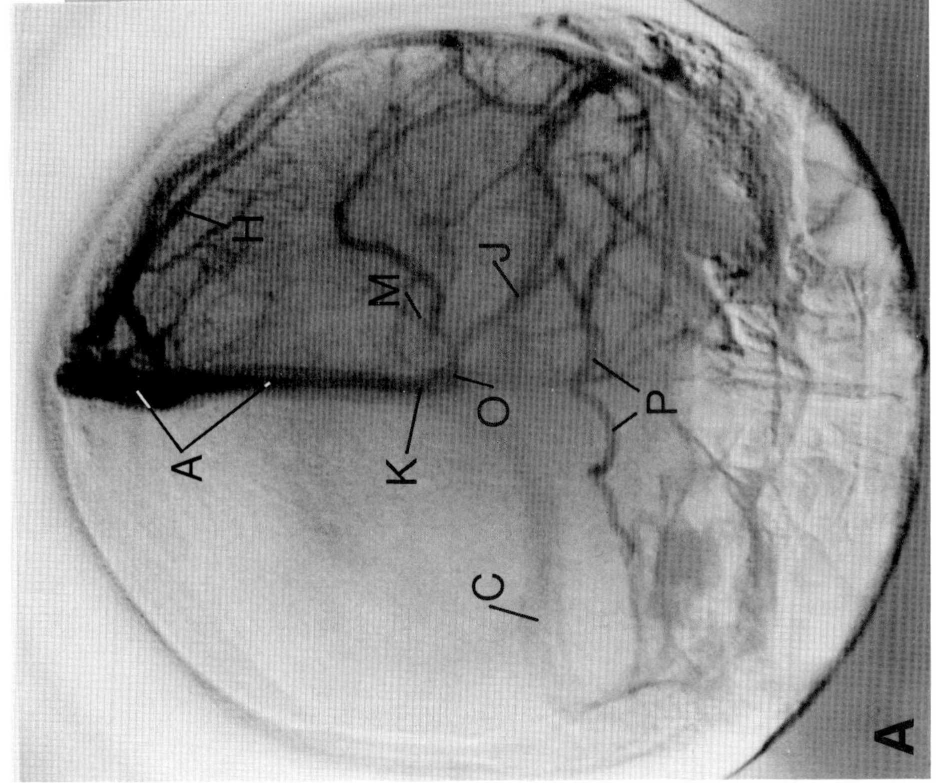
A
N
M
R
K
O
L
H
J
I
Q
G
E
C
D
F
B
B

SECTIONAL ANATOMY

15° AXIAL

Lettered symbols serve for gross and CT together. (Some symbols may pertain only to gross or to CT scan.)

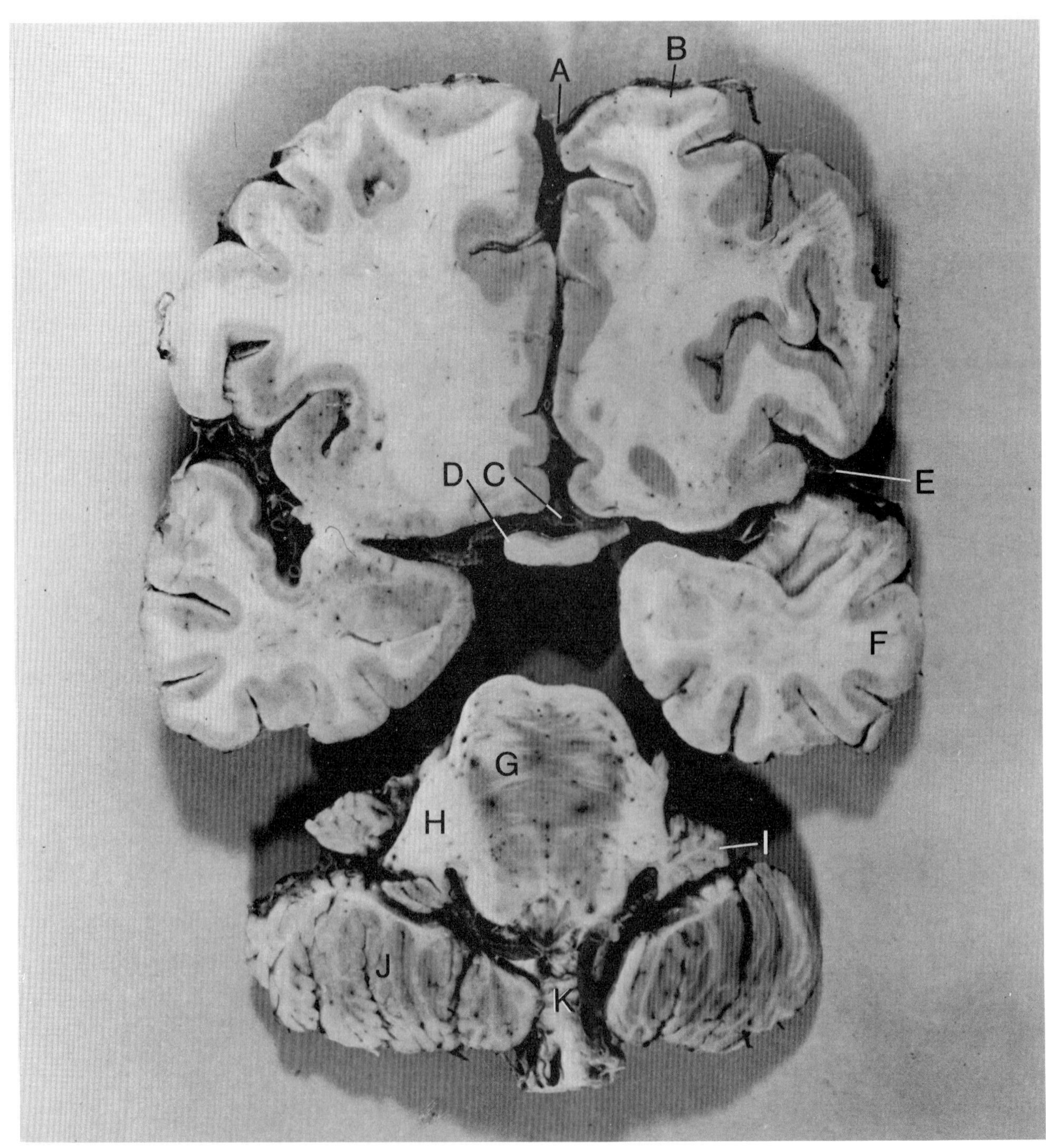

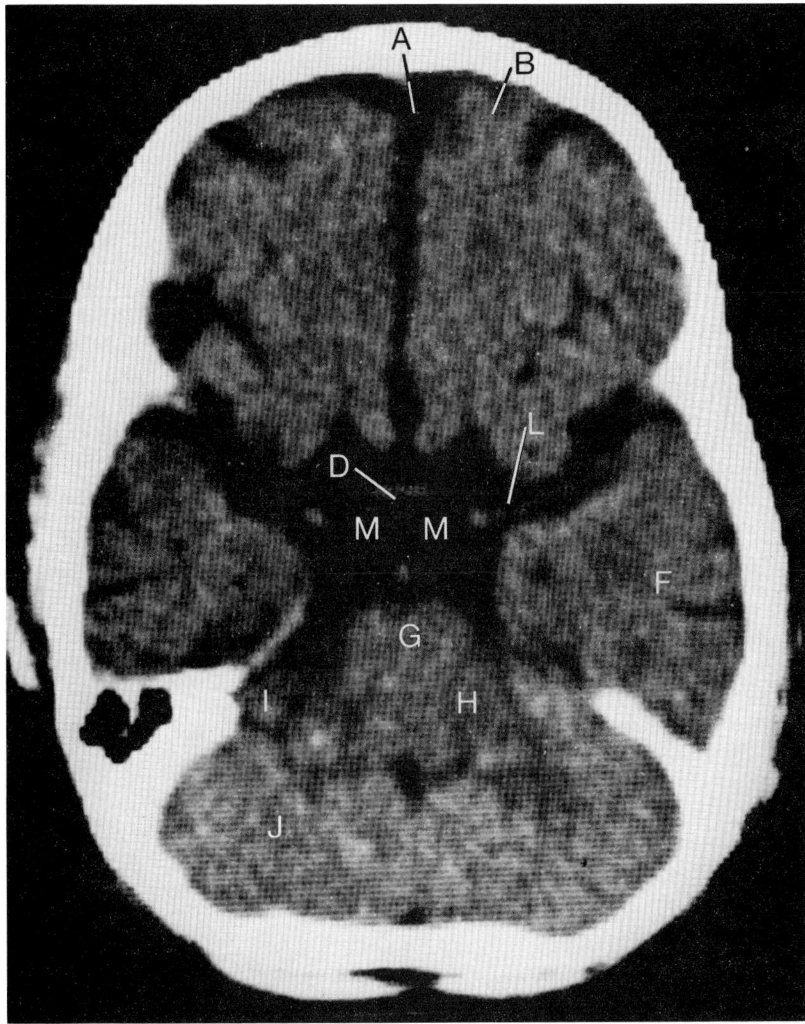

Figure 9-1-1, 2. **Level #1.**

A. Longitudinal fissure.

B. Frontal pole and lobe.

C. Anterior communicating artery.

D. Optic chiasm.

E. Lateral sulcus, containing middle cerebral artery (division).

F. Temporal lobe.

G. Pons.

H. Middle cerebellar peduncle.

I. Flocculus.

J. Cerebellar hemisphere.

K. Junction of medulla with cervical spinal cord.

L. Middle cerebral artery in cistern of the same name.

M. Chiasmatic (suprasellar) cistern.

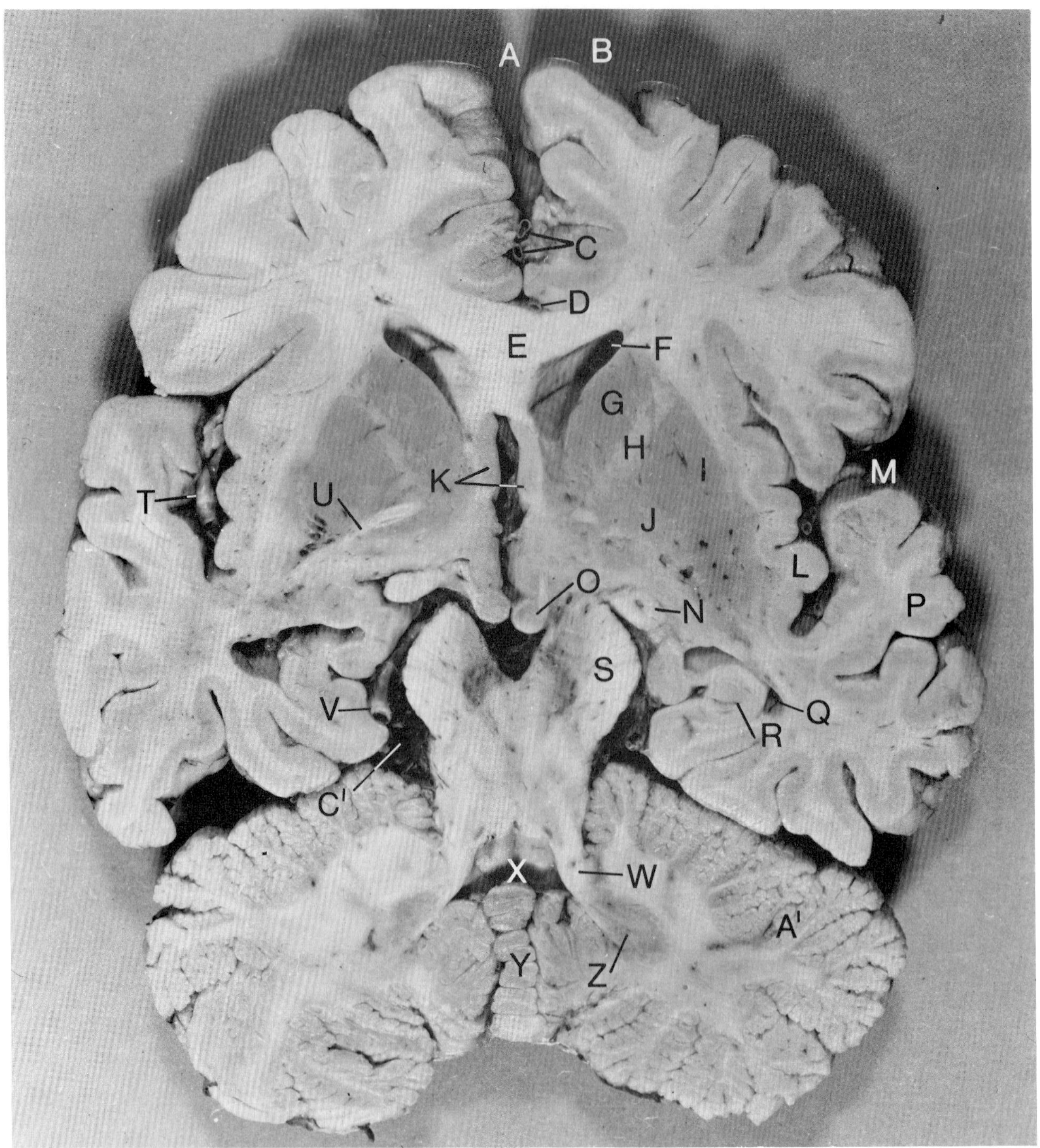

Figure 9-2-1, 2. **Level #2. Axial Series.**

A. Longitudinal fissure.

B. Frontal pole and lobe.

C, D. The variability of arrangement of arteries is illustrated. In C, the upper (more
    anterior) vessel shows the right callosomarginal artery at point of branching. The
    lower vessel (more posterior) is the left anterior cerebral artery, situated farther
    than usual from the corpus callosum, and not yet having contributed the
    callosomarginal artery (in keeping with the larger caliber of the vessel). D is the
    continuation of the right anterior cerebral artery (having early given off the calloso-
    marginal, C) as the supracallosal. See also Figures 7-14 and 8-13.

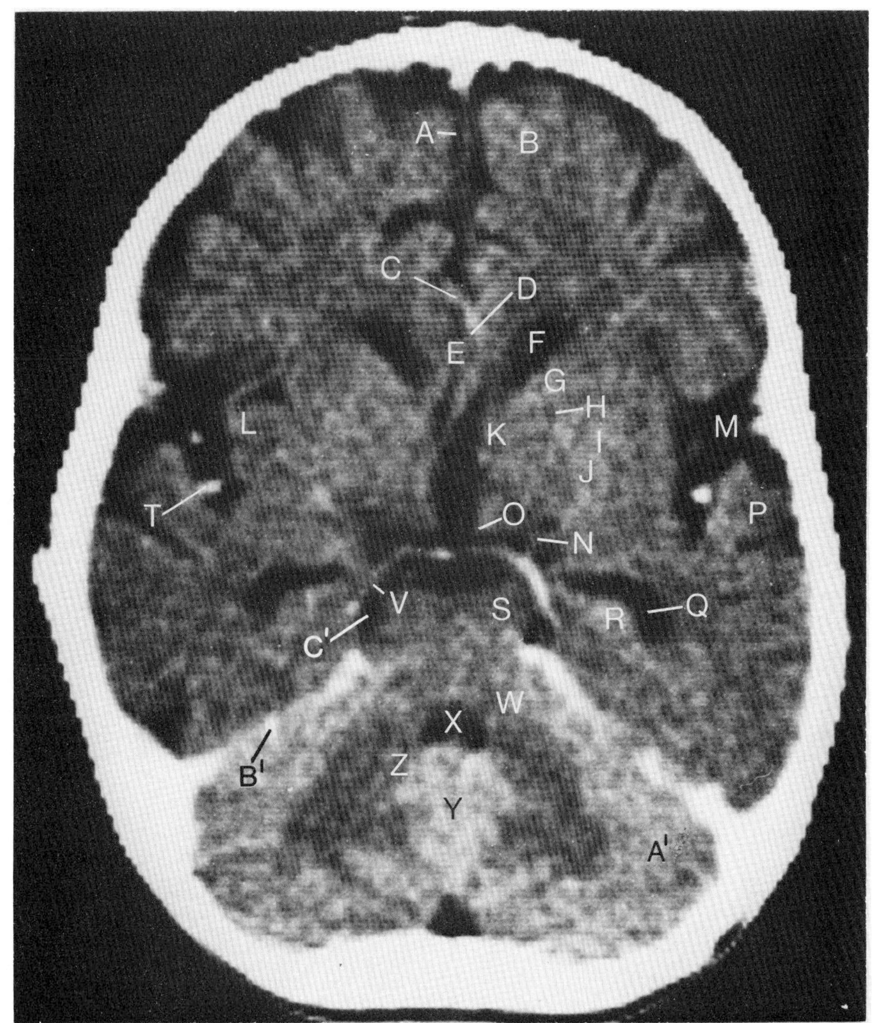

E. Corpus callosum.
F. Anterior horn of lateral ventricle.
G. Head of caudate nucleus.
H. Anterior limb of internal capsule.
I. Putamen.
J. Globus pallidus.
K. Subcallosal gyrus (paraolfactory area).
L. Insula.
M. Lateral sulcus.
N. Optic tract.
O. Mammillary body.
P. Temporal lobe.
Q. Inferior horn of lateral ventricle.
R. Hippocampus.
S. Cerebral peduncle.
T. Middle cerebral artery in suprainsular sulcus. The artery shows patchy sclerosis.
U. Anterior commissure.
V. Posterior cerebral artery. It also shows sclerosis.
W. Superior cerebellar peduncle.
X. Fourth ventricle.
Y. Vermis.
Z. Dentate nucleus.
A'. Cerebellar hemisphere.
B'. Tentorial blush (CT only).
C'. Perimesencephalic cistern.

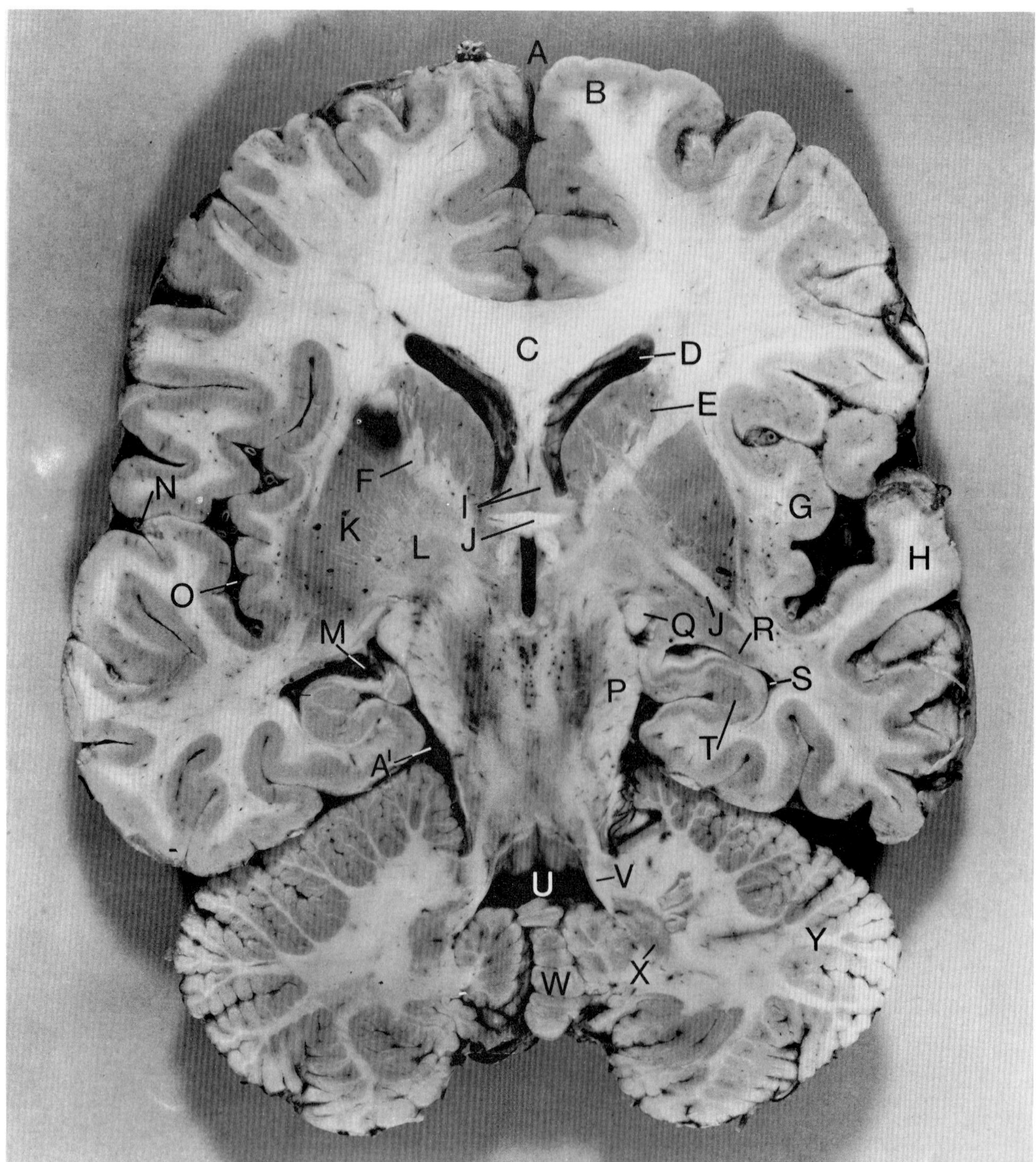

Figure 9-3-1, 2. **Level #3, Axial Series.**

A. Longitudinal fissure.
B. Frontal pole and lobe.
C. Corpus callosum.
D. Anterior horn of lateral ventricle.
E. Head of caudate nucleus.
F. Anterior limb of internal capsule. A focal hemorrhage is seen.
G. Insula.
H. Temporal lobe (primary sensory auditory area).

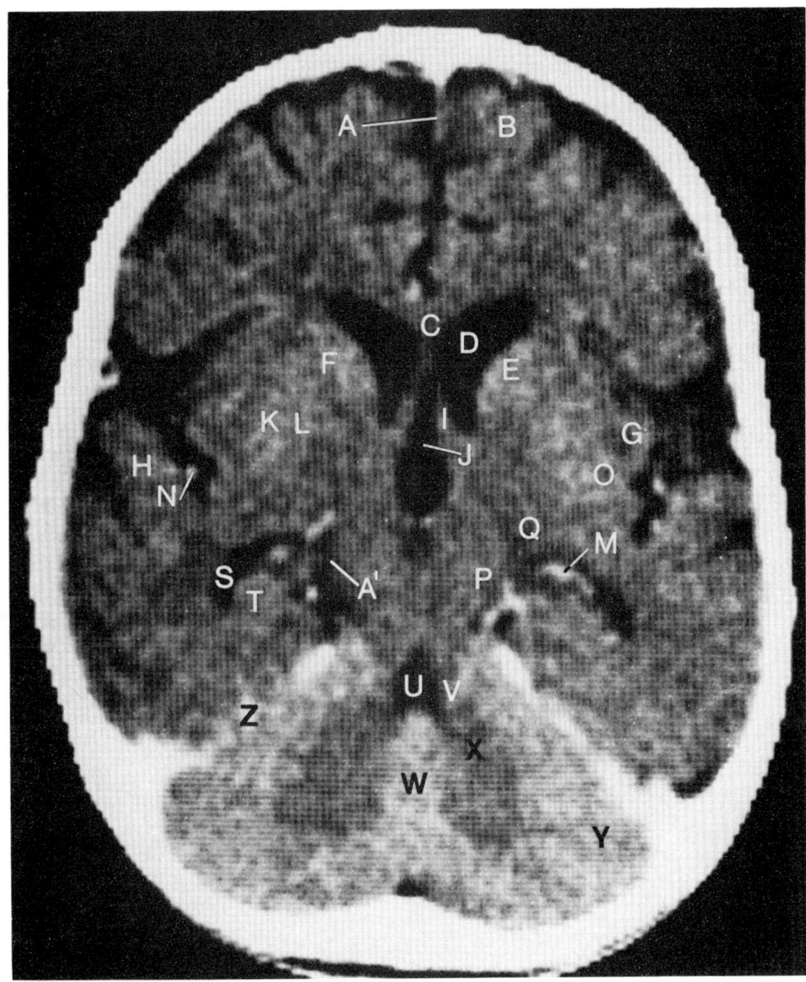

I. Subcallosal gyrus (paraolfactory area).
J. Anterior commissure.
K. Putamen.
L. Globus pallidus.
M. Choroid plexus, in inferior horn of lateral ventricle.
N. Middle cerebral artery branch in lateral sulcus.
O. Suprainsular sulcus containing middle cerebral artery branches.
P. Cerebral peduncle.
Q. Optic tract.
R. Tail of caudate nucleus.
S. Inferior horn of lateral ventricle.
T. Hippocampus.
U. Fourth ventricle.
V. Superior cerebellar peduncle.
W. Vermis.
X. Dentate nucleus.
Y. Cerebellar hemisphere.
Z. Tentorial edge.
A'. Perimesencephalic (ambient) cistern.

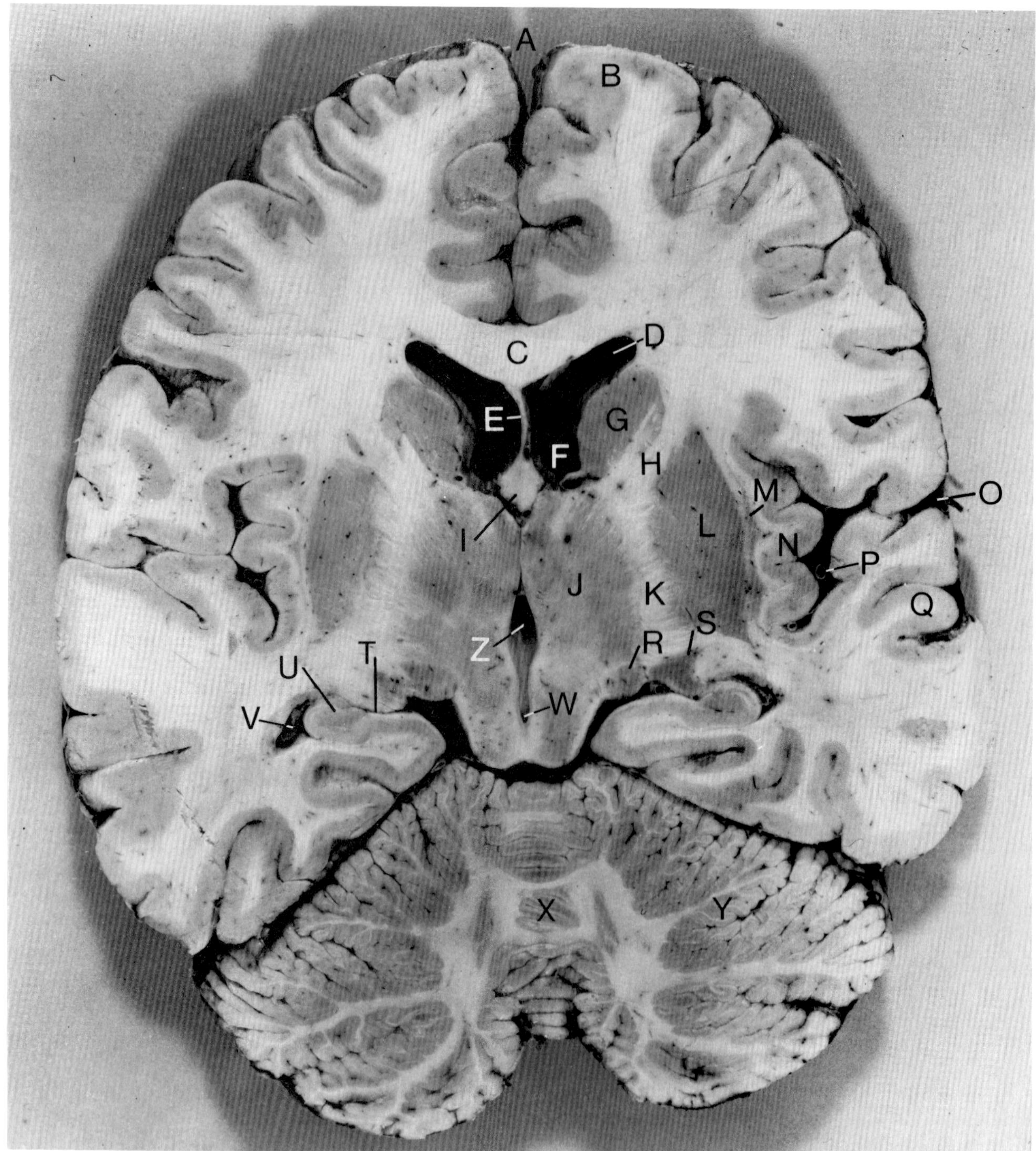

Figure 9-4-1, 2. **Level #4, Axial Series.**

A. Longitudinal fissure.
B. Frontal pole and lobe.
C. Corpus callosum.
D. Anterior horn of lateral ventricle.
E. Septum pellucidum.
F. Body of lateral ventricle.
G. Head of caudate nucleus.
H. Anterior limb of internal capsule.

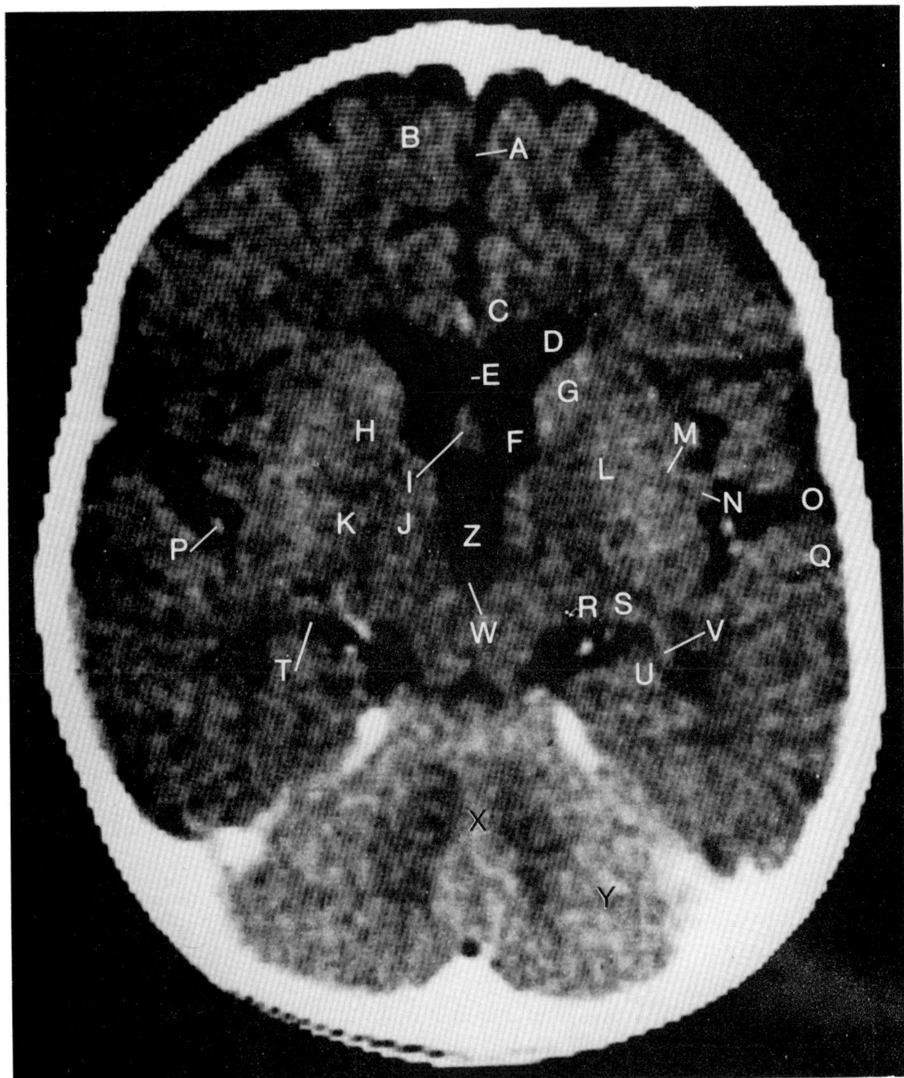

I. Body of fornix.
J. Thalamus.
K. Posterior limb of internal capsule.
L. Lenticular nucleus (putamen).
M. Claustrum.
N. Insula.
O. Lateral sulcus and cistern.
P. Middle cerebral artery branch in suprainsular sulcus.
Q. Temporal lobe.
R. Medial geniculate body.
S. Lateral geniculate body.
T. Choroidal fissure.
U. Hippocampus.
V. Choroid plexus in inferior horn of lateral ventricle.
W. Beginning of cerebral aqueduct.
X. Vermis.
Y. Cerebellar hemisphere.
Z. Third ventricle.

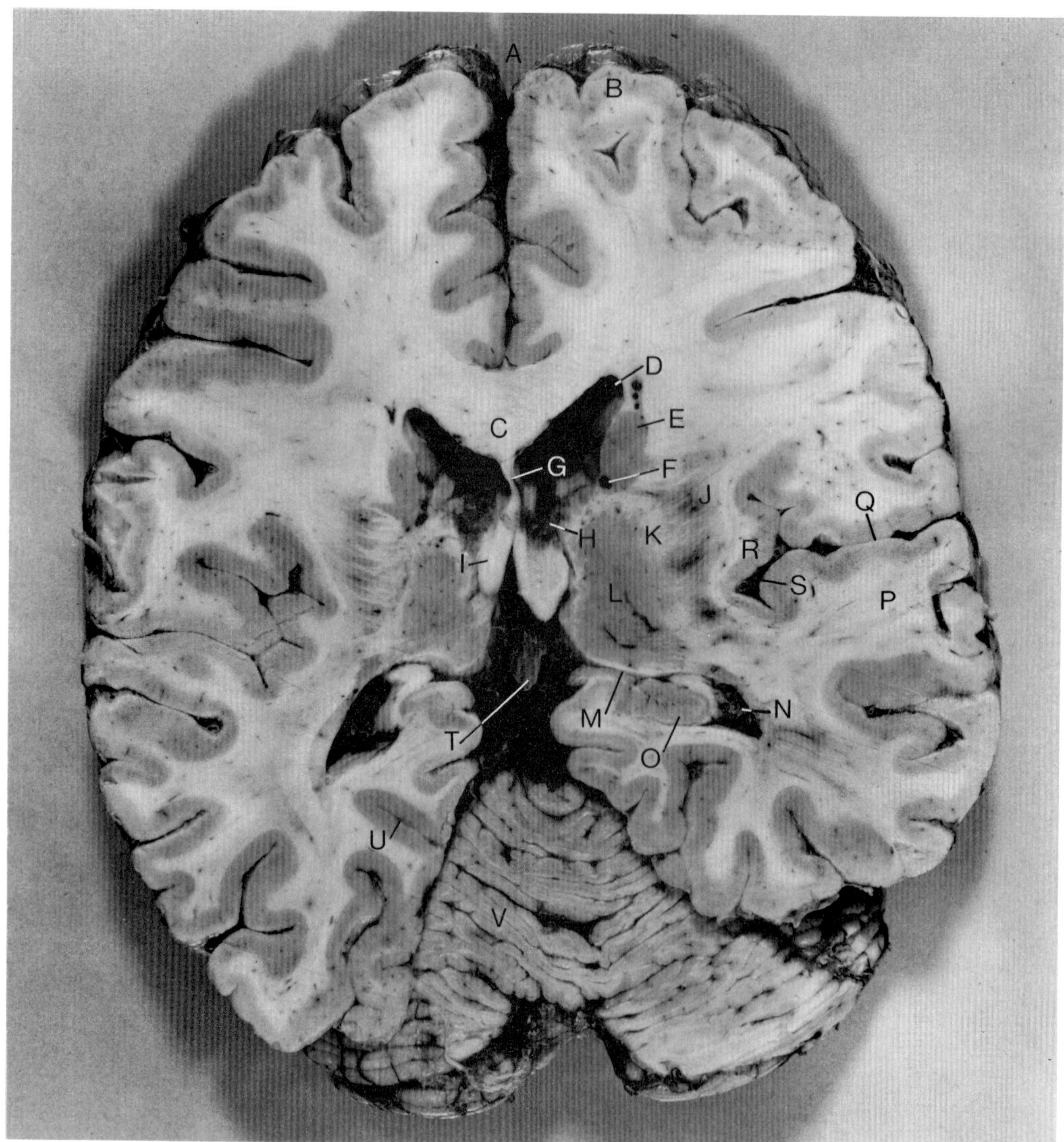

Figure 9-5-1, 2. **Level # 5, Axial Series.**

A. Longitudinal fissure.
B. Frontal pole and lobe.
C. Corpus callosum.
D. Anterior horn of lateral ventricle.
E. Head of caudate nucleus.
F. Thalamostriate vein.
G. Septum pellucidum.
H. Choroid plexus.
I. Column of fornix.
J. Putamen.

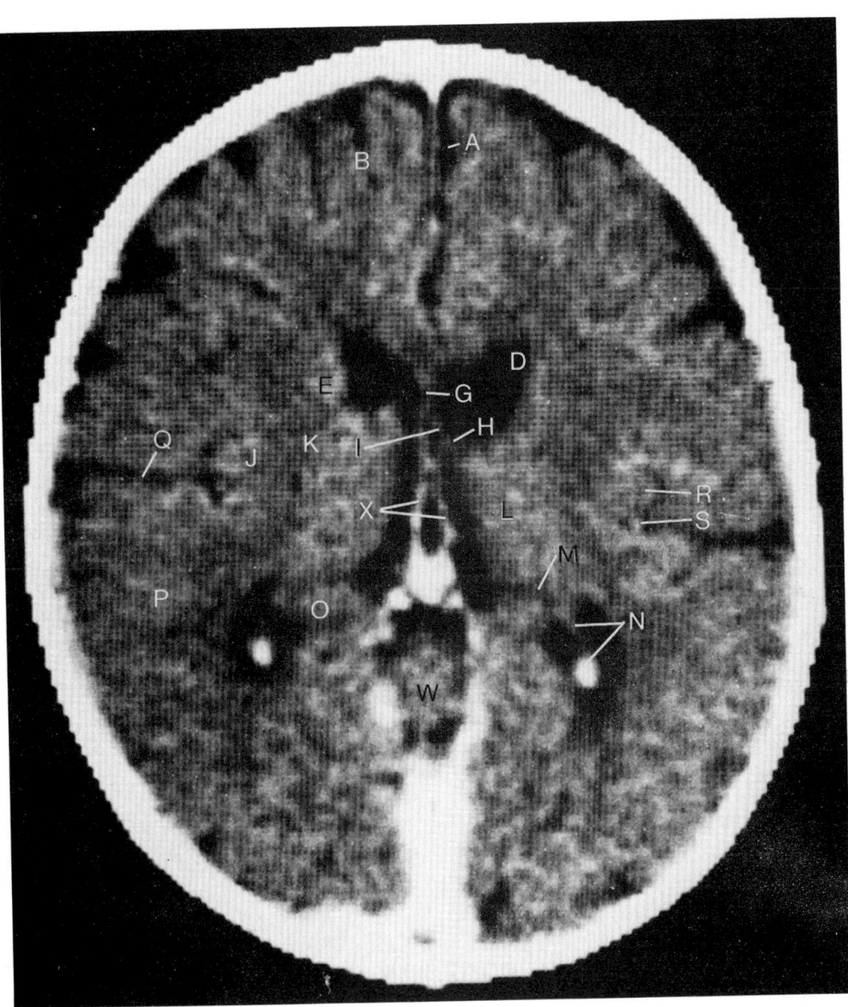

K. Internal capsule.
L. Thalamus.
M. Choroidal fissure.
N. Choroid plexus in inferior horn of lateral ventricle.
O. Hippocampus.
P. Temporal lobe.
Q. Lateral sulcus.
R. Insula.
S. Suprainsular sulcus, containing middle cerebal artery branches.
T. Pineal.
U. Occipitoparietal sulcus.
V. Cerebellar hemisphere.
W. Cerebellar vermis.
X. Internal cerebral veins in roof of third ventricle.

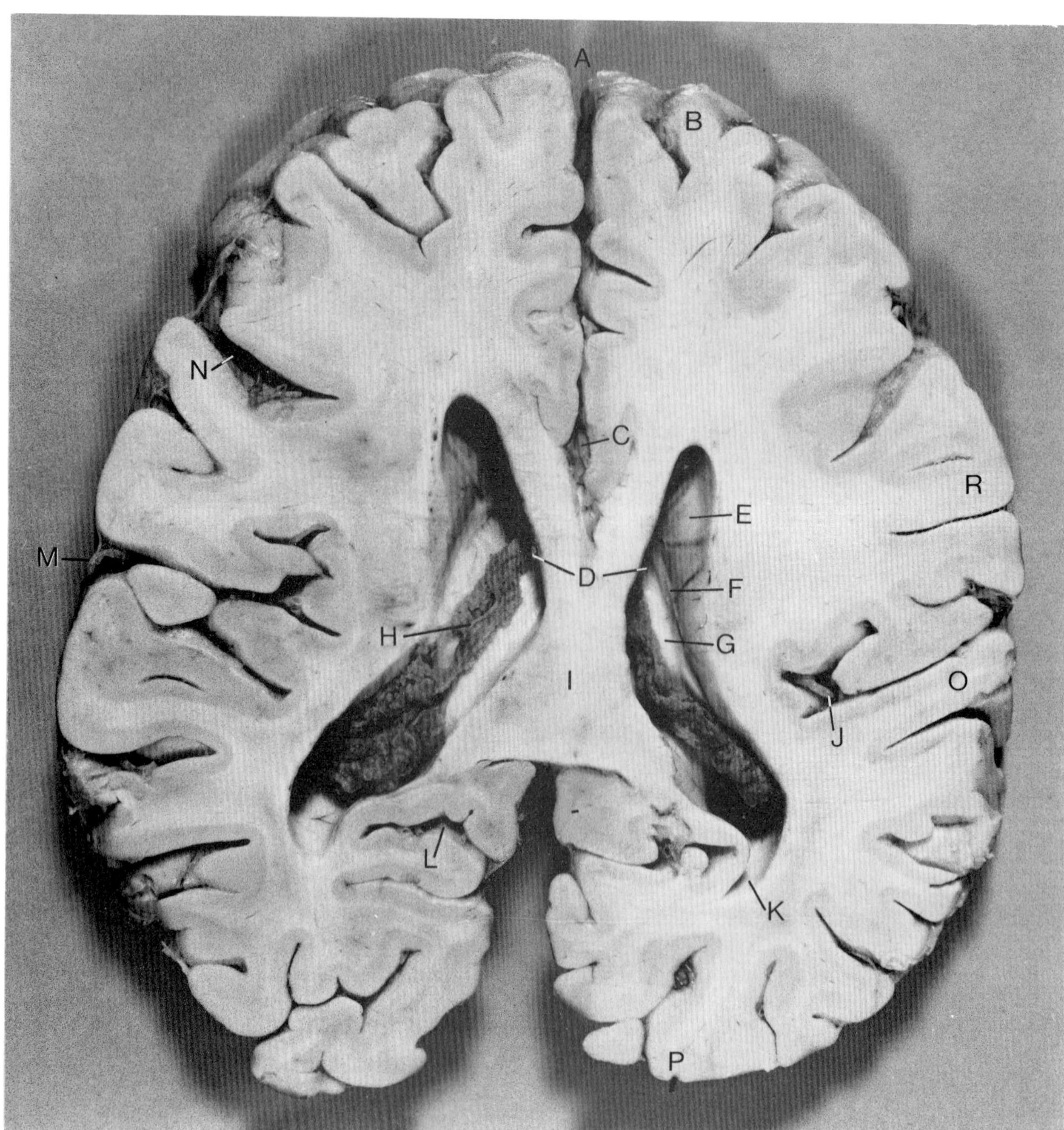

Figure 9-6-1, 2. **Level #6, Axial Series.**

A. Longitudinal fissure.
B. Frontal pole and lobe.
C. Anterior cerebral arteries.
D. Body of lateral ventricle.
E. Caudate nucleus.
F. Thalamostriate vein.
G. Thalamus.
H. Choroidal vein with choroid plexus.
I. Corpus callosum.

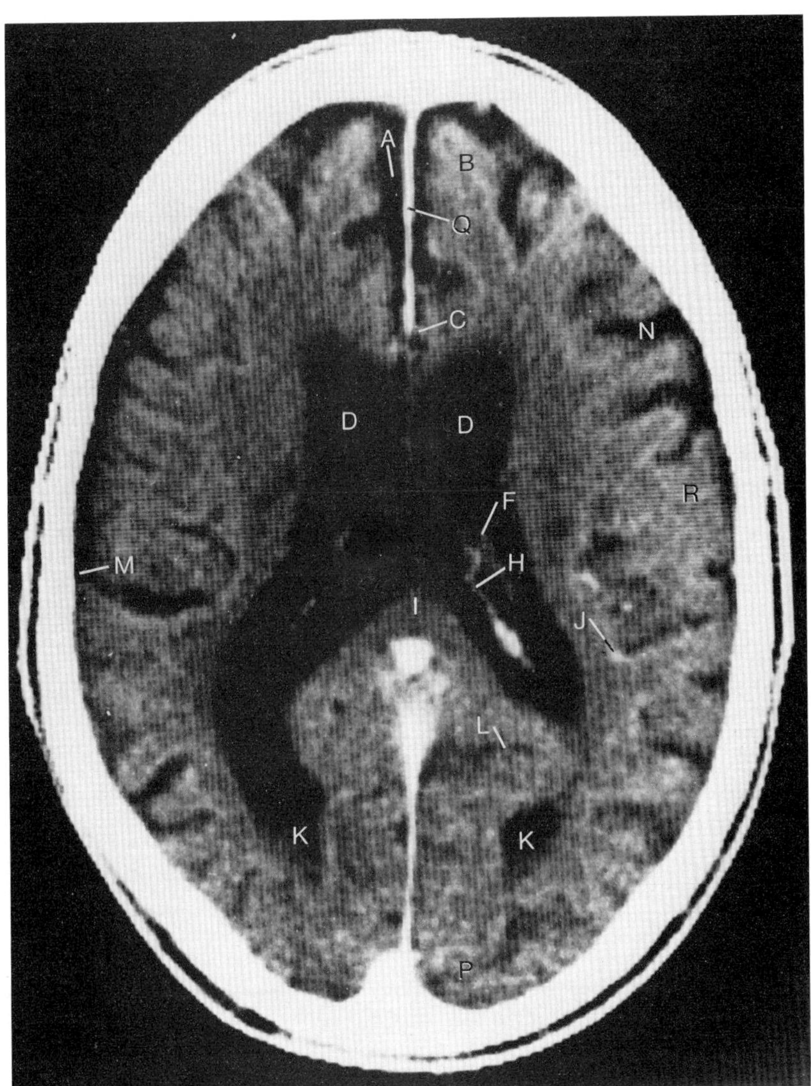

J. Middle cerebral artery at point of junction of lateral and suprainsular sulci.
K. Posterior horn of lateral ventricle.
L. Occipitoparietal sulcus.
M. Arachnoid over cistern of lateral sulcus.
N. Central sulcus.
O. Temporal lobe.
P. Occipital pole and lobe.
Q. Falx cerebri.
R. Parietal lobe.

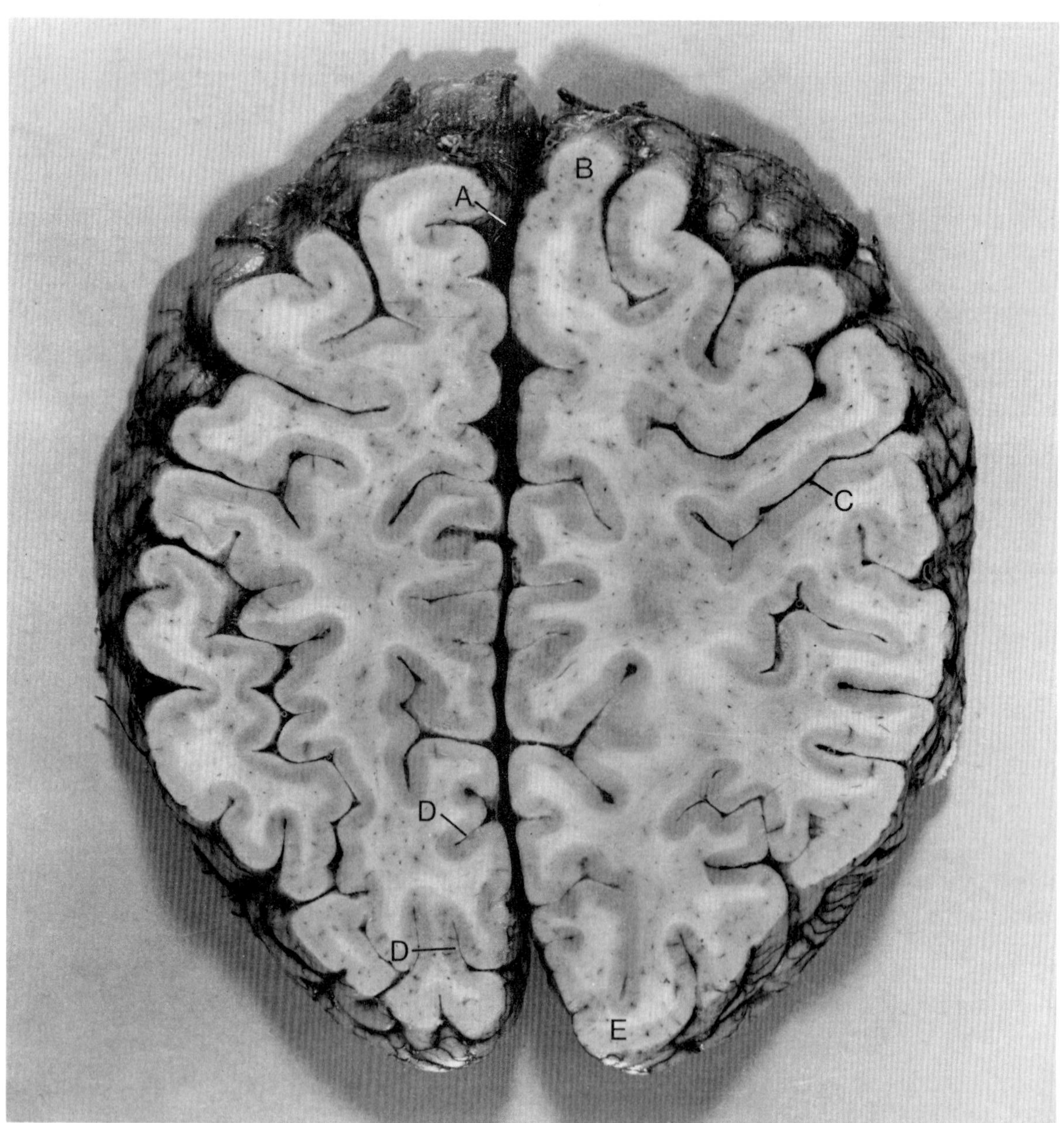

Figure 9-7-1, 2. **Level # 7, Axial Series.**
A. Longitudinal fissure.
B. Frontal pole and lobe.
C. Central sulcus.
D. Calcarine sulcus.
E. Occipital pole and lobe.
F. Falx cerebri.
G. Superior sagittal sinus.

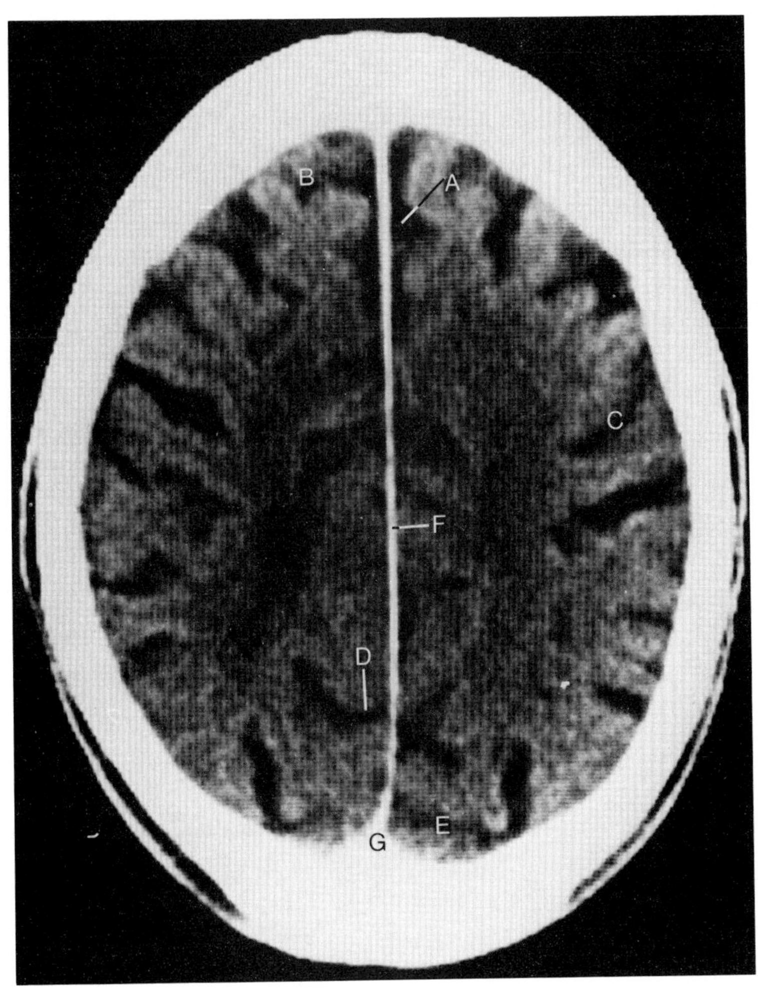

CORONAL

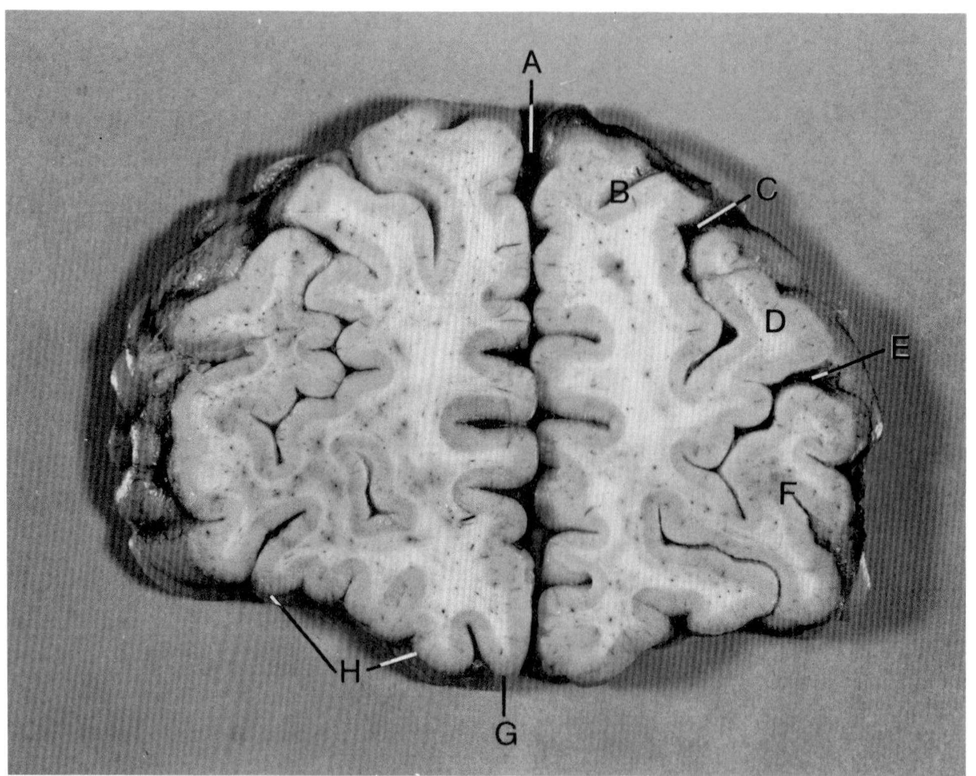

Figure 10-1-1. **Level # 1.**

A. Longitudinal fissure.
B. Superior frontal gyrus.
C. Superior frontal sulcus.
D. Middle frontal gyrus.
E. Inferior frontal sulcus.
F. Inferior frontal gyrus.
G. Gyrus rectus.
H. Orbital gyri.

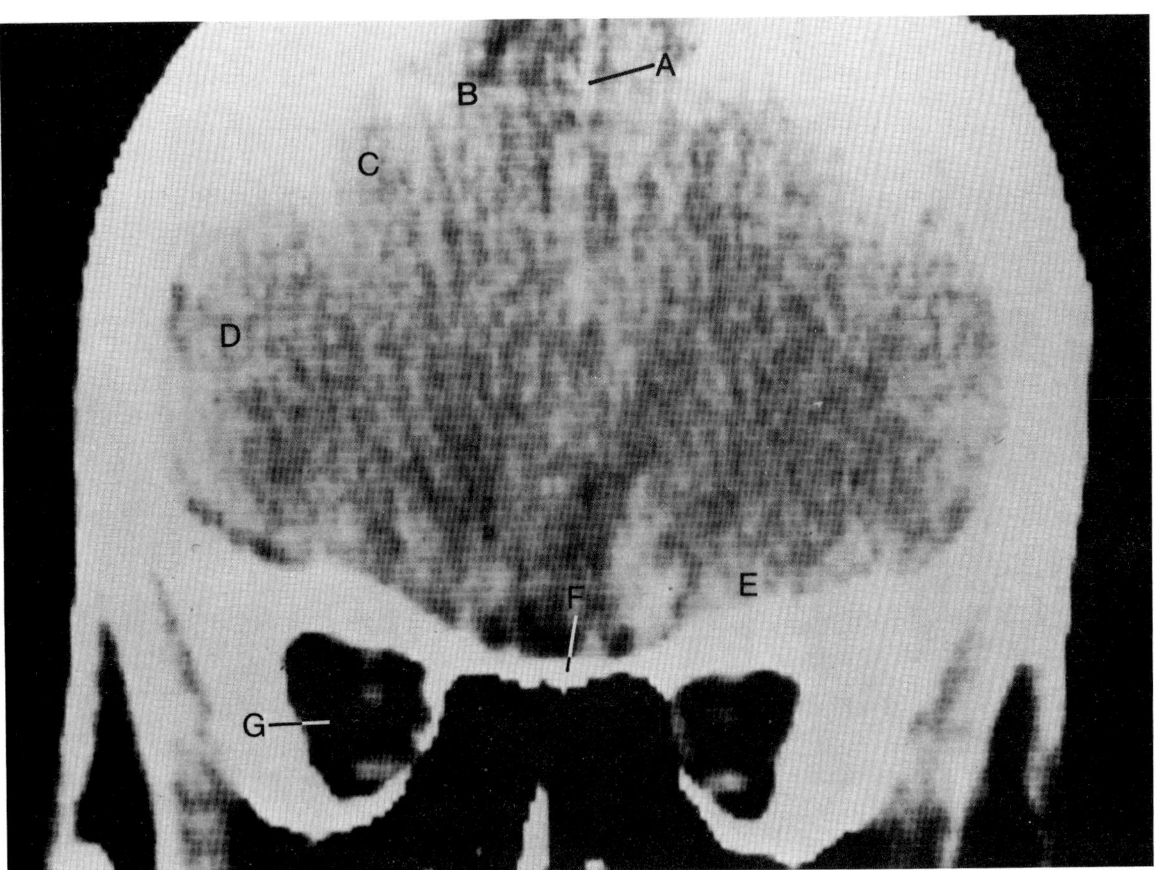

Figure 10-1-2. **Coronal Computed Tomography—Level #1.**
    A. Falx cerebri in longitudinal fissure.
    B. Region of superior frontal gyrus.
    C. Region of superior frontal sulcus.
    D. Middle frontal gyrus.
    E. Orbital gyri.
    F. Planum sphenoidale.
    G. Orbit.

$\rightarrow$

Figure 10-2-1. **Level #2, Coronal Series.**
A. Longitudinal fissure.
B. Corpus callosum.
C. Caudate nucleus. (See C′, below.)
D. Internal capsule.
E. Lenticular nucleus.
F. External capsule.
G. Claustrum.
H. Extreme capsule.
I. Insula.
J. Suprainsular sulcus.
K. Lateral sulcus.
L. Superior temporal gyrus.
M. Middle temporal gyrus.
N. Inferior temporal gyrus.
O. Occipitotemporal gyrus.
P. Collateral sulcus.
Q. Parahippocampal gyrus.
R. Middle cerebral artery.
S. Optic nerve.
T. Optic chiasm.
U. Subcallosal gyrus (paraolfactory area).
V. Anterior commissure.
W. Superior frontal gyrus.
X. Superior frontal sulcus.
Y-Y′. Middle frontal gyrus. This relatively broad gyrus, as occurs in the present
    instance, may be divided into two portions by a middle frontal sulcus (Z).
Z. Middle frontal sulcus.
A′. Inferior frontal sulcus.
B′. Inferior frontal gyrus.
C′. Caudate nucleus. This portion is supplied by the anterior cerebral artery through the
    medial striate, and survives infarction of region supplied by the middle cerebral
    artery (see Fig. 7-10).
D′. Arachnoid covering superior temporal sulcus.

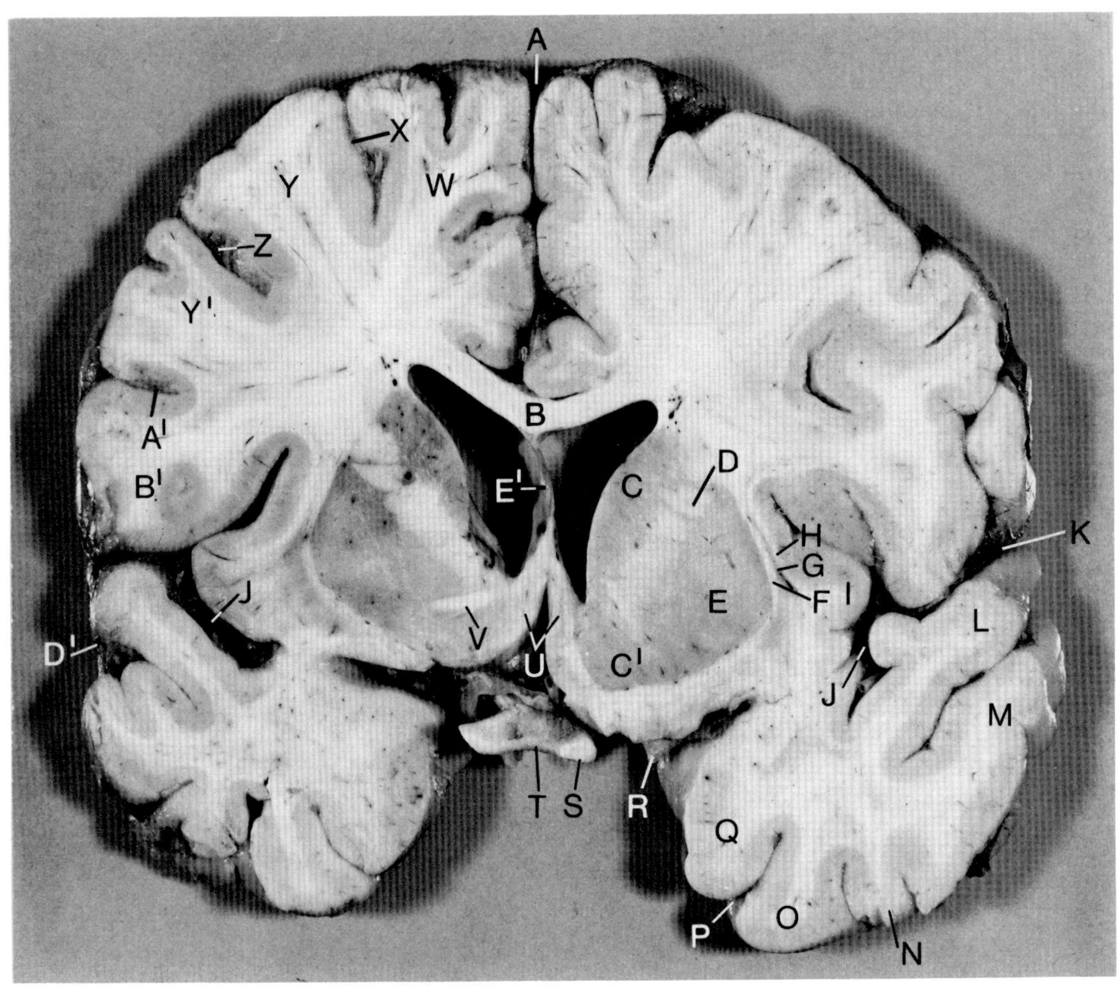
A
X
Y
W
Z
Y'
B
A'
E'
C
D
B'
H
G
E
F
I
K
J
D'
V
V
L
U
C'
J
T
S
R
Q
M
P
O
N

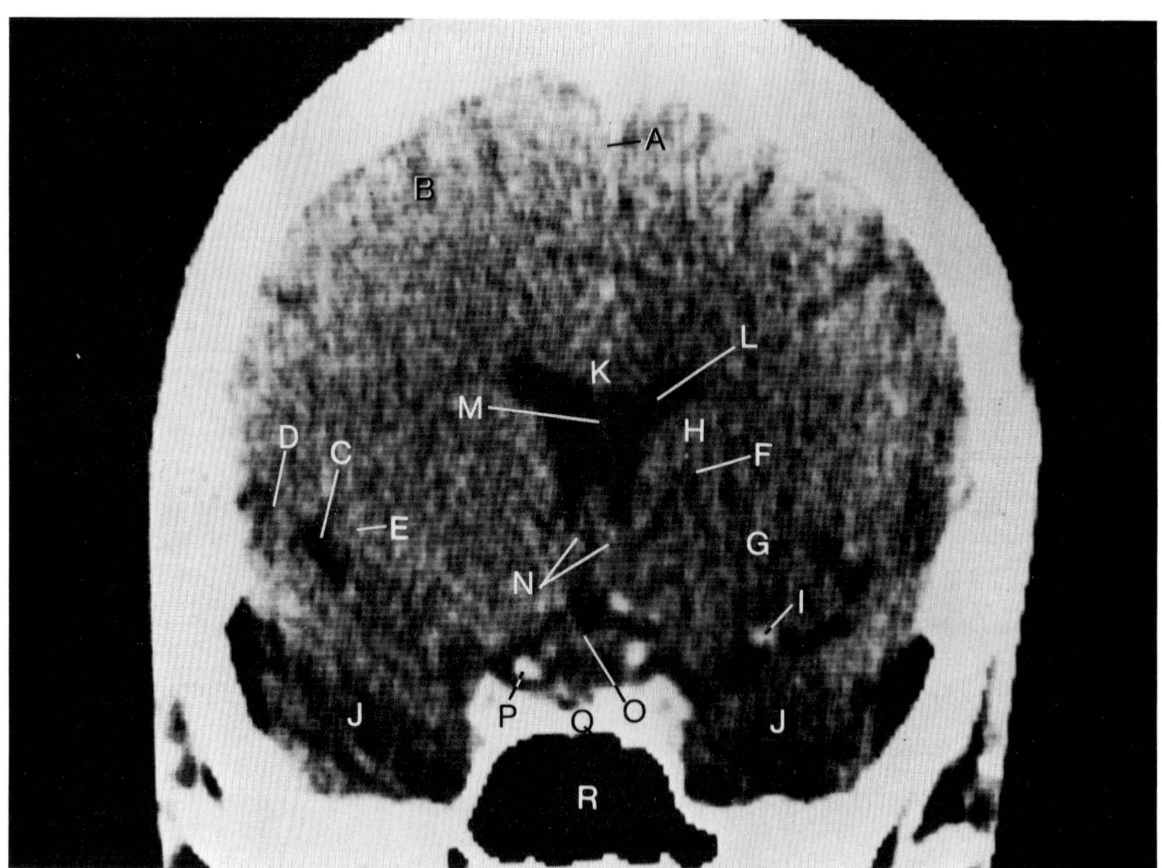

Figure 10-2-2. **Coronal CT Level #2.**

A. Falx in longitudinal fissure.
B. Region of middle frontal gyrus.
C. Suprainsular sulcus.
D. Lateral sulcus.
E. Insula.
F. Internal capsule.
G. Lenticular nucleus.
H. Caudate nucleus.
I. Portion of middle cerebral artery in cistern of middle cerebral artery.
J. Temporal lobe.
K. Corpus callosum.
L. Lateral ventricle.
M. Septum pellucidum.
N. Paraolfactory (subcallosal) area.
O. Optic chiasm.
P. Internal carotid artery.
Q. Region of tuberculum sella.
R. Sphenoid sinus.

Figure 10-3-1. **Level #3, Coronal Series.** (See pages 132 and 133).

$\longrightarrow$

Figure 10-3-1. **Level #3, Coronal Series.**
A. Longitudinal fissure.
B. Superior frontal gyrus.
C. Middle frontal gyrus.
D. Inferior frontal gyrus.
E. Lateral sulcus and its cistern, covered by arachnoid.
F. Suprainsular sulcus.
G. Claustrum.
H. Extreme capsule.
I. External capsule.
J. Putamen.
K. Globus pallidus.
L. Anterior commissure.
M. Amygdala.
N. Collateral sulcus.
O. Optic tract.
P. Mammillary bodies.
Q. Inferior horn of lateral ventricle.
R. Parahippocampal gyrus.
S. Occipitotemporal gyrus.
T. Inferior temporal gyrus.
U. Middle temporal gyrus.
V. Superior temporal gyrus.
W. Middle cerebral artery branch.
X. Internal capsule.
Y. Caudate nucleus.
Z. Junction of fornix (below) with septum pellucidum (above).
A'. Corpus callosum.
B'. Cingulate gyrus.
C'. Cingulate sulcus.
D'. Lateral ventricle.
E'. Thalamostriate vein.

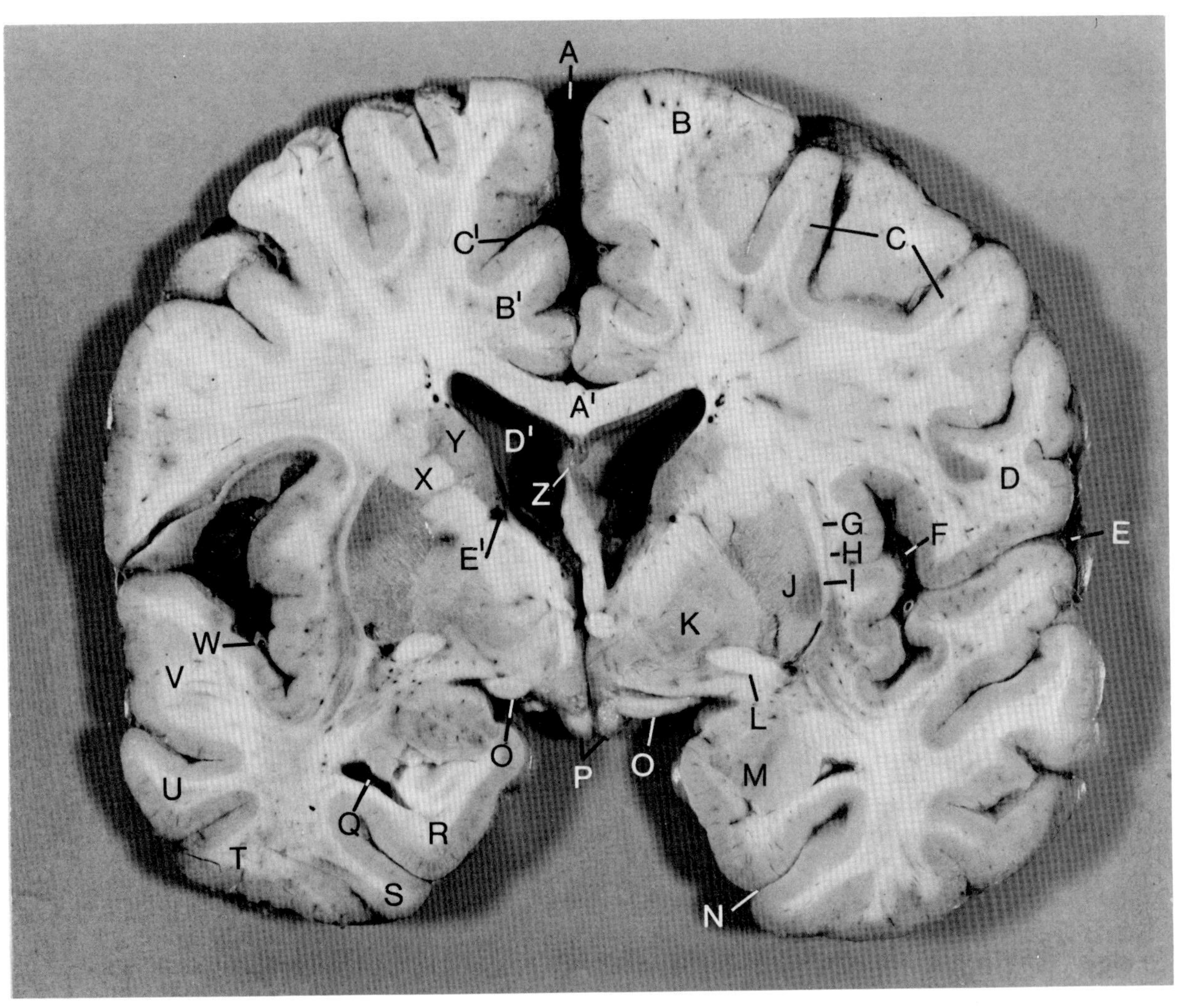
A
B
C'
C
B'
A'
D'
Y
X
Z
D
G
F
H
E
I
E'
J
W
K
L
V
M
U
O
Q
P
O
R
L
T
S
N

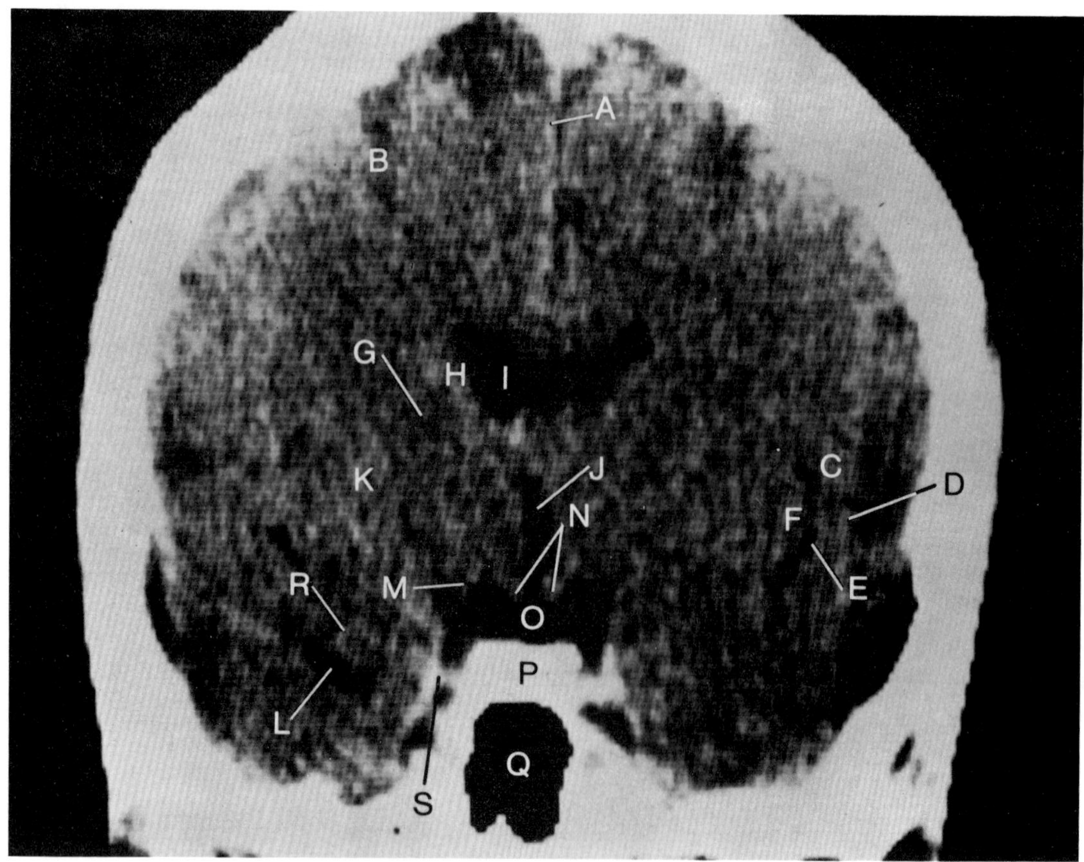

Figure 10-3-2. **Coronal CT, Level #3.**

III. A. Falx in longitudinal fissure.
    B. Region of middle frontal gyrus.
    C. Inferior frontal gyrus.
    D. Lateral sulcus and cistern.
    E. Supracallosal sulcus and cistern.
    F. Insula.
    G. Anterior capsule.
    H. Caudate.
    I. Lateral ventricle.
    J. Third ventricle.
    K. Lenticular nucleus.
    L. Inferior horn of lateral ventricle.
    M. Optic tract.
    N. Mammillary bodies.
    O. Suprasellar cistern.
    P. Dorsum sella.
    Q. Sphenoid sinus.
    R. Amygdala.
    S. Posterior cavernous sinus.

Figure 10-4-1. **Level #4, Coronal Series.** (See pages 136 and 137.)

Figure 10-4-1. **Level #4, Coronal Series.**   →

A. Longitudinal fissure.
B. Precentral gyrus.
C. Central sulcus.
D. Postcentral gyrus.
E. Postcentral sulcus.
F. Inferior, and portion of superior, parietal lobules. There is variation from average in formation of gyrus and sulcus.
G. Arachnoid over cistern of lateral sulcus.
H. Lateral sulcus and cistern.
I. Suprainsular sulcus.
J. Insula.
K. Extreme capsule.
L. Claustrum.
M. External capsule.
N. Inferior horn of lateral ventricle.
O. Tail of caudate nucleus.
P. Optic tract.
Q. Mammillary bodies.
R. Posterior cerebral artery.
S. Basilar artery.
T. Pons.
U. Hippocampus.
V. Parahippocampal gyrus.
W. Occipitotemporal gyrus.
X. Inferior temporal gyrus.
Y. Middle temporal gyrus.
Z. Superior temporal gyrus.
A'. Corpus callosum.
B'. Cingulate gyrus.
C'. Cingulate sulcus.
D'. Junction of septum pellucidum (above) with fornix (below).
E'. Lateral ventricle.
F'. Caudate nucleus, posterior part of head.
G'. Putamen.
H'. Globus pallidus.
I'. Internal capsule.
J'. Thalamus.
K'. Third ventricle.
L'. Mammillothalamic tract.
M'. Middle cerebral artery, branch.

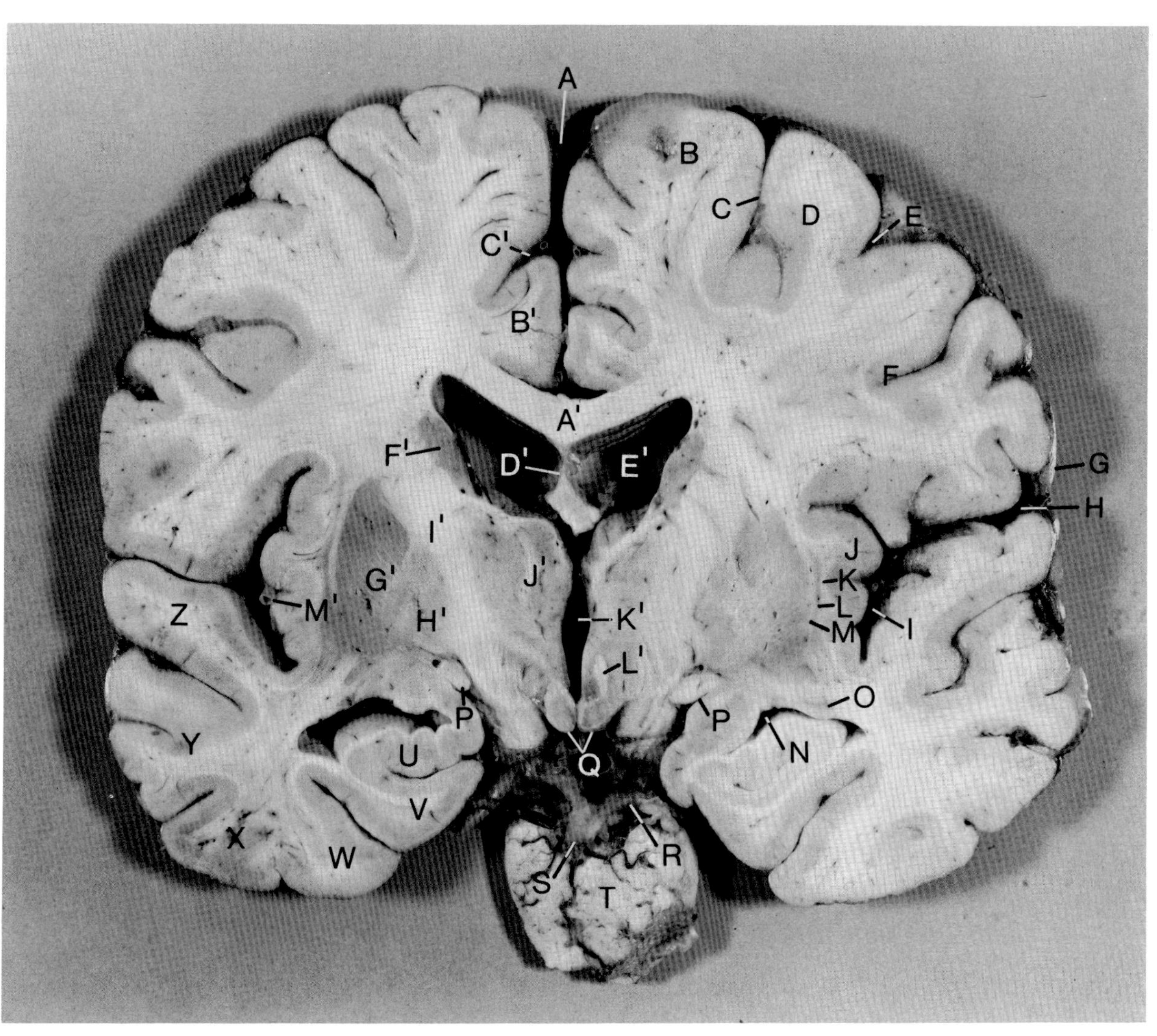
A
B
C
D
E
C'
B'
F
A'
F'
D'
E'
G
H
I'
J
G'
J'
K
M'
L
Z
H'
K'
M
I
L'
O
P
P
Y
U
Q
N
V
X
R
W
S
T

$\longrightarrow$

Figure 10-4-2. **Coronal CT Level #4.**
A. Falx in longitudinal fissure.
B. Corpus callosum.
C. Lateral ventricle.
D. Postcentral gyrus.
E. Lateral sulcus and cistern.
F. Suprainsular sulcus and cistern.
G. Third ventricle.
H. Optic tract.
I. Parahippocampal gyrus and hippocampus.
J. Inferior horn of lateral ventricle.
K. Upper clivus.
L. Internal capsule.
M. Lenticular nucleus.
N. Caudate nucleus.

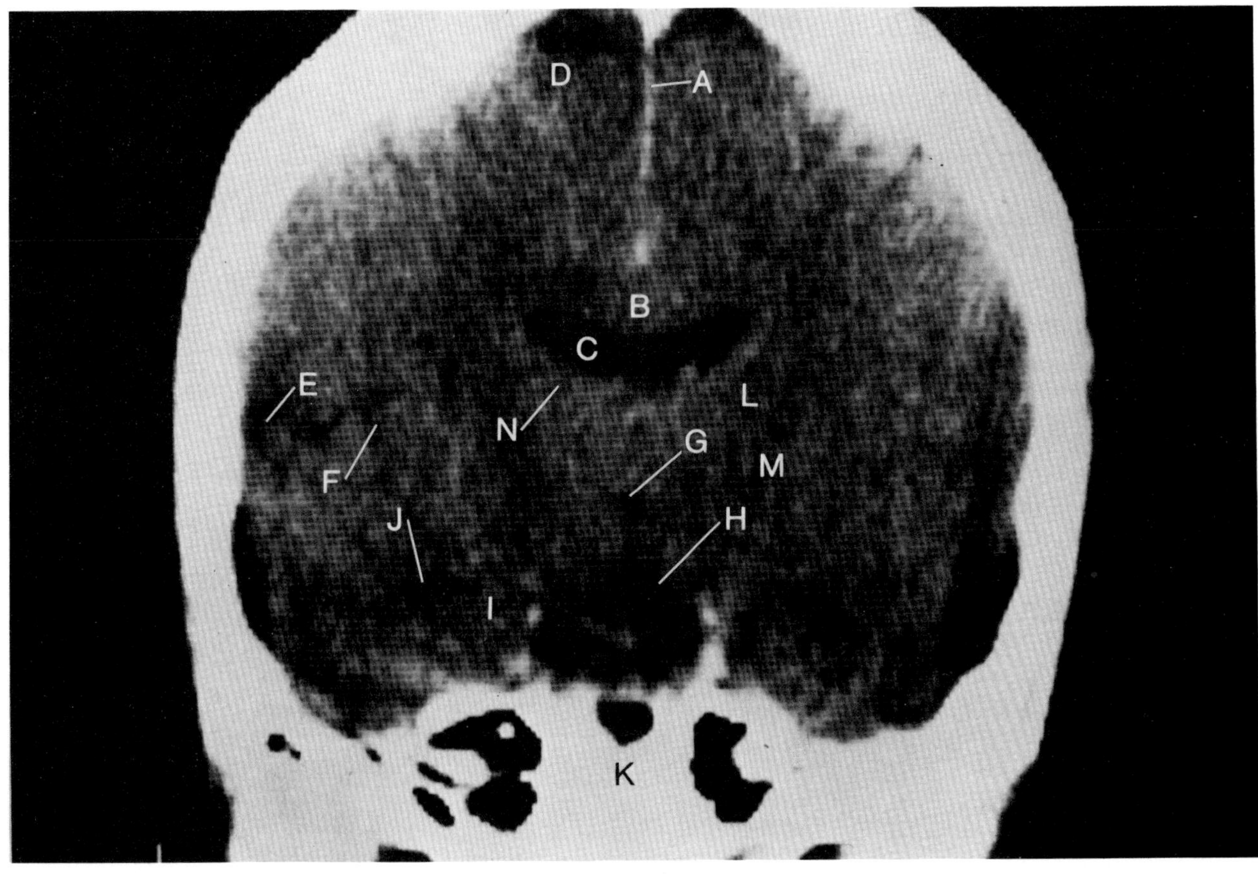

D
A
B
C
E
N
L
G
M
F
J
H
I
K

→

Figure 10-5-1. **Level #5, Coronal Series.**
A. Longitudinal fissure.
B. Precentral gyrus.
C. Central sulcus.
D. Postcentral gyrus.
E. Inferior, and portion of superior, parietal lobules. There was variation from average in formation of gyrus and sulcus.
F. Lateral sulcus.
G. Superior temporal gyrus.
H. Middle temporal gyrus.
I. Inferior temporal gyrus. The variability of gyri is again shown; compare with opposite hemisphere.
J. Occipitotemporal gyrus.
K. Parahippocampal gyrus.
L. Hippocampus.
M. Inferior horn of lateral ventricle.
N. Choroidal fissure.
O. Posterior cerebral artery.
P. Pons.
Q. Interpeduncular fossa and cistern.
R. Basis pedunculi.
S. Third ventricle.
T. Thalamus.
U. Internal capsule.
W. Insula.
X. Suprainsular sulcus.
Y. Extreme capsule.
Z. Claustrum.
A'. External capsule.
B'. Caudate nucleus, region of transition between head and tail.
C'. Lateral ventricle.
D'. Choroid plexus in interventricular foramen.
E'. Corpus callosum.
F'. Cingulate gyrus.
G'. Cingulate sulcus.
H'. Subthalamic nucleus.
I'. Substantia nigra.

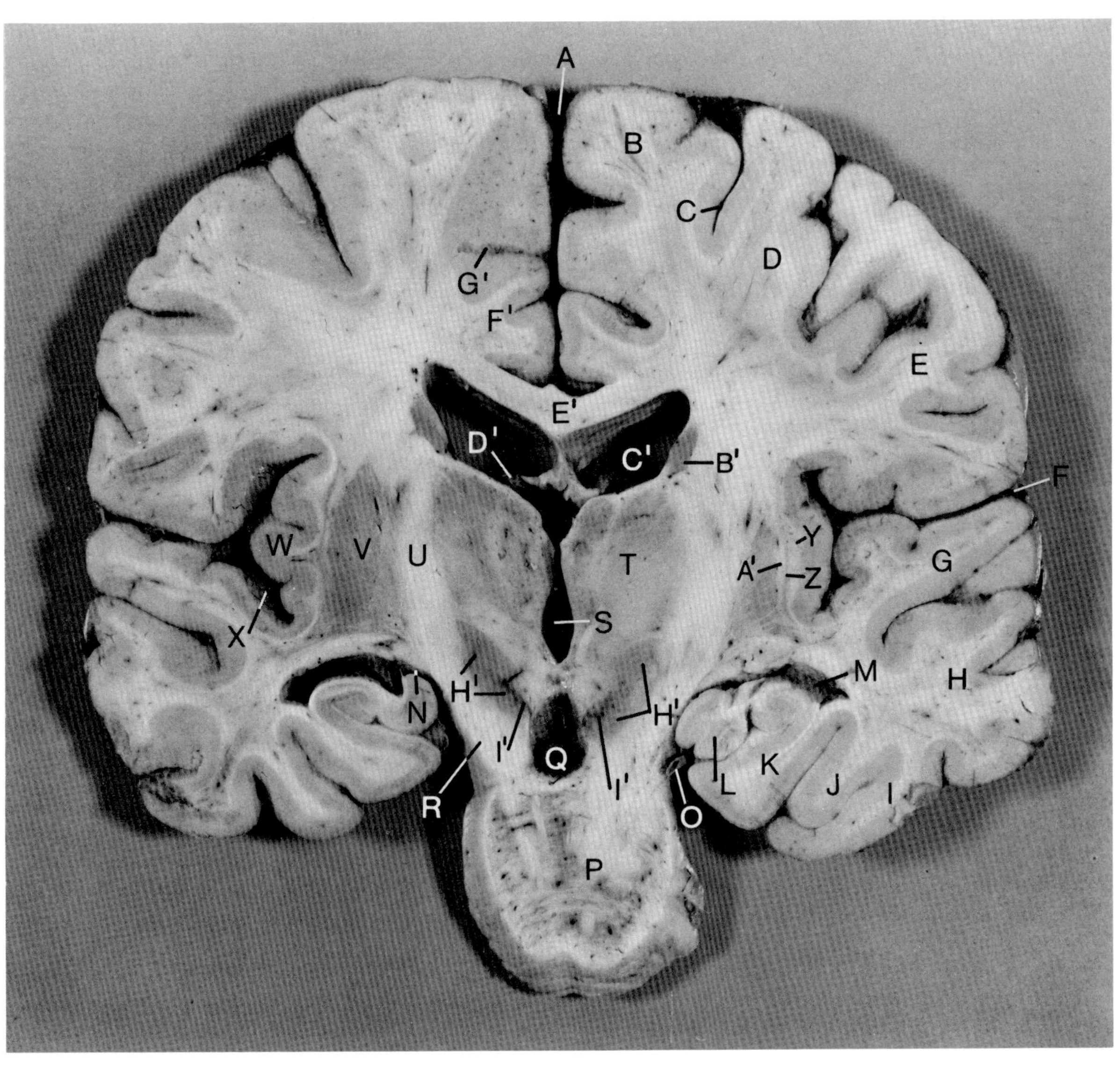

A
B
C
D
G'
F'
E
E'
D'
C'
B'
F
W
V
U
Y
Z
A'
G
X
T
S
M
H
N
H'
H'
I'
I'
Q
R
L
K
J
I
O
P

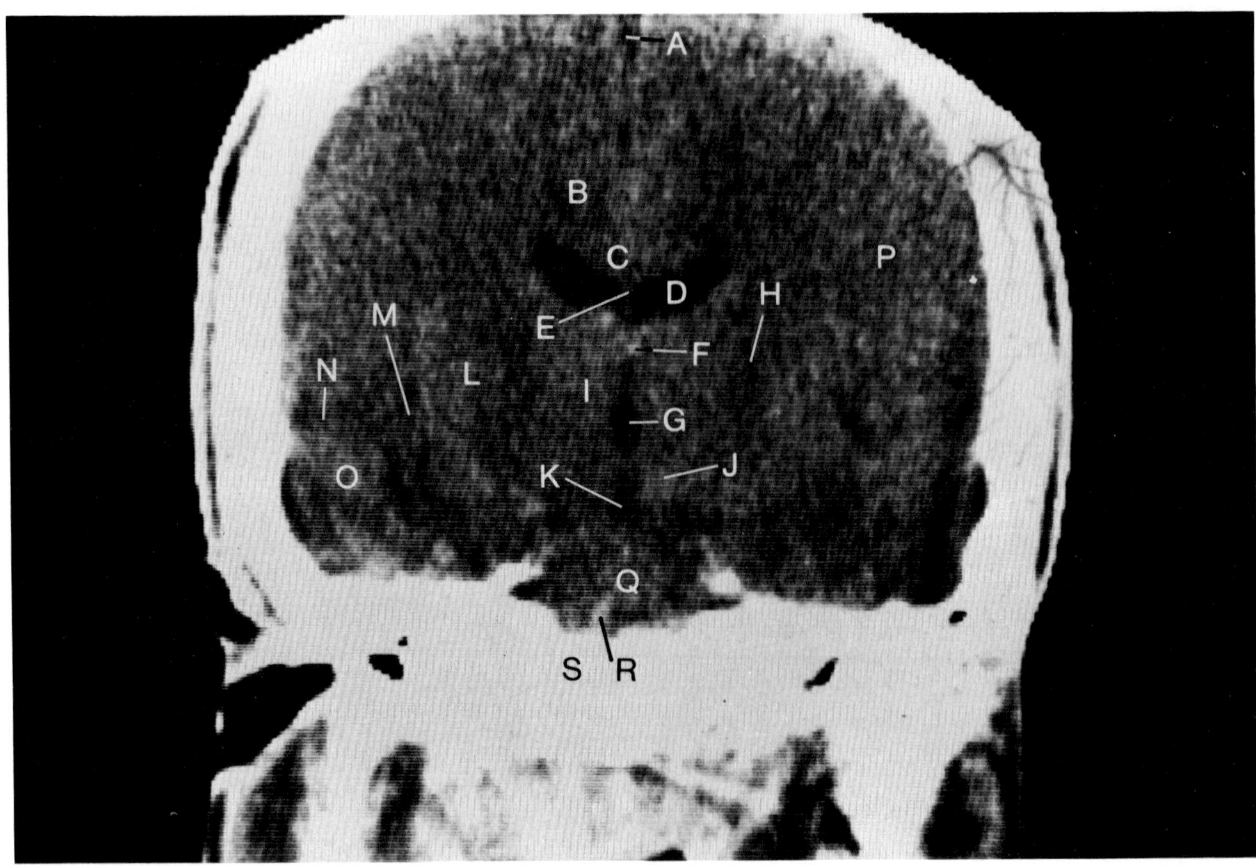

Figure 10-5-2. Coronal Computed Tomography, **Level #5.**

A. Longitudinal fissure.
B. Cingulate gyrus.
C. Corpus callosum.
D. Lateral ventricle.
E. Septum pellucidum.
F. Internal cerebral vein in roof of third ventricle.
G. Third ventricle.
H. Internal capsule.
I. Thalamus.
J. Subthalamic nuclei.
K. Interpeduncular fossa and cistern.
L. Lenticular nucleus.
M. Insula.
N. Lateral sulcus and cistern.
O. Temporal lobe.
P. Parietal lobe.
Q. Pons.
R. Basilar artery.
S. Lower clivus.

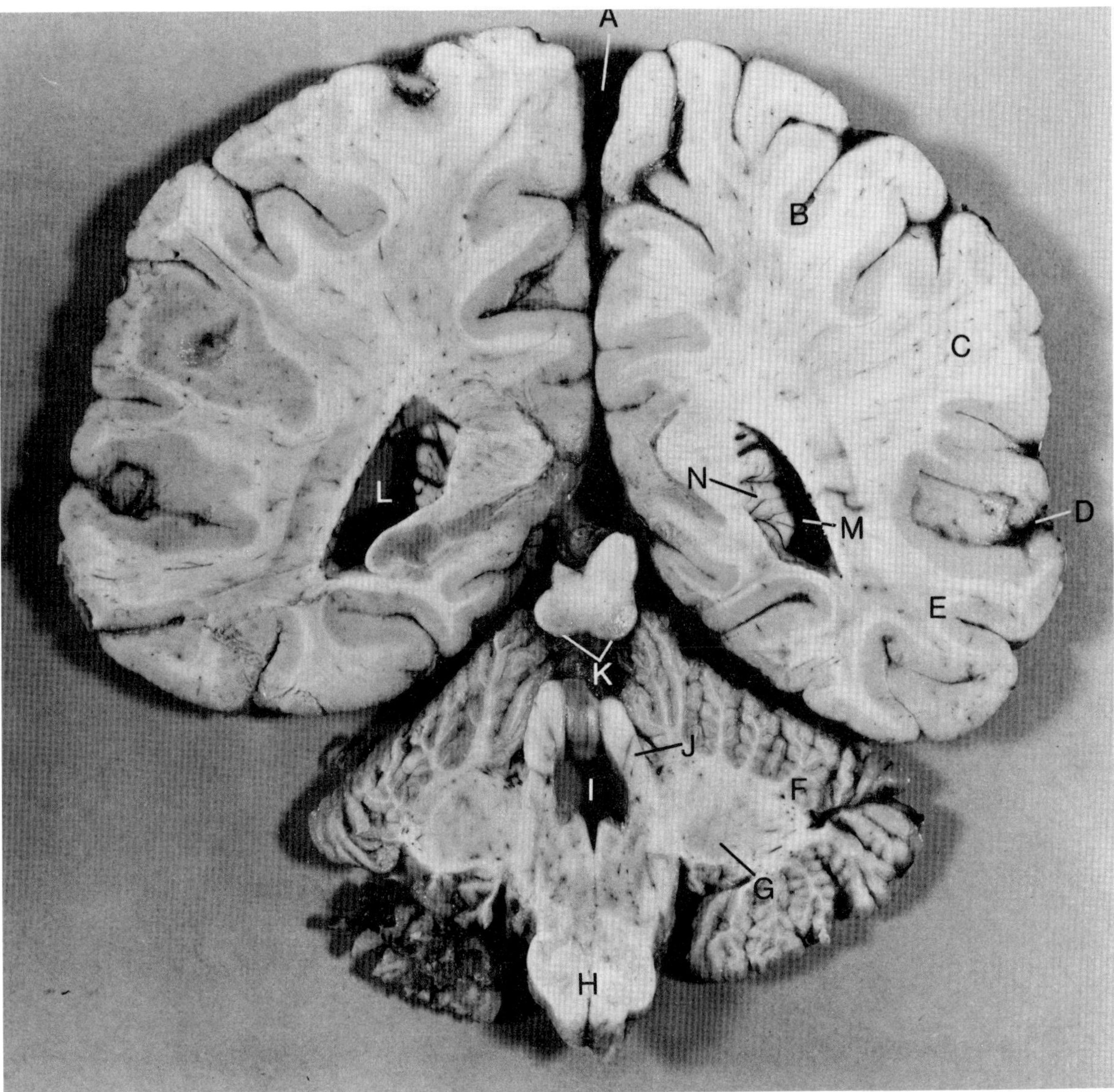

Figure 10-6-1. **Level #6, Coronal Series.**
A. Longitudinal fissure.
B. Superior parietal lobule.
C. Inferior parietal lobule.
D. Lateral sulcus.
E. Temporal lobe.
F. Cerebellar hemisphere.
G. Dentate nucleus.
H. Medulla.
I. Fourth ventricle.
J. Superior cerebellar peduncle.
K. Inferior colliculi and added portion of midbrain.
L. Atrium of lateral ventricle.
M. Beginning of posterior horn of lateral ventricle.
N. Calcar avis.

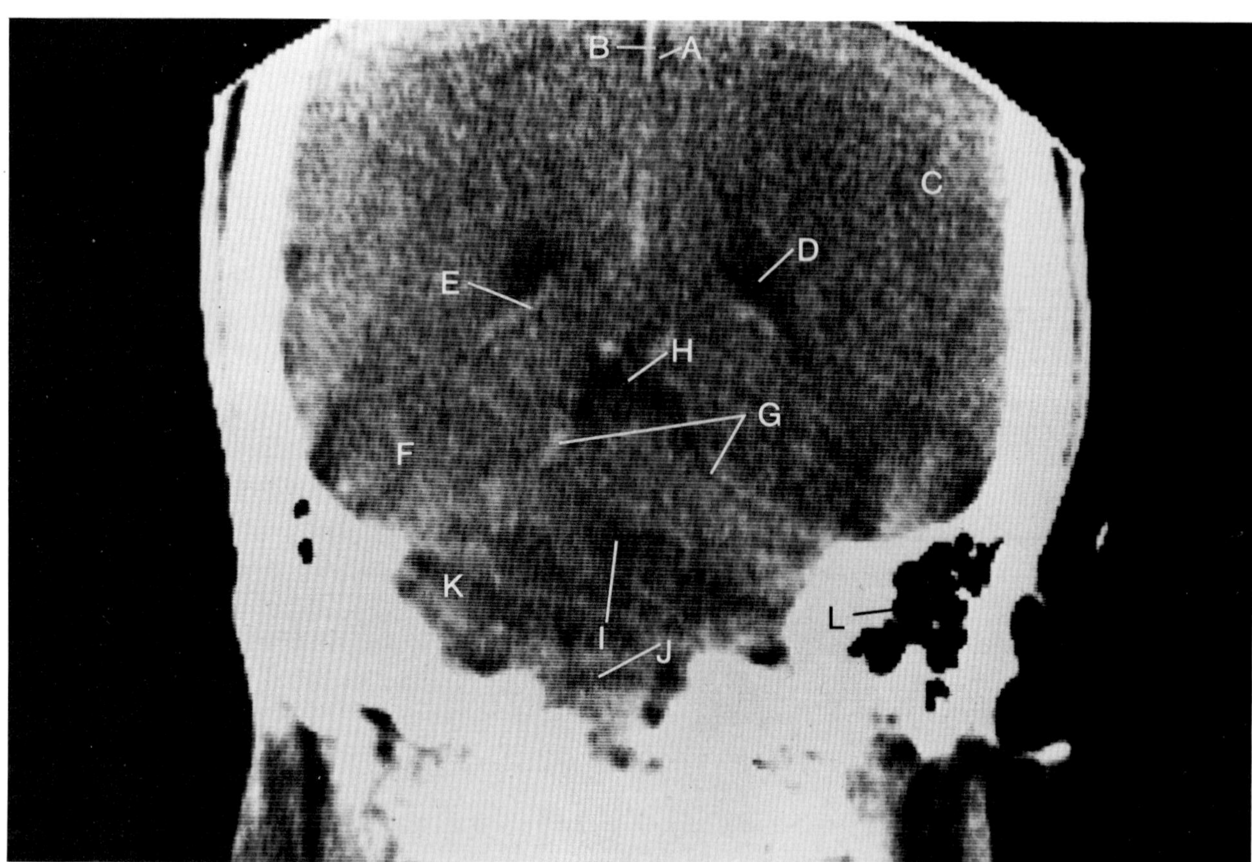

Figure 10-6-2. **Coronal Computed Tomography, Level #6.**
A. Longitudinal fissure.
B. Falx cerebri.
C. Parietal lobe.
D. Atrium of lateral ventricle.
E. Choroid plexus of lateral ventricle atrium.
F. Temporal lobe.
G. Contrast enhancement of the tentorium cerebelli.
H. Inferior collicular cistern.
I. Fourth ventricle.
J. Medulla.
K. Cerebellum.
L. Mastoid air cells.

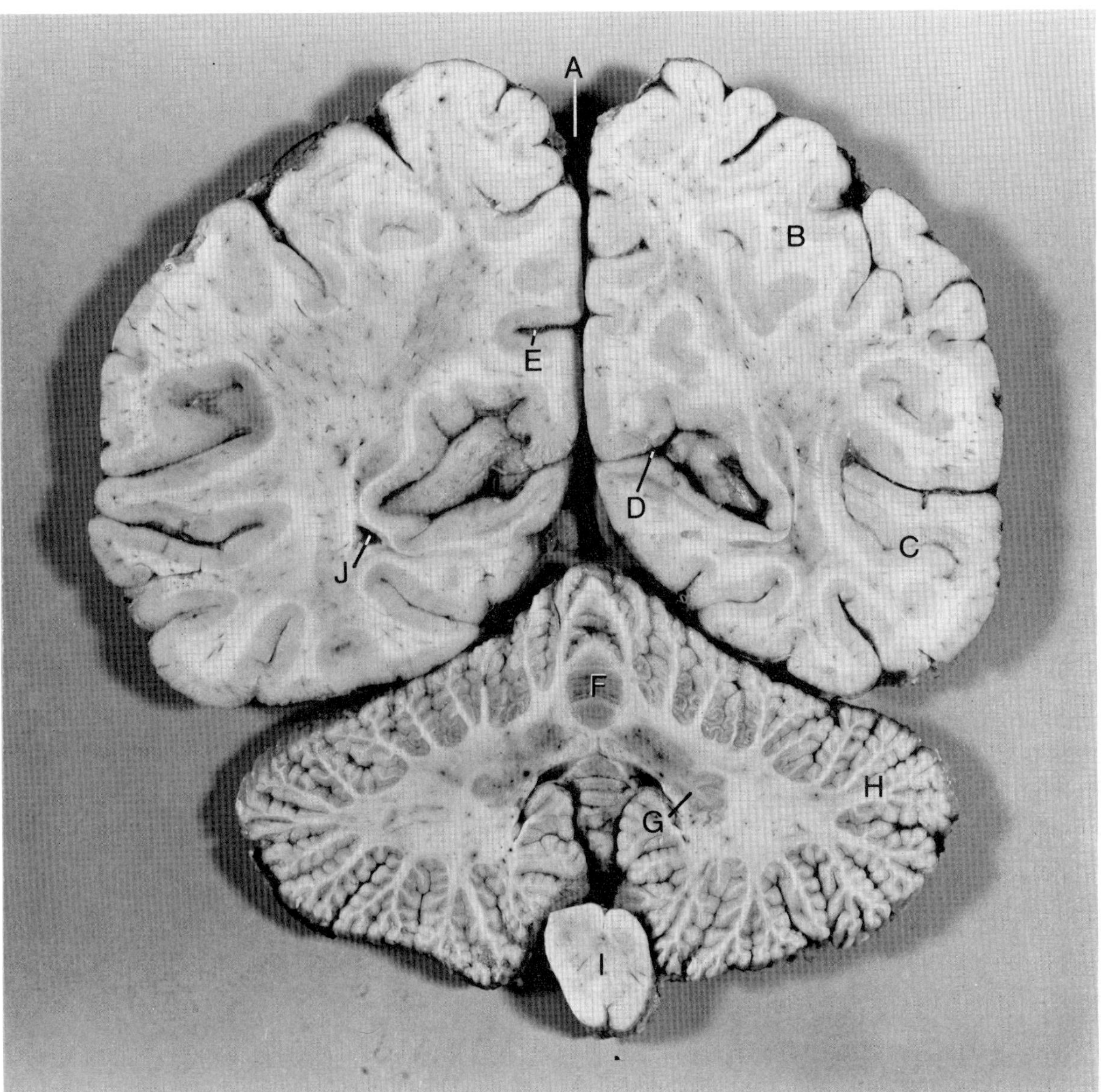

Figure 10-7-1. **Level #6, Coronal Series.**
A. Longitudinal fissure.
B. Parietal lobe, posterior portion.
C. Occipital lobe, anterior portion.
D. Calcarine sulcus.
E. Occipitoparietal sulcus.
F. Vermis of cerebellum.
G. Dentate nucleus.
H. Cerebellar hemisphere.
I. Medulla.
J. Posterior extremity of posterior horn of lateral ventricle.

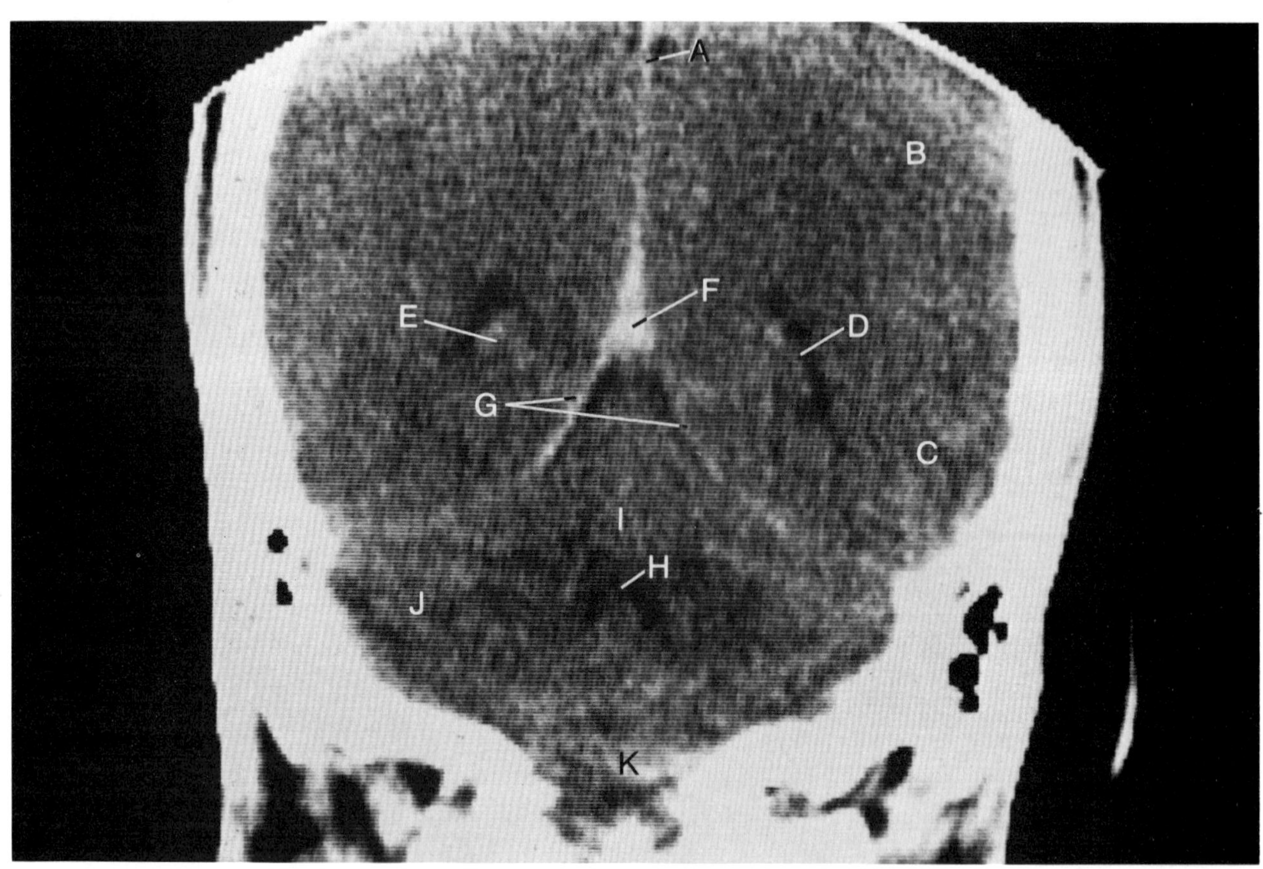

Figure 10-7-2. **Coronal Computed Tomography, Level #7.**
A. Falx cerebri in longitudinal fissure.
B. Parietal lobe, posterior portion.
C. Occipital lobe, anterior portion.
D. Posterior atrium lateral ventricle.
E. Choroid, posterior atrium lateral ventricle.
F. Straight sinus.
G. Tentorium cerebelli.
H. Fourth ventricle.
I. Cerebellar vermis.
J. Cerebellar hemisphere.
K. Medulla.

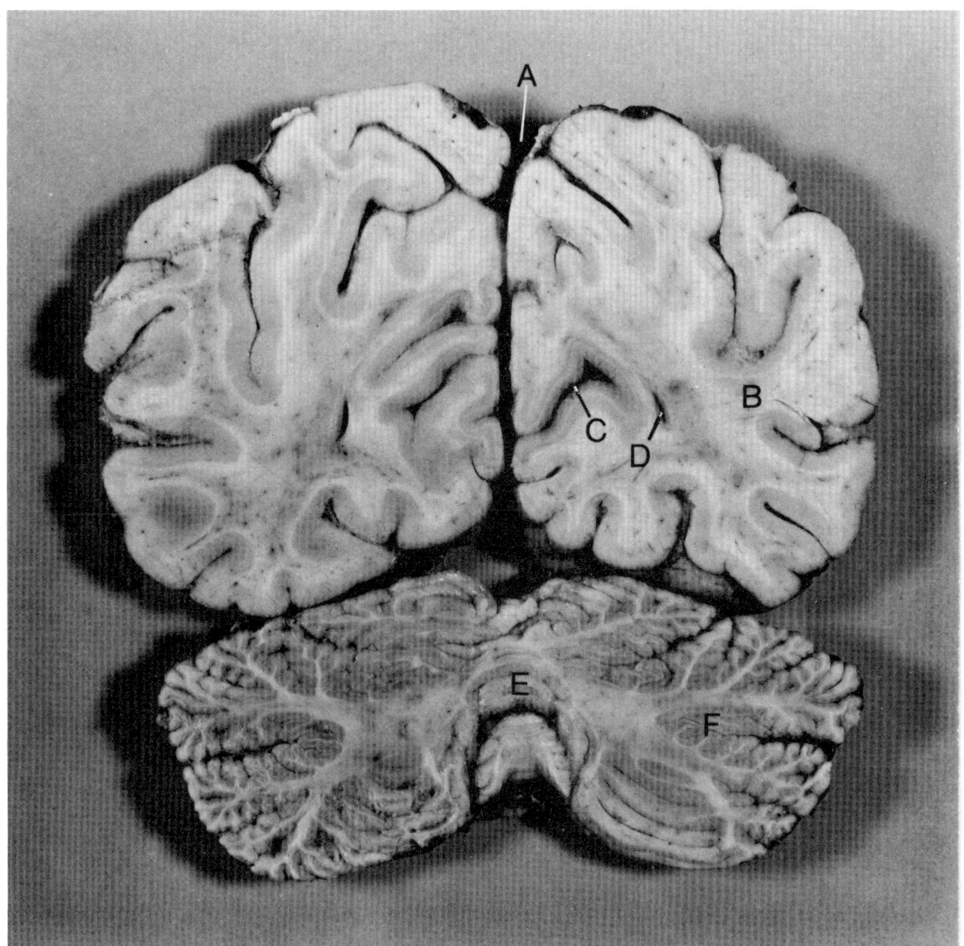

Figure 10-8-1. **Level #8, Coronal Series.**
A. Longitudinal fissure.
B. Occipital lobe.
C. Calcarine sulcus.
D. Posterior tip of posterior horn of lateral ventricle.
E. Vermis of cerebellum.
F. Cerebellar hemisphere.

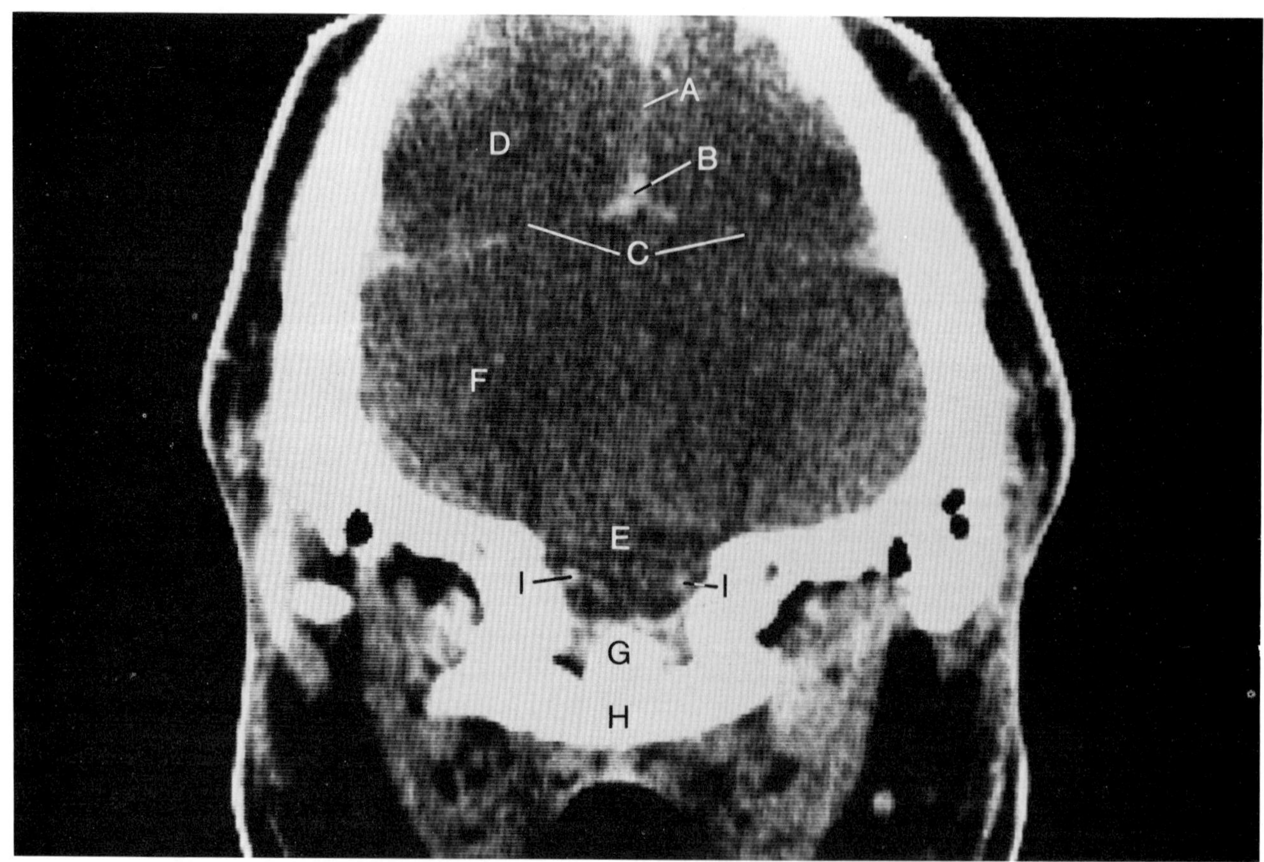

Figure 10-8-2. **Coronal Computed Tomography, Level #8.**
A. Falx cerebri longitudinal fissure.
B. Straight sinus.
C. Tentorium cerebelli.
D. Occipital lobe.
E. Combination of medulla and inferior vermis.
F. Cerebellar hemisphere.
G. Odontoid (dens).
H. Anterior arch of C1.
I. Lateral margin foramen magnum.

SAGITTAL

Figure 11-1-1. **Midsagittal Section (Level #1).** (See pages 150 and 151.)

$\longrightarrow$

Figure 11-1-1. **Midsagittal Section (Level #1).**

A. A. Frontal pole.
B. Occipital pole.
C. Temporal pole.
D. Internal carotid artery.
E. Striate arteries.
F. Basilar artery.
G. Vertebral artery.
H. Calcarine sulcus.
I. Calcarine artery (illustrates variability of arrangement; the artery usually is found in the mouth of the sulcus).
J. Parieto-occipital sulcus and artery (the former, the boundary between parietal and occipital lobes).
K. Callosomarginal artery.
L. Pericallosal artery.
M. Superior frontal gyrus.
N. Cingulate gyrus.
O. Anterior frontal artery.
P. Frontopolar artery.
Q. Orbital artery.
R. Splenium of corpus callosum.
S. Septum pellucidum. (The opening is artifact.)
T. Body of corpus callosum.
U. Genu of corpus callosum.
V. Thalamus.
W. Opening of cerebral aqueduct.
X. Pineal.
Y. Anterior medullary velum.
Z. Fourth ventricle.
A' to I' — Divisions of vermis of cerebellum.
A'. Lingula.
B'. Central lobule.
C'. Culmen.
D'. Declive.
E'. Folium.
F'. Tuber.
G'. Pyramis.
H'. Uvula.
I'. Nodule.
J'. Posterior inferior cerebellar artery.

B. A. Fornix.
B. Choroid plexus.
C. Interventricular foramen.
D. Lamina terminalis.
E. Optic recess.
F. Optic chiasm, from which the nerve extends anterolaterally.
G. Infundibulum.
H. Infundibular recess.
I. Mammillary body.
J. Superior and inferior colliculi.
K. Posterior commissure.
L. Habenula.
M. Precentral cerebellar vein.
N. Great cerebellar vein.
O. Internal cerebral vein.

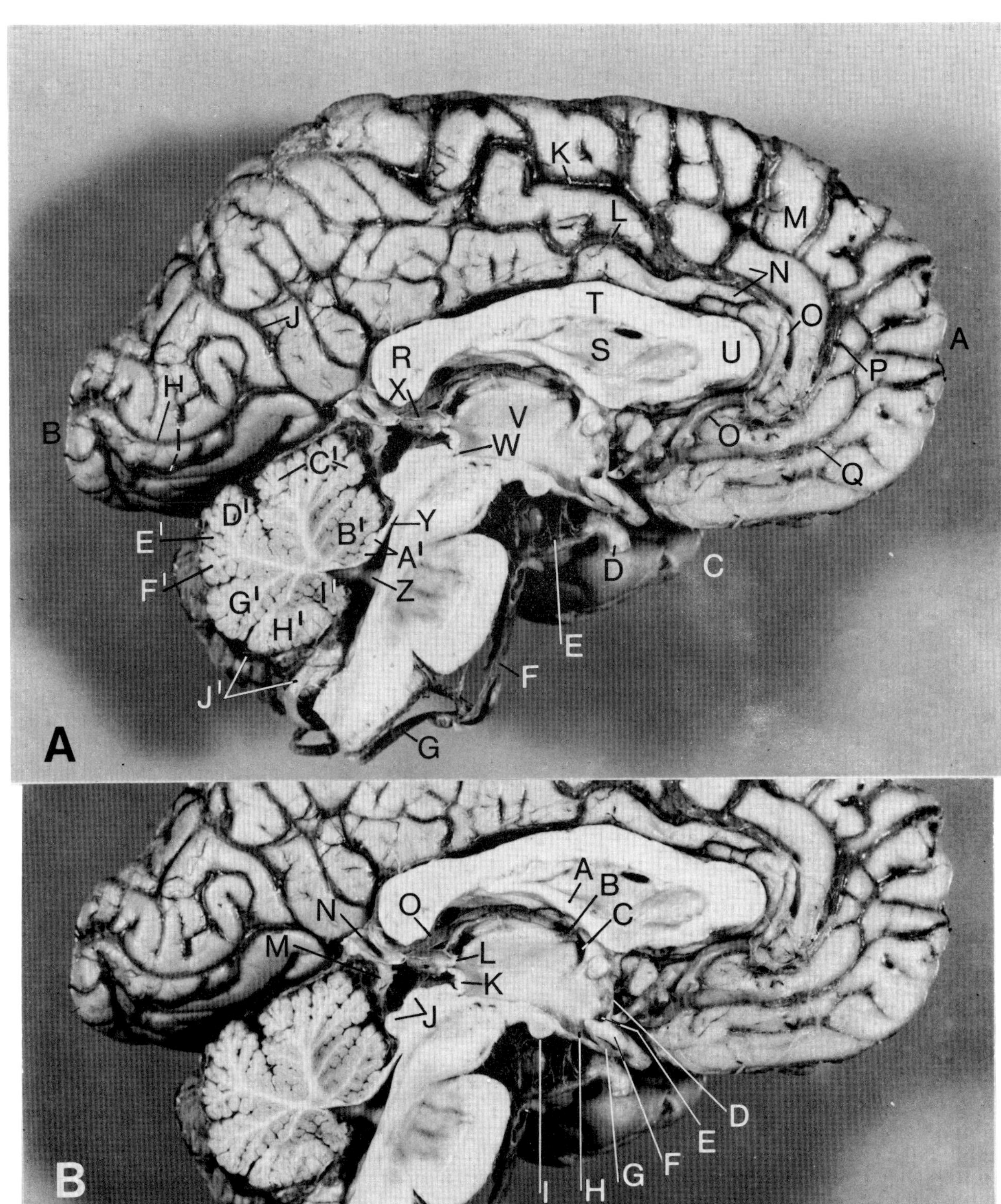

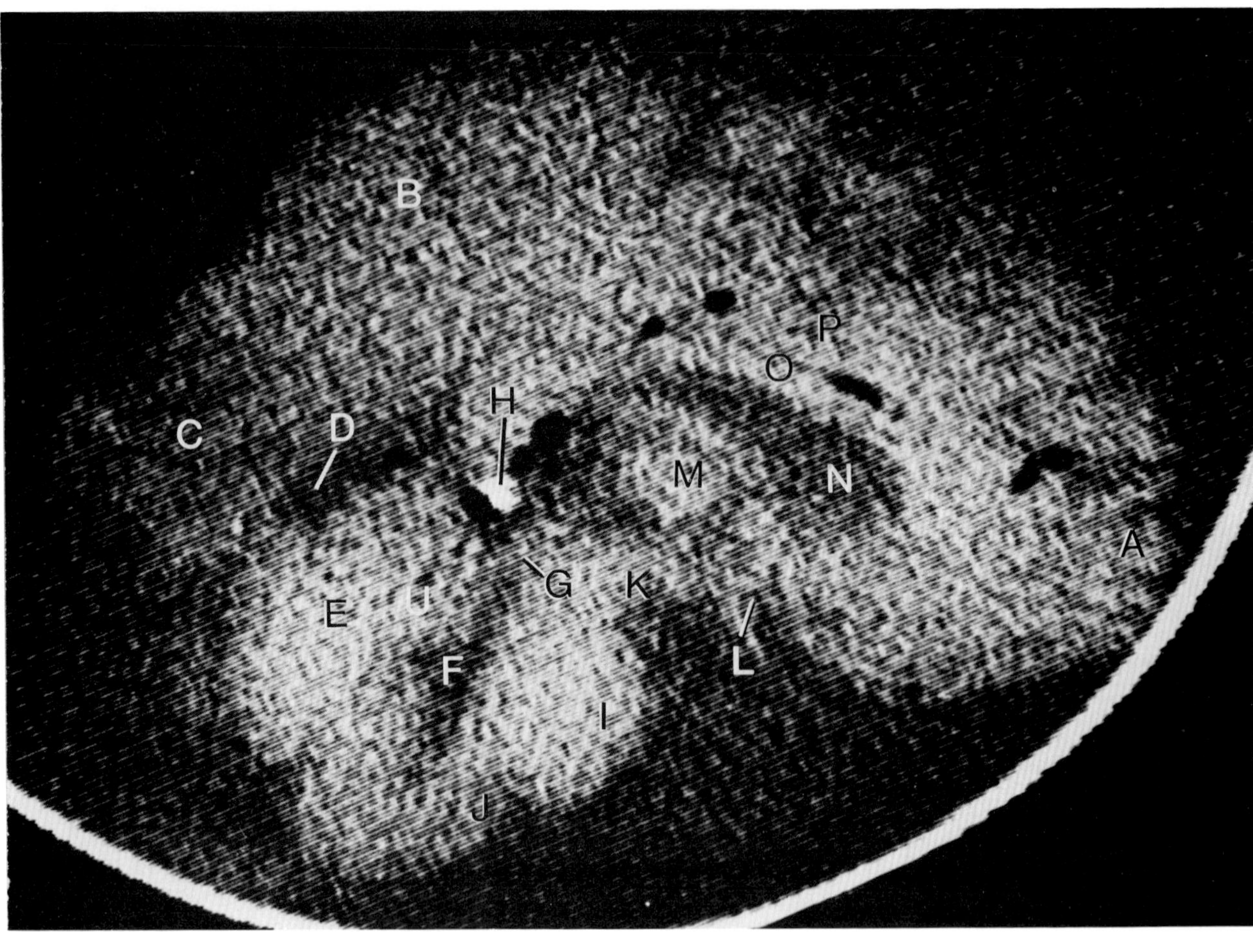

Figure 11-1-2. **Midsagittal CT Section.**

A. Frontal pole and lobe.
B. Parietal lobe.
C. Occipital pole and lobe.
D. Space occupied by tentorium.
E. Cerebellum.
F. Fourth ventricle.
G. Quadrigeminal plate.
H. Calcified pineal gland.
I. Pons.
J. Medulla.
K. Cerebral peduncles.
L. Optic chiasm.
M. Interthalamic connection.
N. Third ventricle.
O. Corpus callosum.
P. Cingulate gyrus.

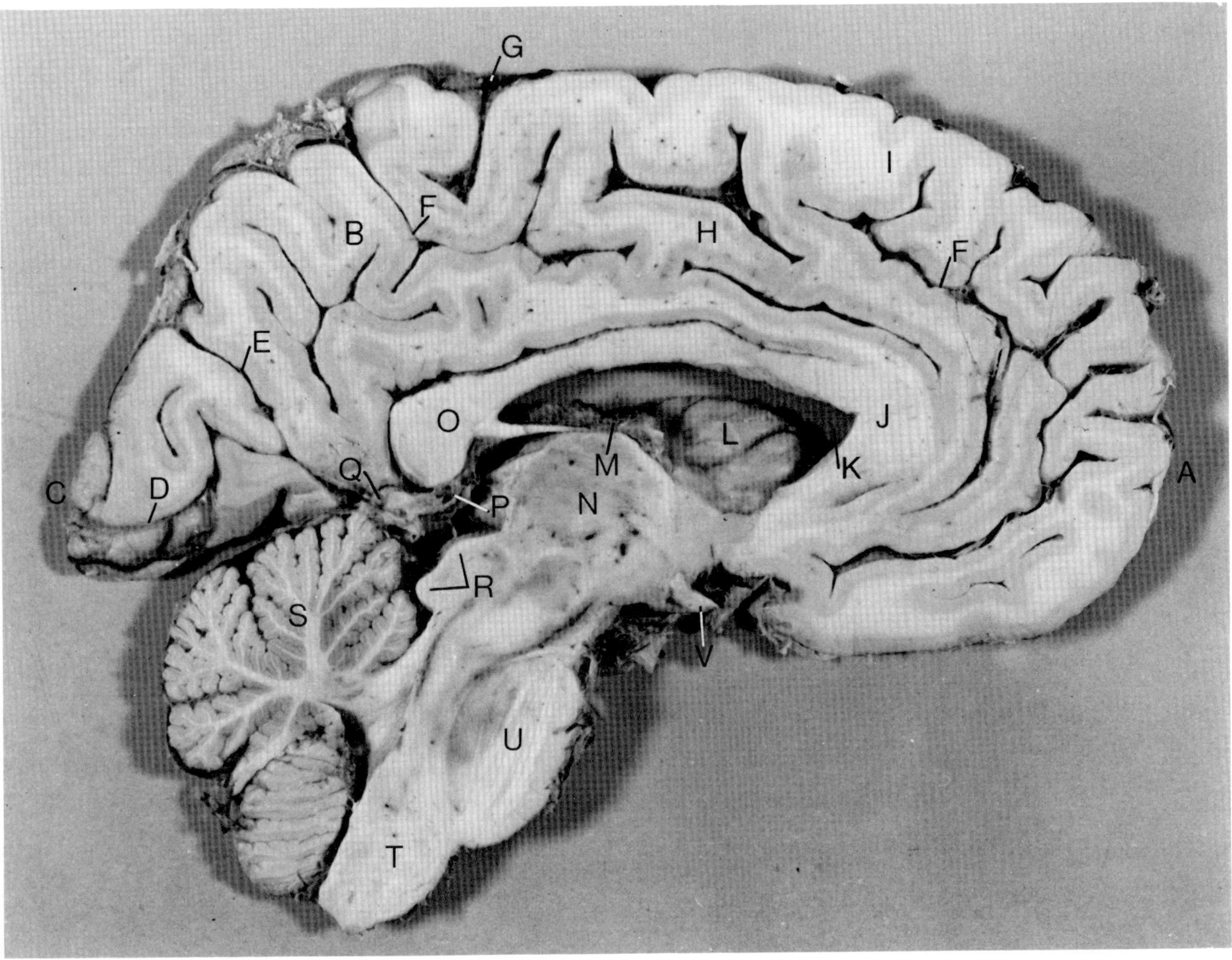

Figure 11-2-1. **Section #2, Sagittal Series.**
A. Frontal pole and lobe.
B. Parietal lobe.
C. Occipital pole and lobe.
D. Calcarine sulcus.
E. Occipitoparietal sulcus.
F. Cingulate sulcus.
G. Central sulcus.
H. Cingulate gyrus.
I. Superior frontal gyrus.
J. Genu of corpus callosum.
K. Lateral ventricle.
L. Caudate nucleus. Subependymal veins course over it.
M. Choroid plexus.
N. Thalamus.
O. Splenium of corpus callosum.
P. Internal cerebral vein.
Q. Great cerebral vein.
R. Superior and inferior colliculi.
S. Vermis of cerebellum. (See Fig. 11-1-1 for further detail.)
T. Medulla.
U. Pons.
V. Optic chiasm.

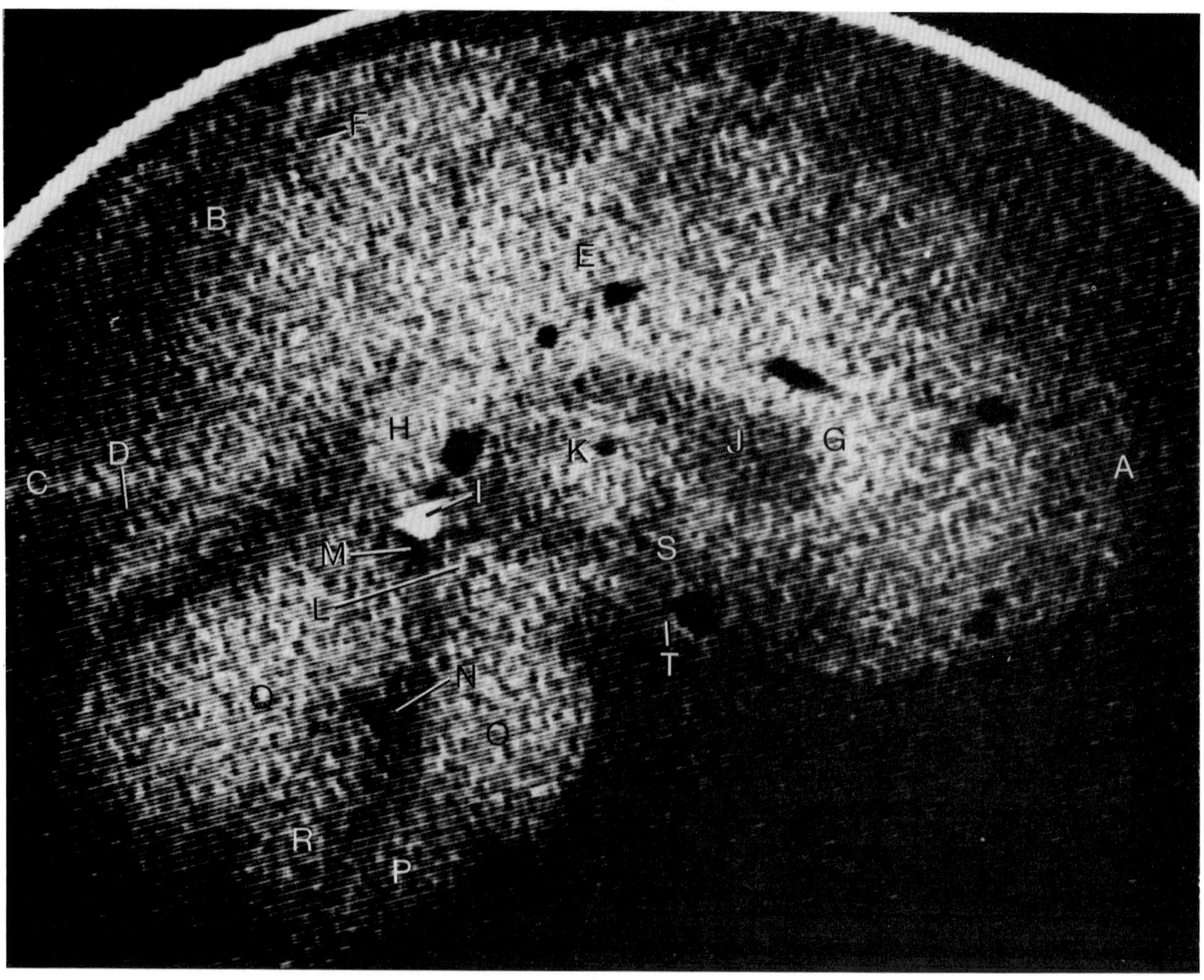

Figure 11-2-2. **Sagittal CT Series, Level #2.**

A. Frontal pole and lobe.
B. Parietal lobe.
C. Occipital pole and lobe.
D. Calcarine sulcus.
E. Cingulate gyrus.
F. Occipitoparietal sulcus.
G. Genu of corpus callosum.
H. Splenium of corpus callosum.
I. Calcified pineal.
J. Lateral ventricle.
K. Thalamus.
L. Collicular plate.
M. Collicular cistern.
N. Fourth ventricle.
O. Pons.
P. Medulla.
Q. Cerebellum.
R. Cerebellar tonsil.
S. Inferior recess of third ventricle.
T. Optic chiasm.

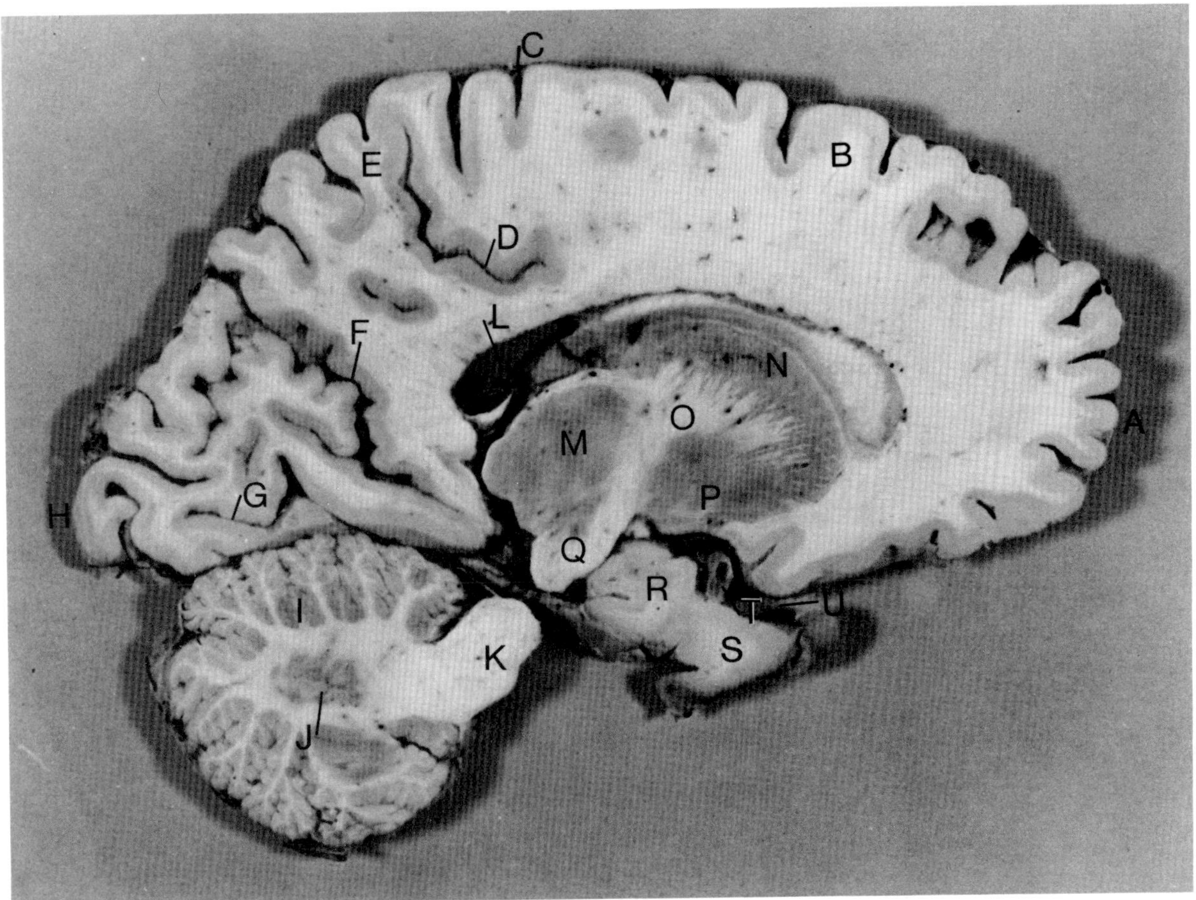

Figure 11-3-1. **Level #3, Sagittal Series.**

A. Frontal pole and lobe.
B. Superior frontal gyrus.
C. Central sulcus.
D. Cingulate sulcus.
E. Parietal lobe.
F. Occipitoparietal sulcus.
G. Calcarine sulcus.
H. Occiptal pole and lobe.
I. Cerebellar hemisphere.
J. Dentate nucleus.
K. Middle cerebellar peduncle.
L. Lateral ventricle.
M. Thalamus.
N. Caudate nucleus.
O. Internal capsule.
P. Globus pallidus.
Q. Cerebral peduncle.
R. Hippocampus.
S. Uncus.
T. Middle cerebral artery.
U. Lateral sulcus.

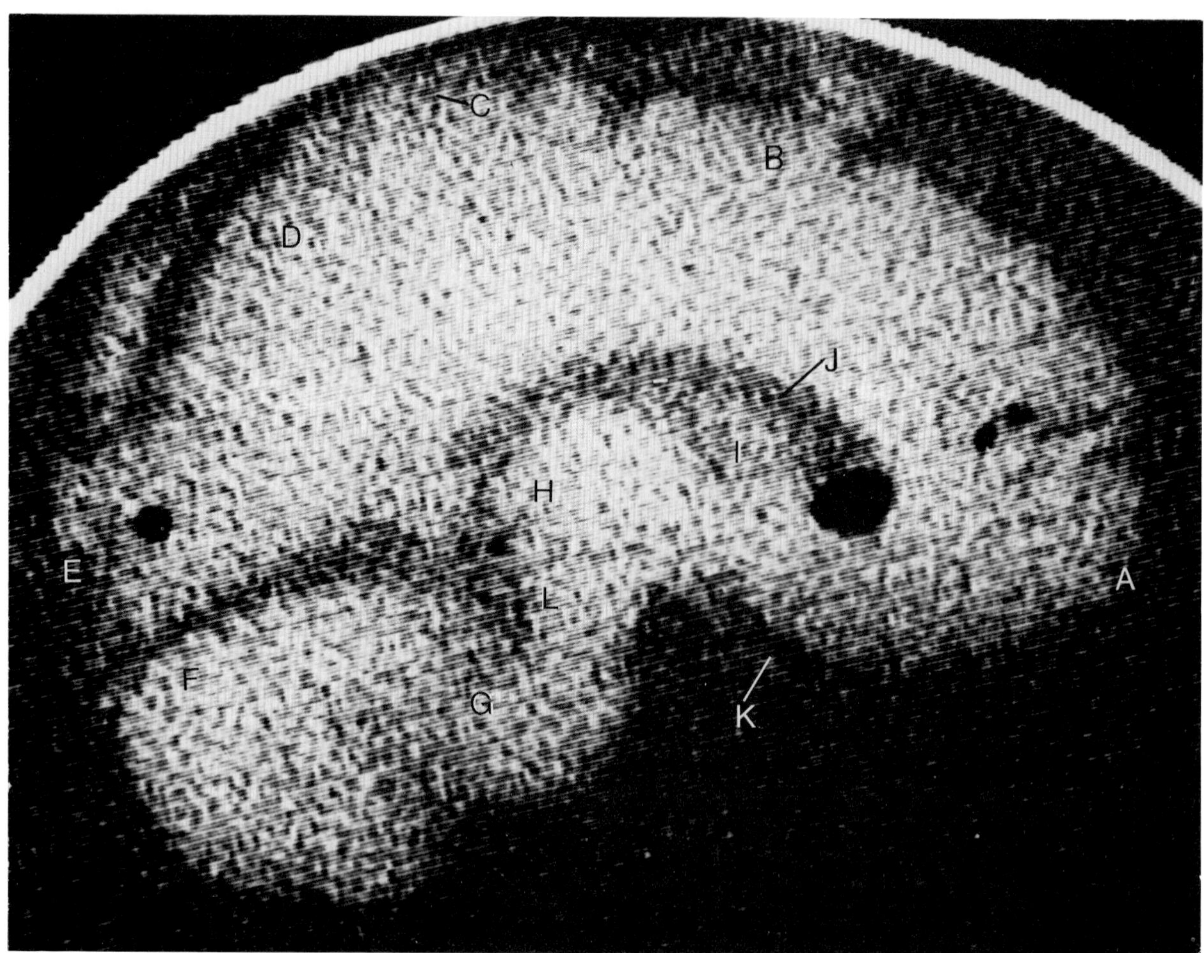

Figure 11-3-2. **Sagittal CT Series, Level #3.**
A. Frontal pole and lobe.
B. Superior frontal gyrus.
C. Central sulcus.
D. Parietal lobe.
E. Occipital pole and lobe.
F. Cerebellar hemisphere.
G. Middle cerebral peduncle.
H. Thalamus.
I. Caudate nucleus.
J. Lateral ventricle.
K. Portion of middle cerebral artery.
L. Cerebral peduncle.

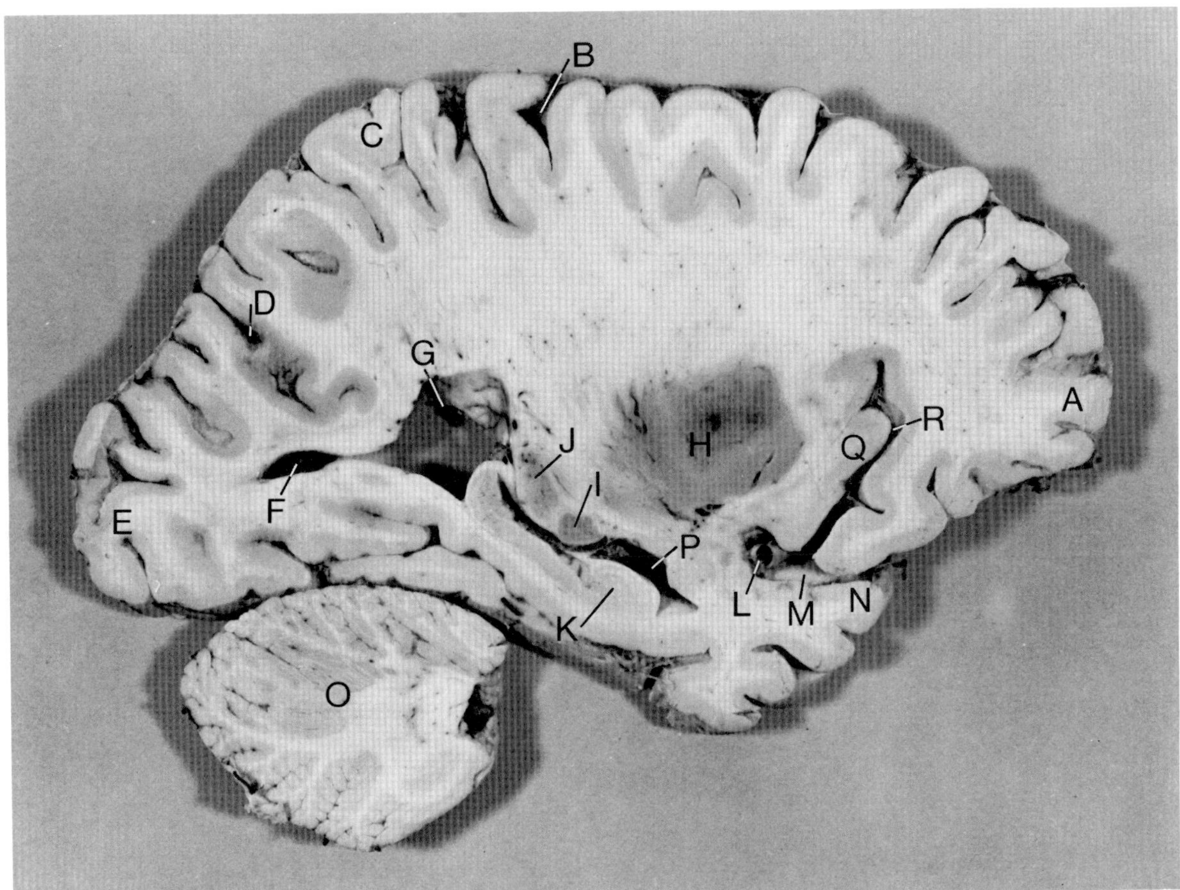

Figure 11-4-1. **Level #4, Sagittal Series.**

A. Frontal pole and lobe.
B. Central sulcus.
C. Parietal lobe.
D. Occipitoparietal sulcus.
E. Occipital pole and lobe.
F. Posterior horn of lateral ventricle.
G. Atrium of lateral ventricle.
H. Lenticular nucleus.
I. Lateral geniculate body.
J. Marginal portion of pulvinar.
K. Hippocampus.
L. Middle cerebral artery in lateral sulcus.
M. Anterior oblique gyrus (primary auditory area).
N. Superior temporal gyrus.
O. Cerebellar hemisphere.
P. Inferior horn of lateral ventricle.
Q. Insula.
R. Suprainsular sulcus.

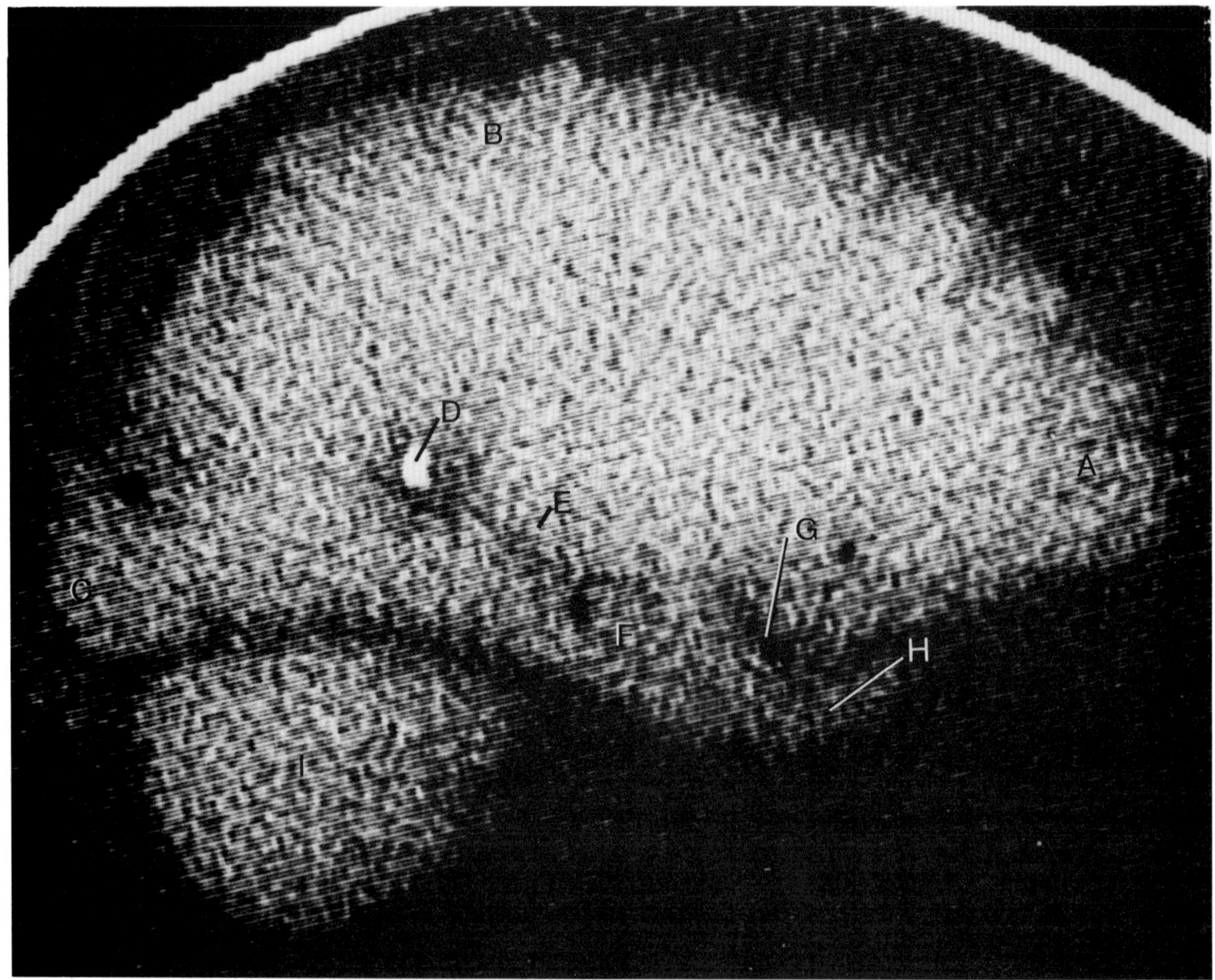

Figure 11-4-2. **Sagittal CT Series, Level #4.**
A. Frontal pole and lobe.
B. Parietal lobe.
C. Occipital pole and lobe.
D. Calcified choroid plexus, in atrium of lateral ventricle.
E. Pulvinar of thalamus.
F. Inferior horn, lateral ventricle.
G. Lateral sulcus.
H. Superior temporal gyrus.
I. Cerebellar hemisphere.

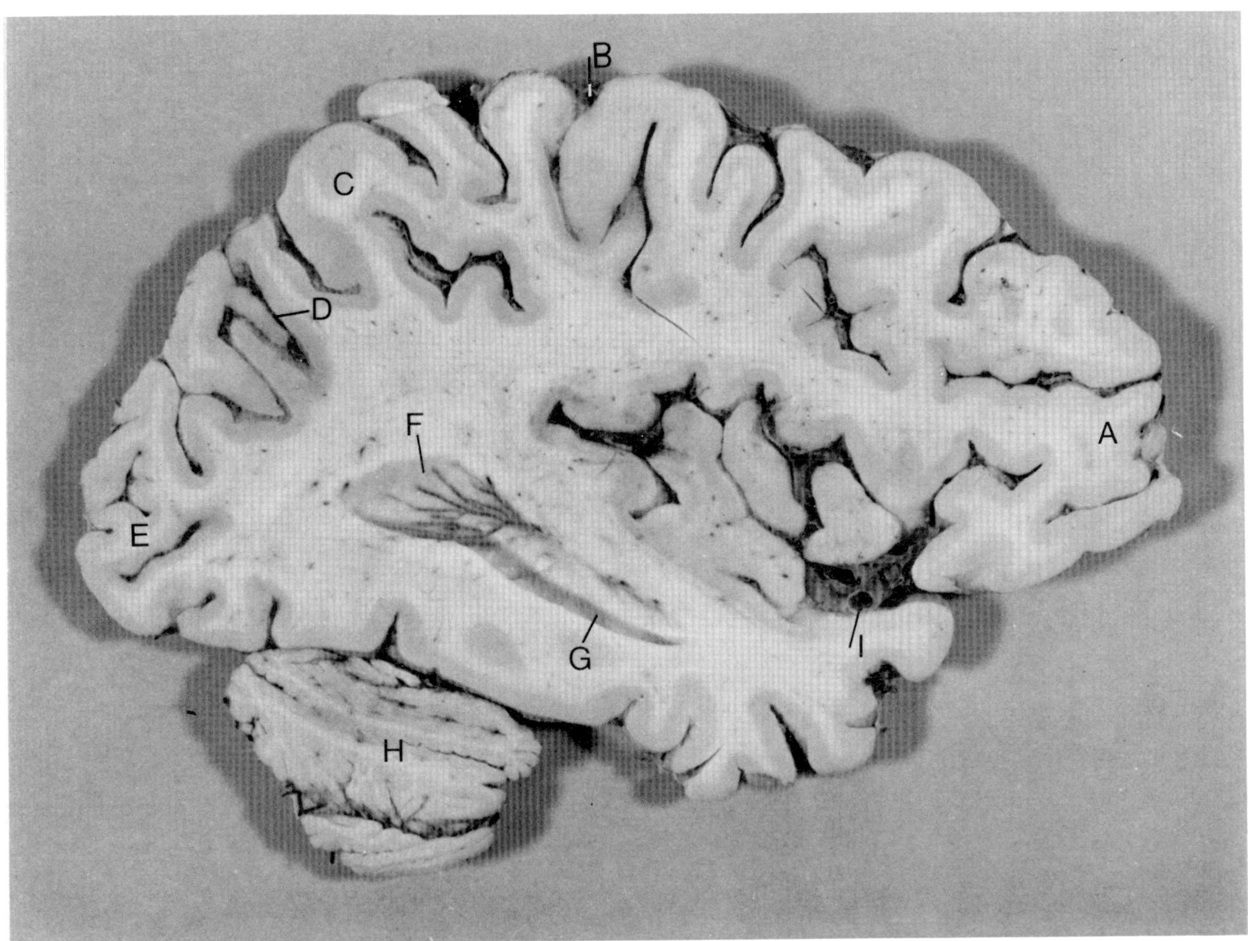

Figure 11-5-1. **Level #5, Sagittal Series.**
A. Frontal lobe.
B. Central sulcus.
C. Parietal lobe.
D. Occipitoparietal sulcus.
E. Occipital lobe.
F. Atrium of lateral ventricle.
G. Inferior horn of lateral ventricle.
H. Cerebellar hemisphere.
I. Middle cerebral artery in lateral sulcus.

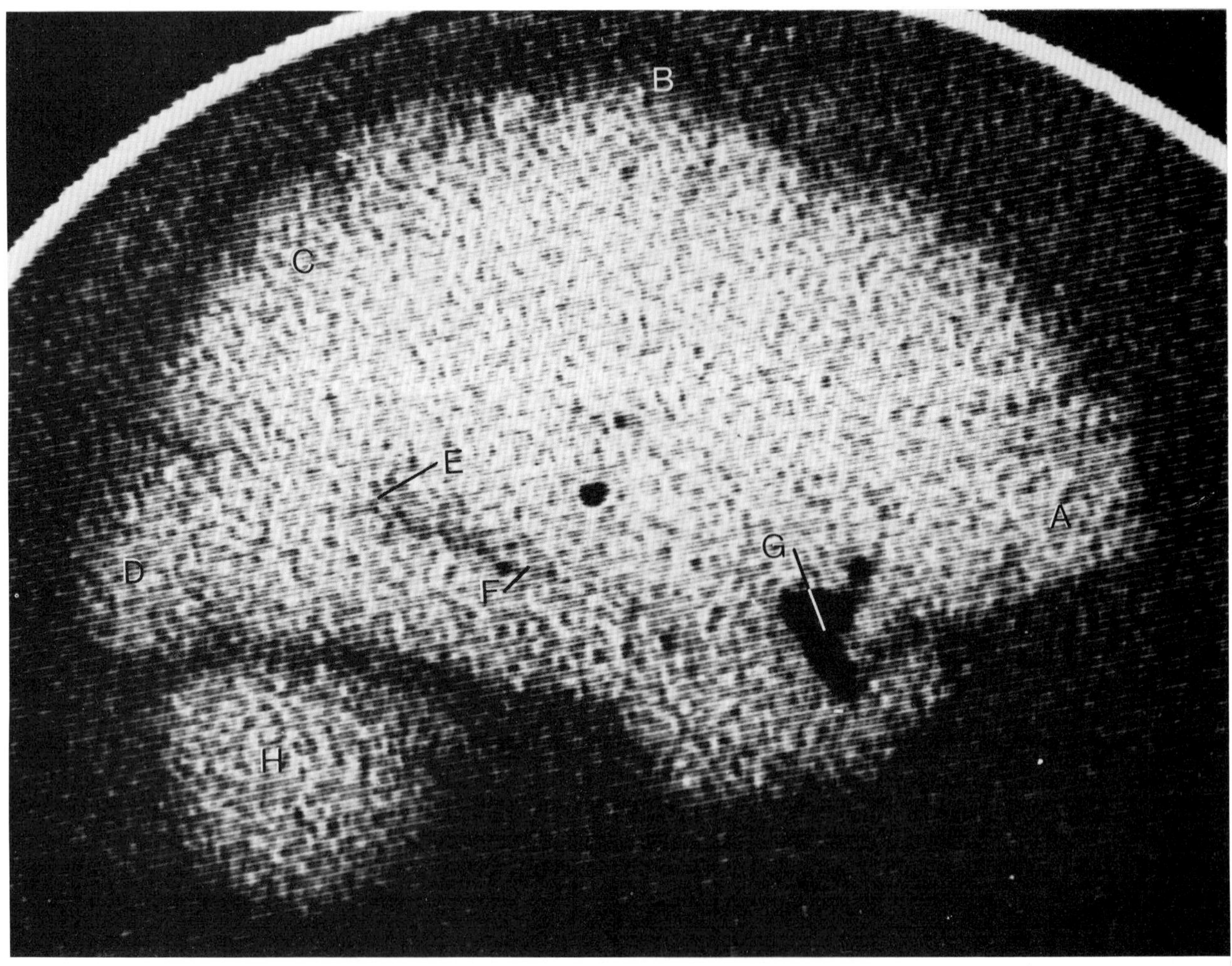

Figure 11-5-2. **Sagittal CT Series, Level #5.**

A. Frontal lobe.
B. Occipitoparietal sulcus.
C. Parietal lobe.
D. Occipital lobe.
E. Atrium of lateral ventricle.
F. Inferior horn lateral ventricle.
G. Lateral sulcus.
H. Cerebellar hemisphere.

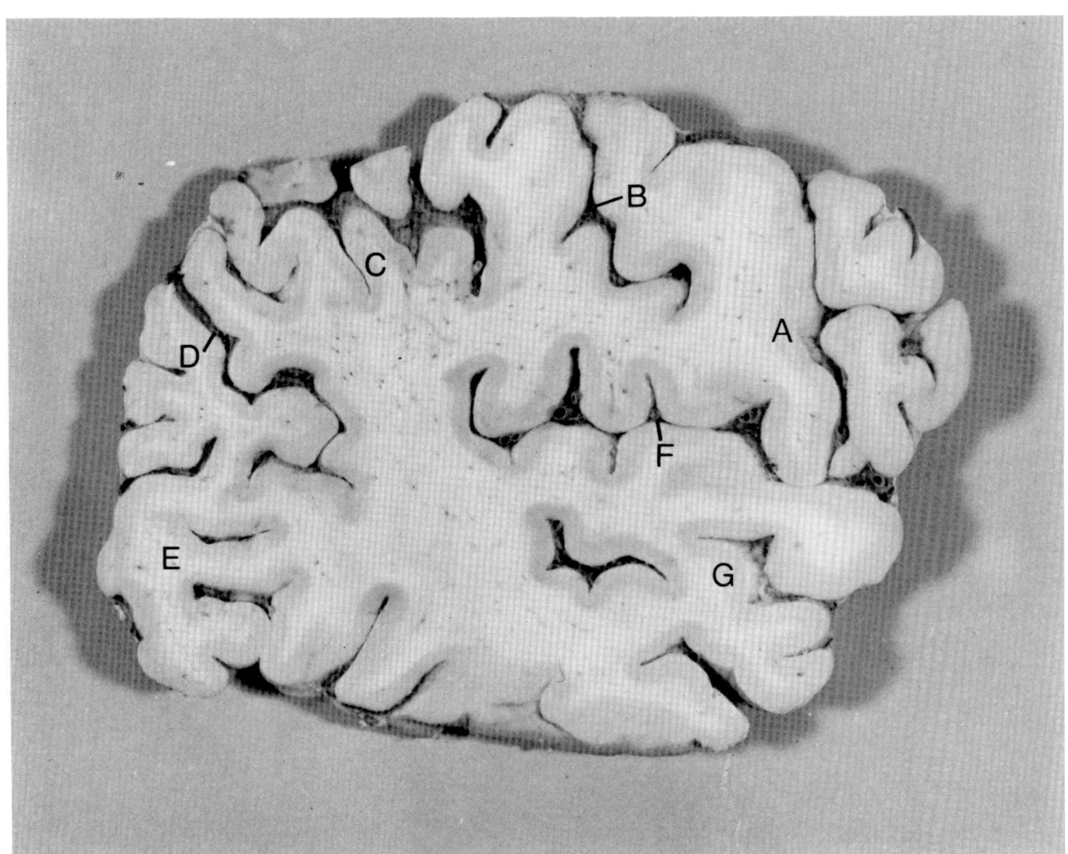

Figure 11-6-1. **Level #6, Sagittal Series.**
A. Frontal lobe.
B. Central sulcus.
C. Parietal lobe.
D. Occipitoparietal sulcus.
E. Occipital lobe.
F. Lateral sulcus.
G. Temporal lobe.

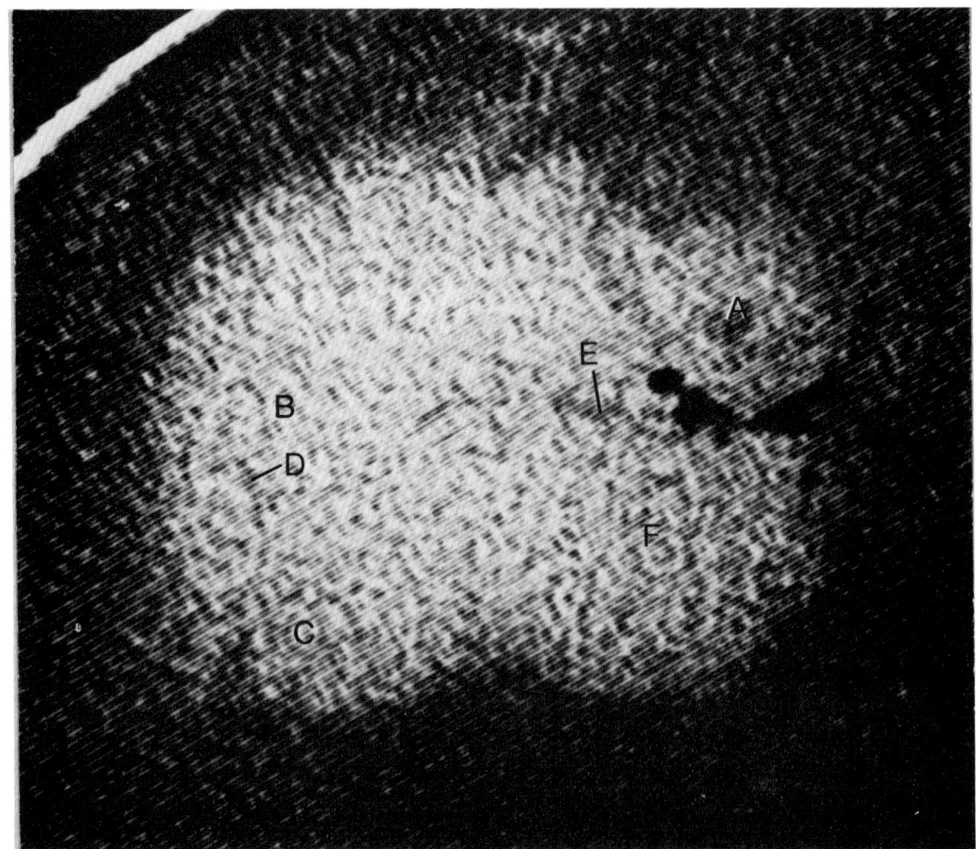

Figure 11-6-2. **Sagittal CT Series, Level #6.**
A. Frontal lobe.
B. Parietal lobe.
C. Occipital lobe.
D. Occipitoparietal sulcus.
E. Lateral sulcus.
F. Temporal lobe.

Chapter Three

Congenital Malformations

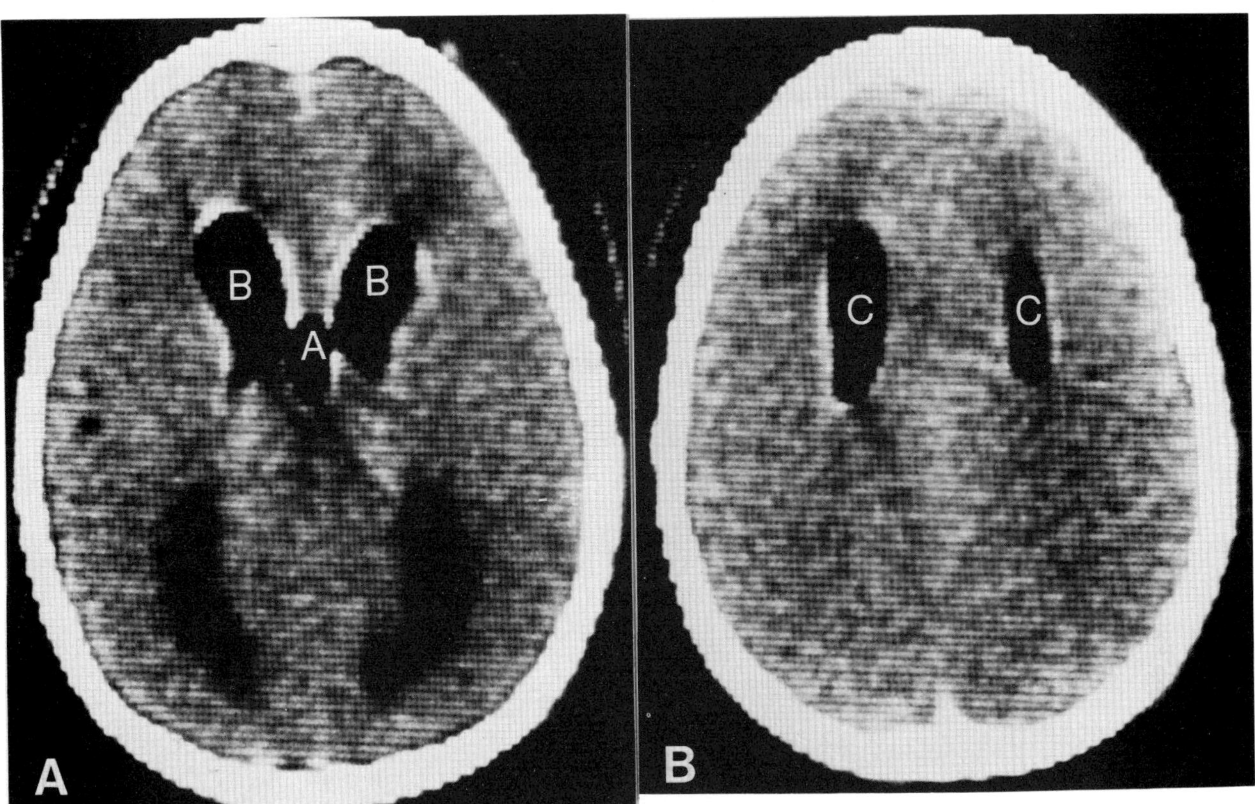

Figure 12-1-1. **Computed Tomography of Agenesis of the Corpus Callosum.**
Following a pneumoencephalogram in this mentally retarded child, two levels from a
CT study demonstrate: in *A*, a dilated third ventricle (A) which is abnormally
positioned cephalad between dilated anterior lateral ventricles (B). Note the air in the
anterior ventricular system, surrounded by high density computer artifact. The
interventricular foramina are more horizontally positioned betwen A and B than is
normally seen. A higher section (*B*) demonstrates widely separated anterior lateral
ventricles (C), again due to the abnormally cephalad positioned third ventricle
secondary to agenesis of the corpus callosum.

While this entity occasionally may be asymptomatic, many of these individuals
are mentally retarded. This condition may be associated with multiple other anomalies
to various degrees, including among others Dandy-Walker syndrome.

Letters in italics refer to larger letters denoting subdivisions of the illustration. Nonitalicized letters refer to smaller letters that indicate individual structures in the illustration.

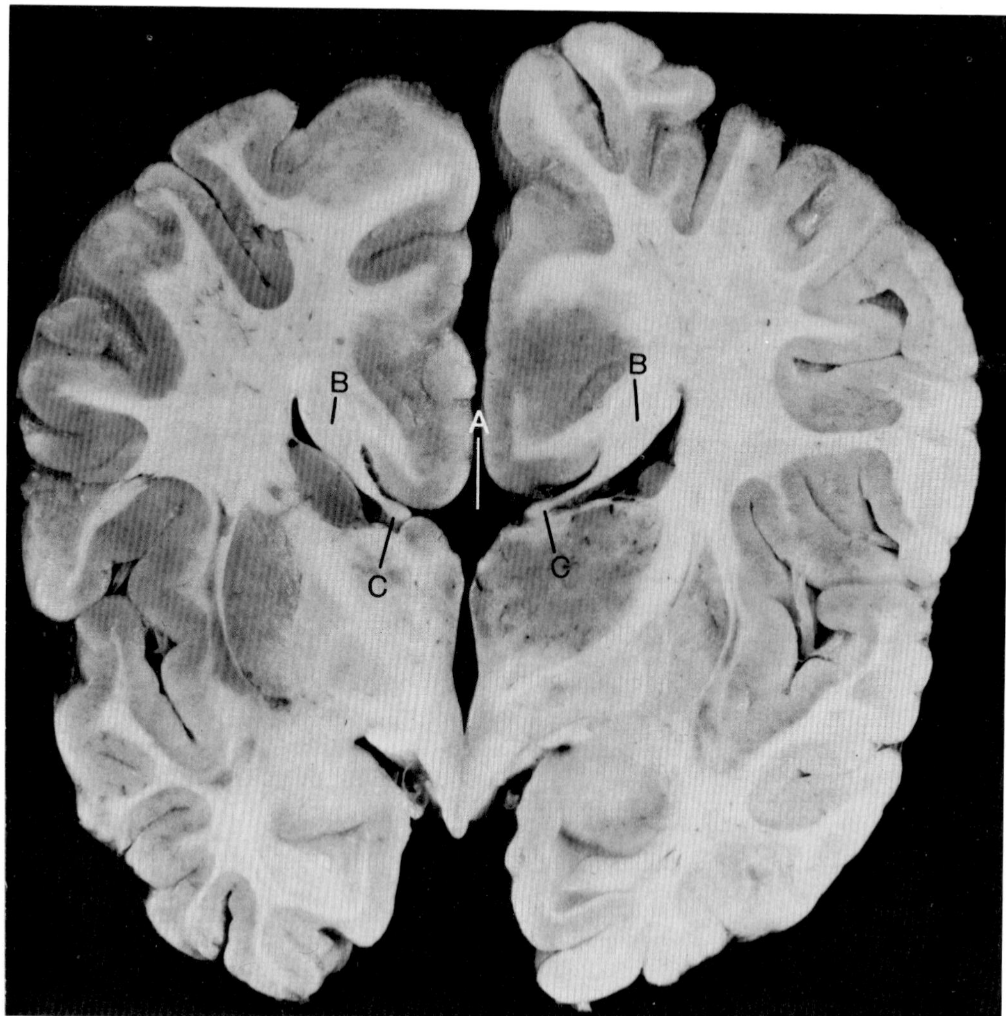

Figure 12-1-2. **Defective Formation of the Corpus Callosum.**

A. Point at which the corpus callosum ordinarily extends across the base of the longitudinal fissure as a commissure between the cerebral hemispheres. There is a disjunction in the present case.

B. There is relatively good formation of the lateral portions of the corpus callosum. As the latter extends medially from each side, it becomes increasingly thinner.

C. Rounded-up medial end-margins of the corpus callosum.

From Dublin, W. B.: *Fundamentals of Neuropathology,* Ed. II, 1967, Charles C Thomas, Springfield, Illinois.

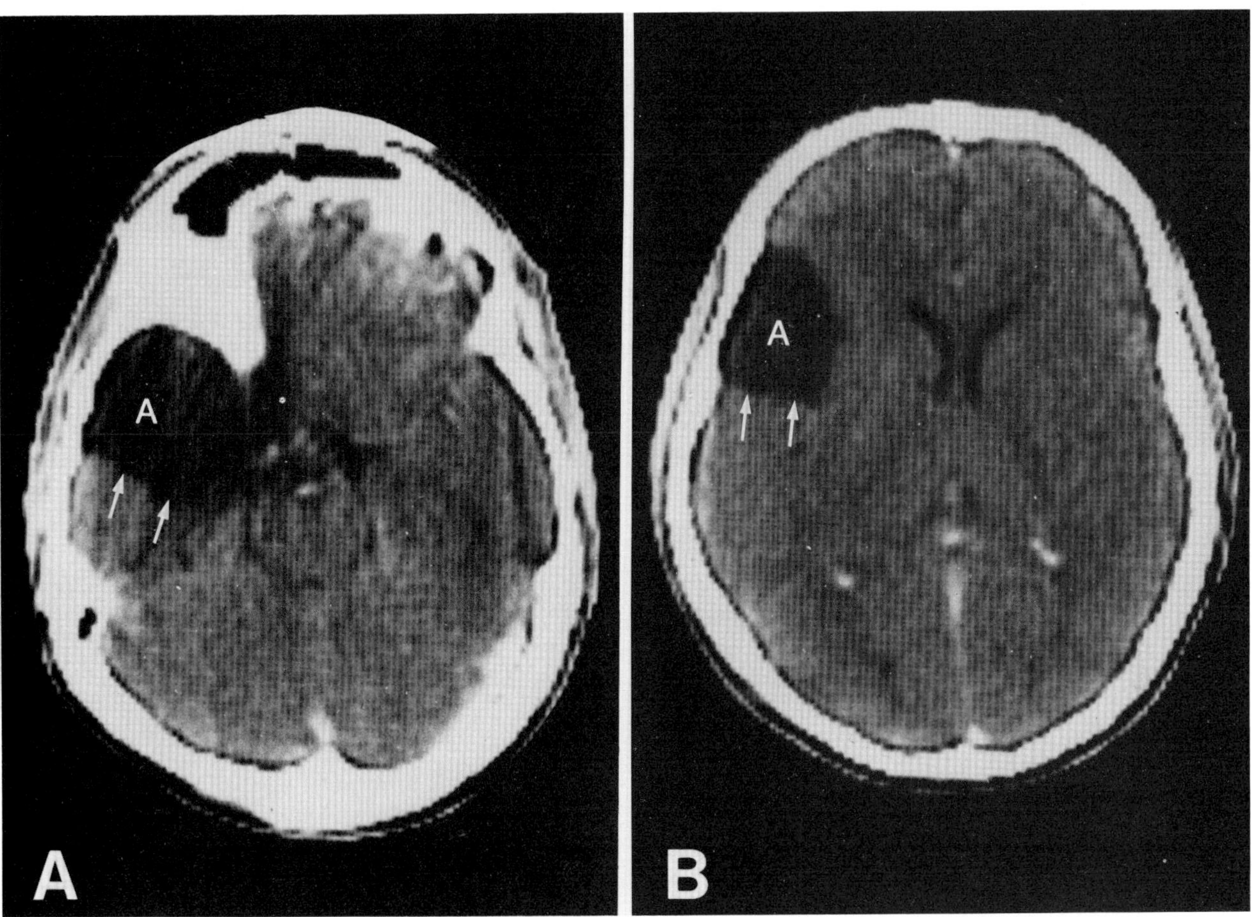

Figure 12-2-1. **Arachnoid Cyst, Middle Fossa.** *A, B:* A CSF density oval lesion is identified extending upwards from the middle fossa (A). The posterior margin of the cyst is flattened (arrows) characteristic of this disorder within the middle fossa. The middle cerebral artery, which can help to classify this as an intra- or extra-axial lesion, is not definitely identified in *A*. Only minimal mass effect upon midline structures (*B*) is noted, consistent with a chronic process. Letters in italics refer to larger letters denoting subdivisions of the illustration. Nonitalicized letters refer to smaller letters that indicate individual structures in the illustration.

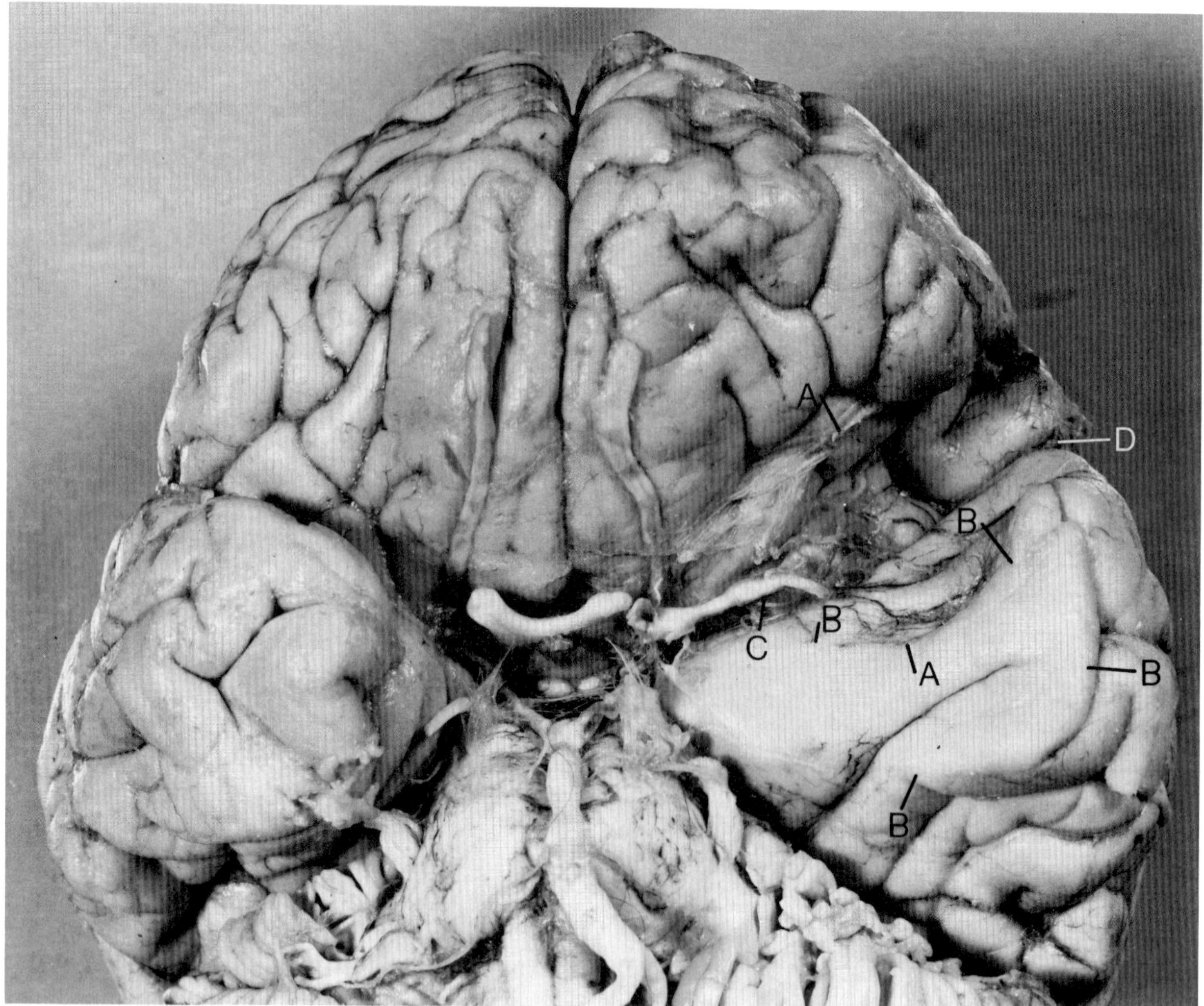

Figure 12-2-2. **Congenital Meningeal Cyst.** (Continuation from 12-2-1.) The cyst
appeared to lie partly between dura and arachnoid, and partly between arachnoid and
pia. The cyst lay in the lateral sulcus, with underformation of adjacent portions of
frontal and temporal lobes.
A–A. The portion of the cyst having deep lining of arachnoid.
B–B. The portion with only pia as deep lining; the surface of this portion is smooth and
         avascular.
C. Middle cerebral artery; the vessel is attenuated and sclerotic.
D. Lateral sulcus.

Figure 12-2-3. Continuation. Cross section levels in the 15° axial plane of the cyst $\rightarrow$
shown in Figure 12-2-2, just preceding.
A. A. The cyst, in the lateral sulcus.
    B. Middle cerebral artery with arachnoid.
    C. Frontal lobe.
    D. Temporal lobe.
    The tissue lining the floor of the lateral sulcus, including the primary acoustic
    area, is underdeveloped.
B. A–D. As in *A.*
    E. Insula.

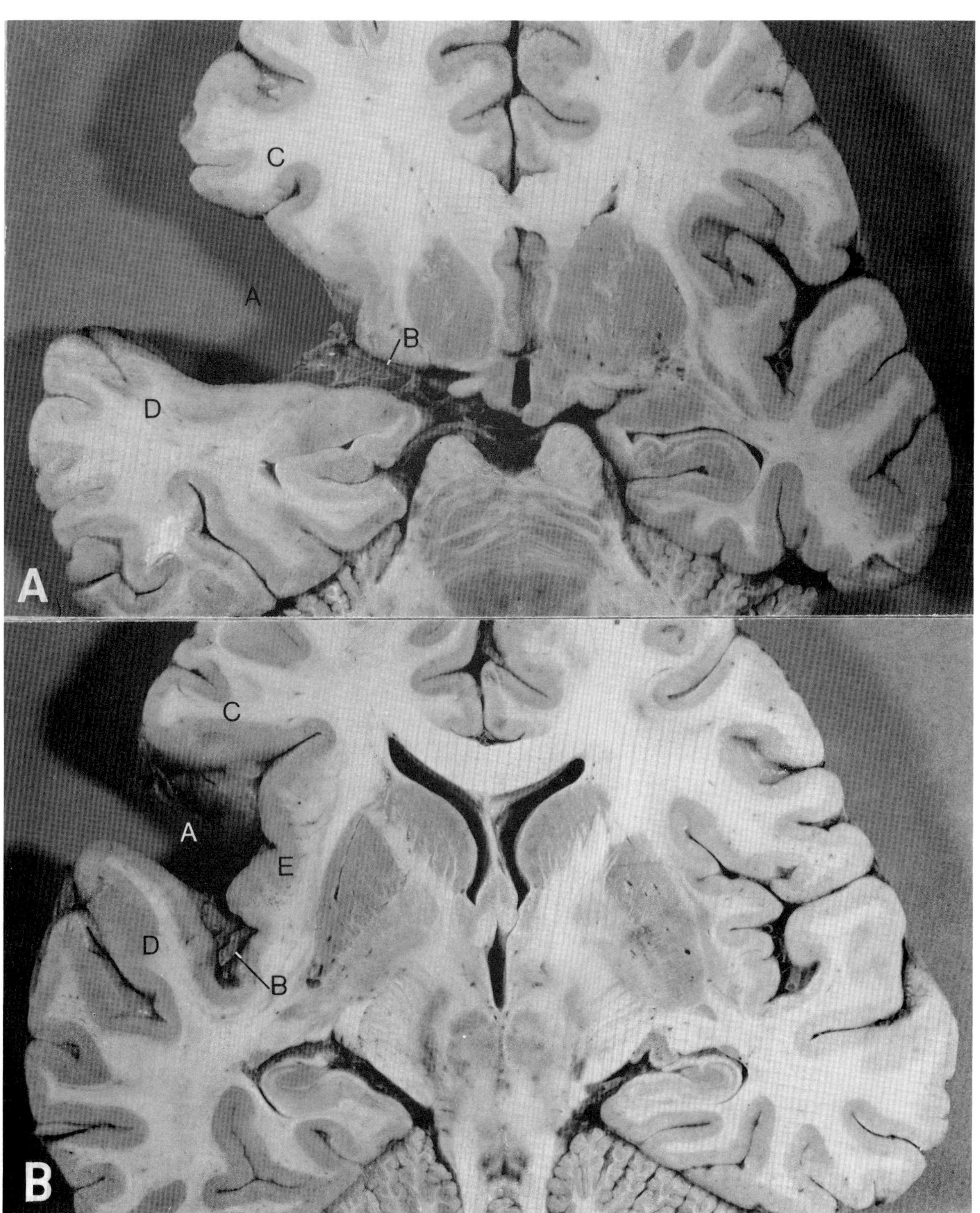
C
A
B
D
A
C
A
E
D
B
B

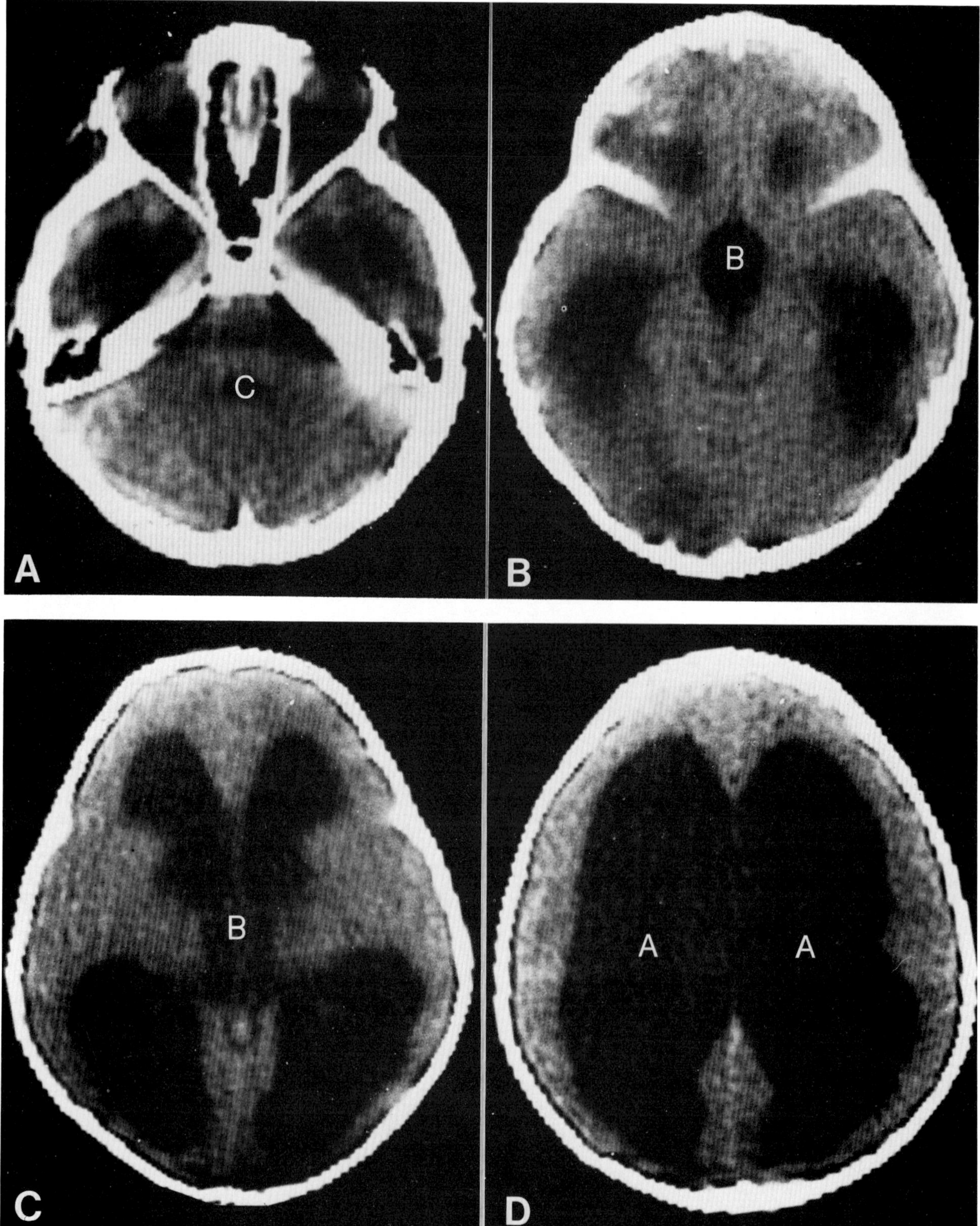

Figure 12-3-1. *(A-D)*. **Aqueductal Stenosis, Computed Tomography.** Greatly dilated lateral (A), and third (B) ventricles are seen, with a small decompressed fourth ventricle (C) typical of aqueductal stenosis. In some cases, the fourth ventricle may be enlarged rather than small. This is due to continued CSF production within this structure and obstruction of flow of the fluid over the convexities due to the lateral ventricular hydrocephalus.

    Letters in italics refer to larger letters denoting subdivisions of the illustration. Non-italicized letters refer to smaller letters that indicate individual structures in the illustration.

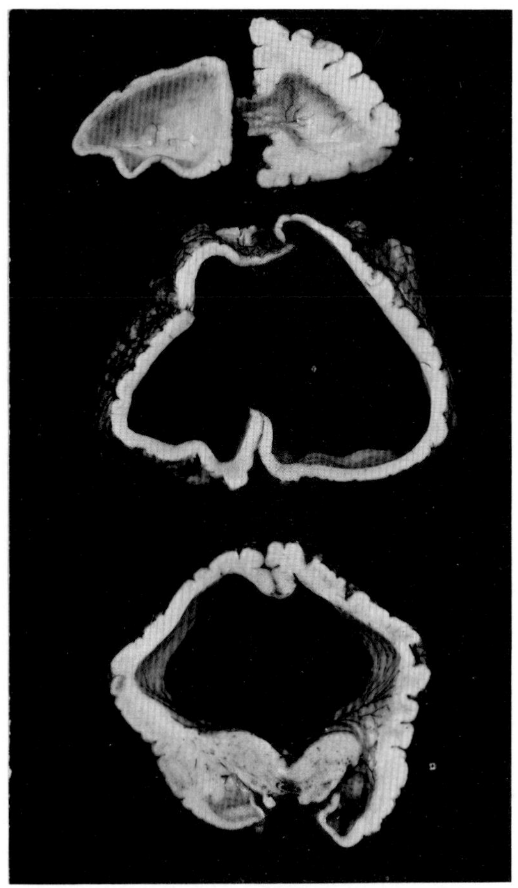

Figure 12-3-2. **Hydrocephalus in Aqueductal Stenosis.**
From Dublin, W.B.: *Fundamentals of Neuropathology,* Ed. II, 1967, Charles C. Thomas, Springfield, Illinois.

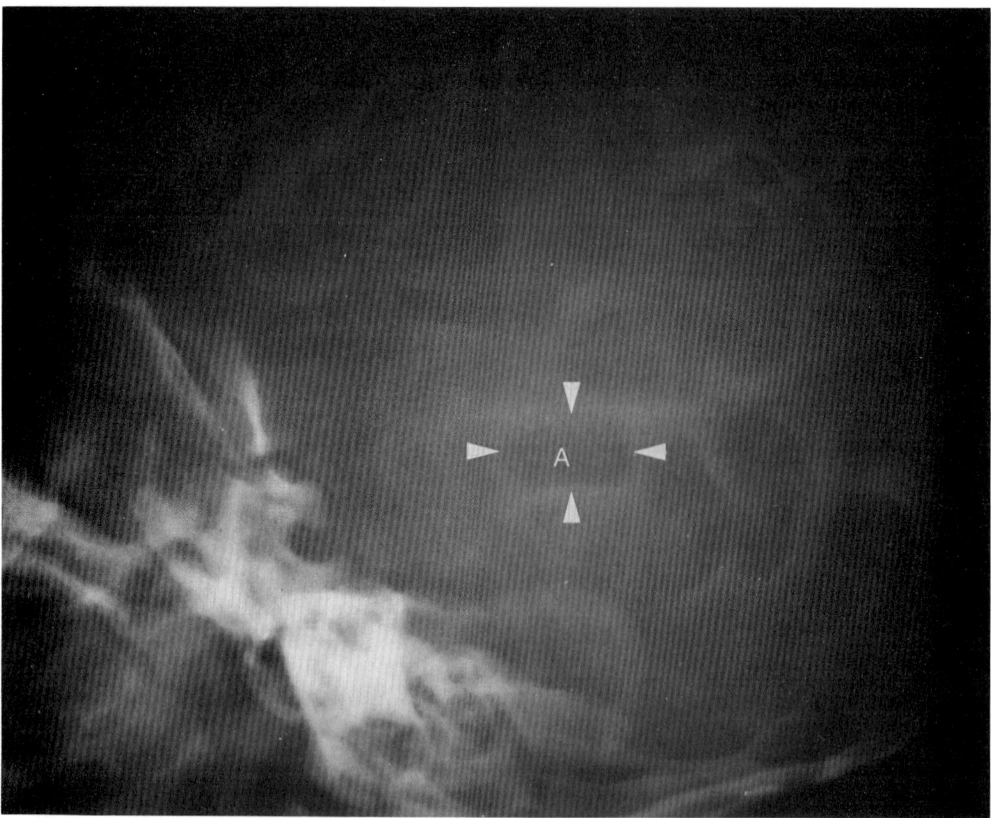

Figure 12-4-1. **Plain Radiographic Appearance of Lacunar Skull (Leukenshädel) and Arnold-Chiari Type II.** A lateral skull film shows a dysplastic area in the skull (A) surrounded by more normal membranous bone (arrowheads) typical of lacunar skull. This pattern is unrelated to the temporal development of hydrocephalus and should not be confused with increased digital marking (beaten silver pattern) caused by increased intracranial pressure.

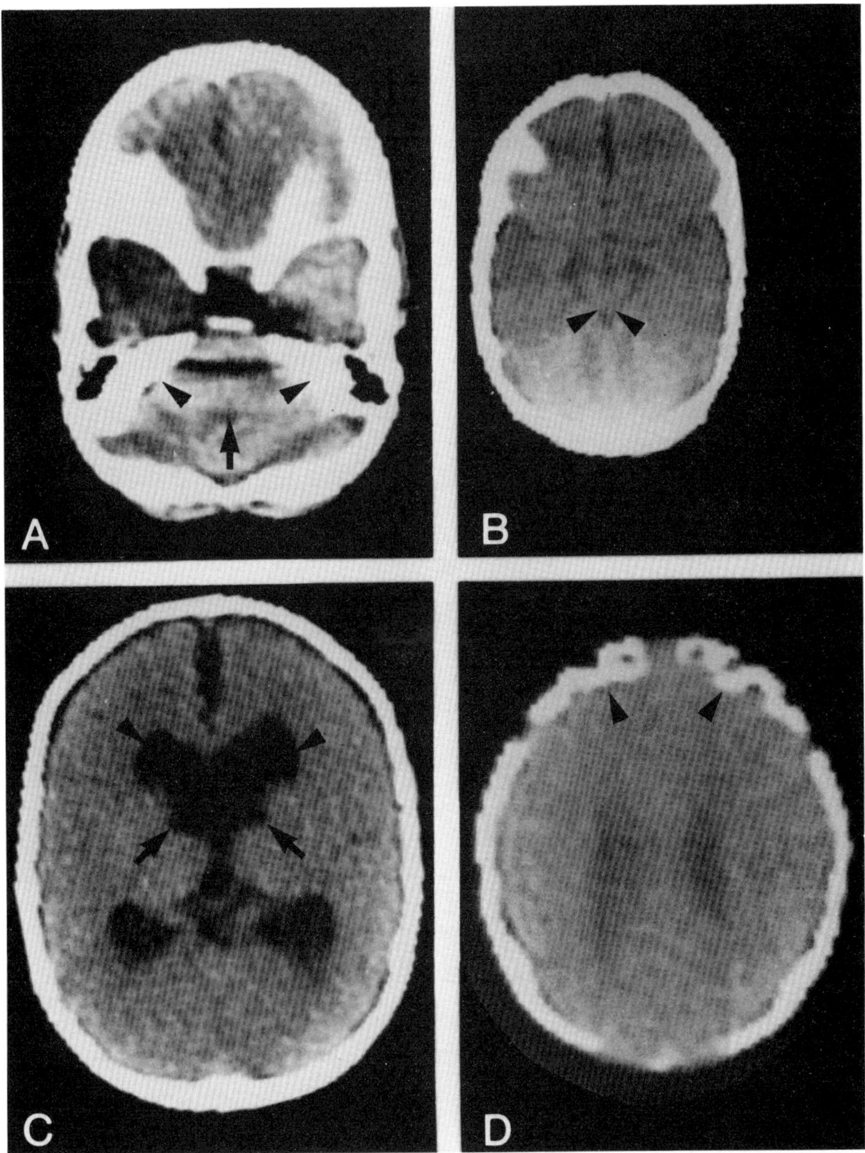

Figure 12-4-2. **Computed Tomographic Findings of Arnold-Chiari Type II Malformation. A.** A small posterior fossa with posteriorly concave petrous bones, and a small caudally displaced fourth ventricle (arrow), are seen. **B.** A higher section of a different patient demonstrates "pointing" or "beaking" posteriorly of the quadrigeminal plate (tectum) (arrowheads). **C.** Hydrocephalic enlargement of the lateral ventricles with flattening of the lateral aspects of the anterior ventricular horns (arrowheads) is identified. A prominent "beak" (arrows) representing an increased cleft between the caudate and thalamic nuclei is visualized. **D.** An undulating "ribbon" appearance of the calvarium anteriorly (arrowheads) is typical of leukenschädel (lacunar skull). The combination of the foregoing findings is pathognomic of Arnold-Chiari Type II.

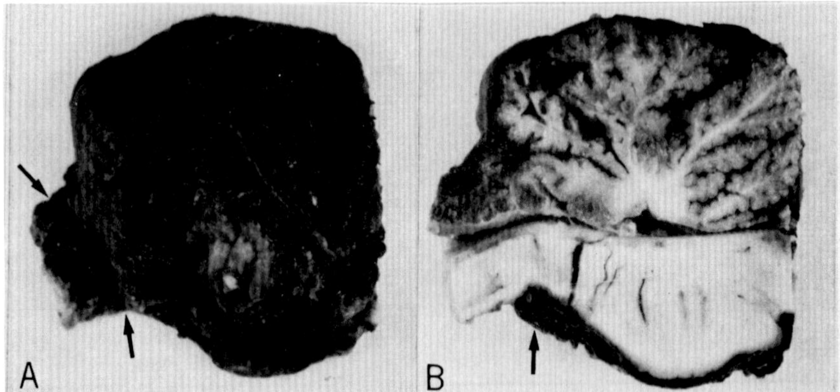

Figure 12-4-3. **Arnold-Chiari Deformity.** This condition consists basically of a developmental malformation of cerebellum and brain stem, resulting in displacement of dysplastic portions of vermis, medulla, and caudal fourth ventricle through the foramen magnum. Pathogenesis is subject to variation of opinion. There usually is associated hydrocephalus. Main types of the syndrome are recognized, although not necessarily with sharp distinction. In type I, hydrocephalus is mild, and the fourth ventricle is not herniated. The condition may be subclinical, being found only at postmortem. In type II, herniation and hydrocephalus are more severe, and tend to be accompanied by spinal meningomyelocele. The latter results from failure of proper closure of the caudal portion of the neural tube.
A. Lateral view of cerebellum and brain stem in a case of Arnold-Chiari deformity in a newborn infant. Line of compression by rim of foramen magnum is shown with arrows.
B. Sagittal view. Portions of vermis and medulla are herniated. There is indentation of the ventral surface of the medulla, constituting a degree of basilar impression. This is pointed out by the arrow; the latter is placed slightly low in order to preserve detail. Although the compression is severe, the case may perhaps be classed as Type I; the fourth ventricle is not severely herniated and is not dilated (hydrocephalus was not present), and there was no meningomyelocele. Illustration from Dublin, W.B.: *Fundamentals of Neuropathology,* Ed. II, 1967, Charles C. Thomas, Springfield, Illinois.

Chapter Four

Infections

This chapter deals with some combined radiologic and pathologic features of infections.

Radionuclide brain scanning may be comparatively sensitive in the early detection of encephalitis and/or meningitis. CT, however, is quite helpful in the evaluation of intracranial infectious disease, particularly when it is focal and deep-seated. Thus, multilocular abscesses may be easily defined; this may be of extreme importance in surgical drainage or extirpation. The feature of multilocularity may not be as clearly demonstrated by radionuclide scanning. In addition, secondary complications such as hydrocephalus can be appreciated best with CT.

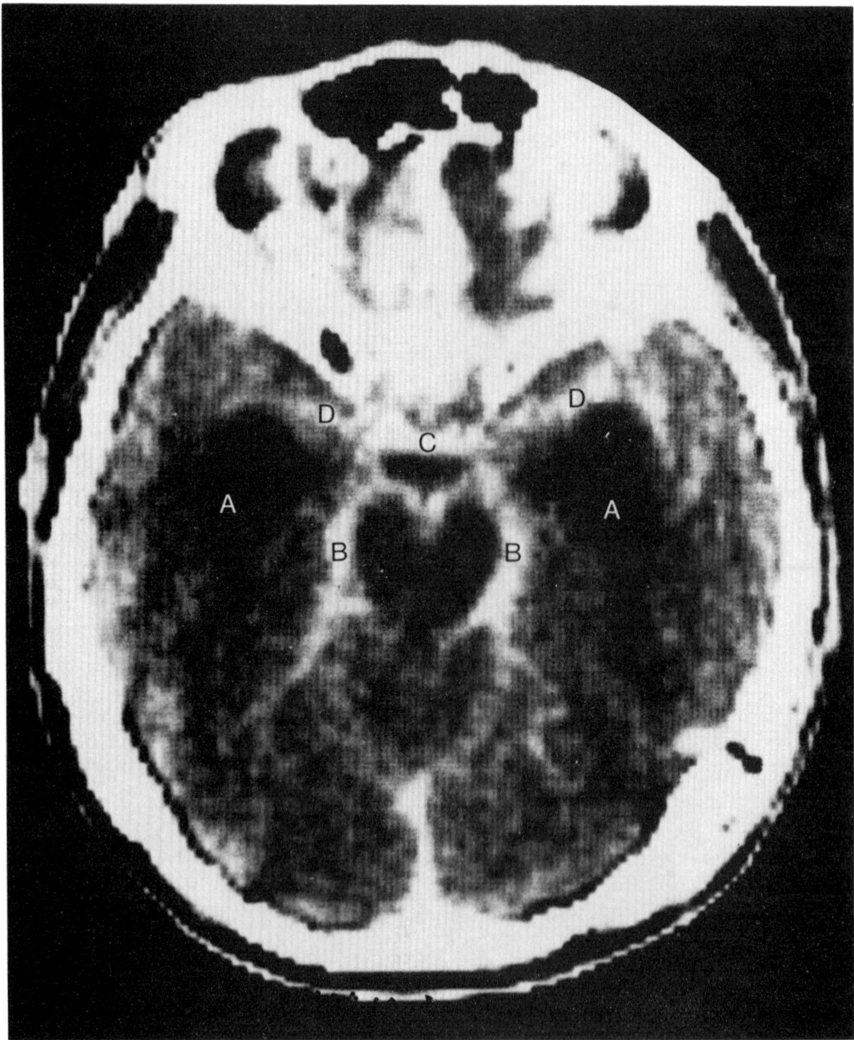

Figure 13-1-1. **Computed Tomography of Meningitis.** Hydrocephalus as evident by enlarged inferior horns (A) is secondary to basal arachnoiditis. Extremely abnormal and prominent enhancement of the basal cisterns representing such arachnoiditis is seen. Cisternal structures including the perimesencephalic (ambient, B), suprasellar (chiasmatic, C), and cistern of the middle cerebral artery (A) are demonstrated. Other entities which may mimic this condition on contrast studies would include intrathecal introduction of agents like metrizamide, and subarachnoid hemorrhage. Abnormal contrast enhancement of this type may be noted also in postsubarachnoid hemorrhage states, and in metastatic involvement of the meninges by tumor.

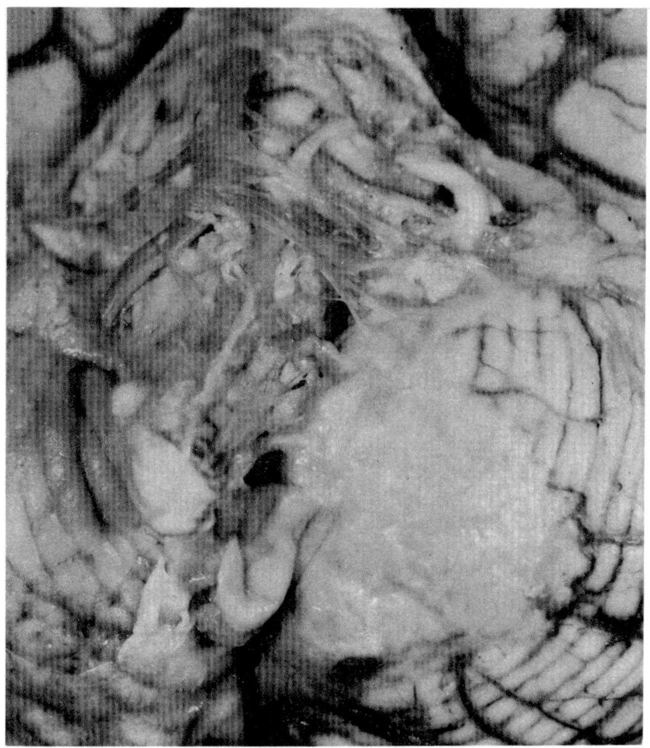

Figure 13-1-2. **Purulent Staphylococcal Meningitis Involving the Base of the Brain.** From Dublin, W. B.: *Fundamentals of Sensorineural Auditory Pathology,* 1976, Charles C Thomas, Springfield, Illinois.

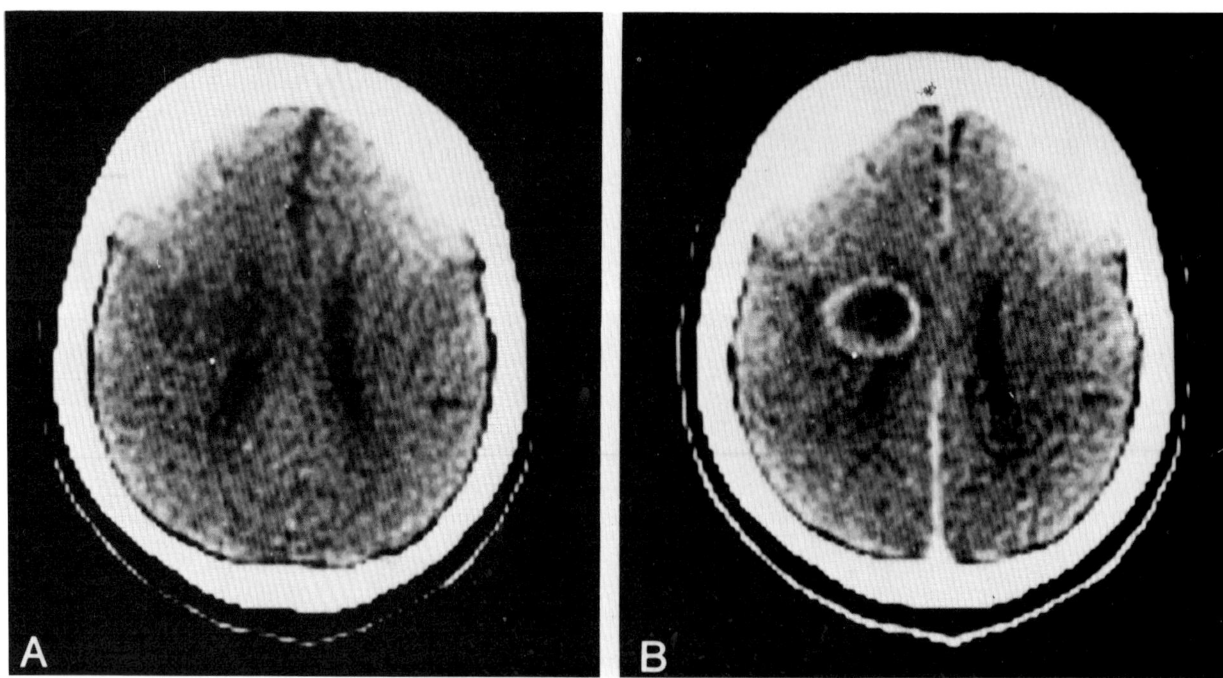

Figure 13-2-1. **Computed Tomography of Intracerebral Abscess.**
A. A noncontrast scan shows an oval area of decreased density adjacent to the lateral ventricle. **B.** A thin "ring" of enhancement is demonstrated. While this ring may be "pencil-thin" or very smooth and regular in an abscess, a "shaggy" or thickened ring may also be seen. Thus, the appearance of ring enhancement is not necessarily a reliable differential point distinguishing a variety of pathological entities, including: abscess, primary and secondary neoplasm, infarct, and hematoma. In secondary neoplasms and abscesses, however, there usually is significant edema surrounding the area of ring enhancement. However, the amount of edema in this particular case is far from impressive. The presence of ring enhancement in an abscess generally implies that a wall about the abscess has started to form. The lesion may not be cavitary. Occasionally, however, the wall may be poorly formed at the time of surgery, and the clinical time course for the patient's illness should be considered when evaluating computed tomographic findings for possible surgical excision and/or drainage of those lesions.

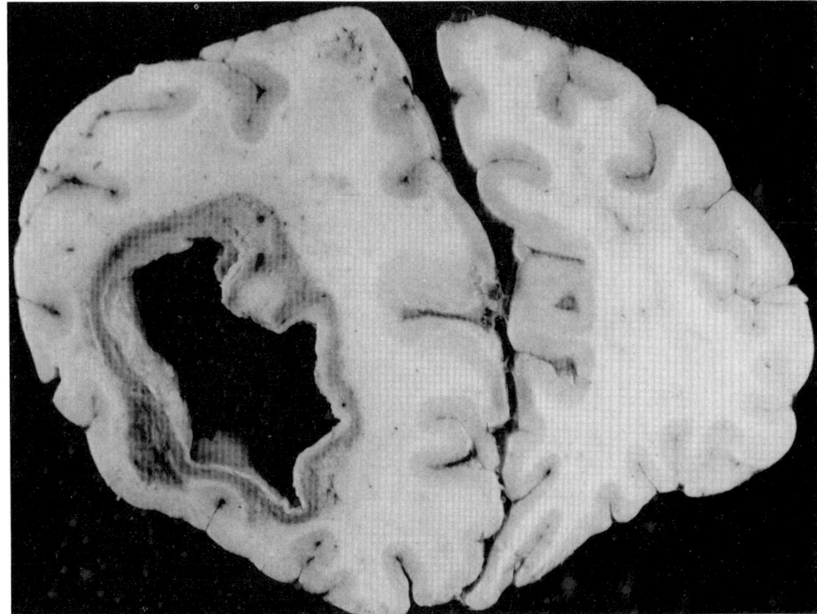

Figure 13-2-2. **Cerebral Abscess.** The lesion is of one month's duration; a cavity has been formed, and there is early encapsulation. The surrounding tissue is edematous, with general expansion of the affected hemisphere, and flattening of convolutions. The capsule of the abscess would correspond to the enhancing ring seen on CT, while the cavity would correspond to the dark central nonenhancing CT region. From Dublin, W. B.: *Fundamentals of Neuropathology,* Ed. II, 1967, Charles C Thomas, Springfield, Illinois.

Chapter Five

Injuries

Computed tomography indisputably is the tool of choice in the evaluation of acute and chronic traumatic intracranial hemorrhage. Paradoxically, it may be found that those with depressed skull fractures may exhibit minimal intracranial hemorrhage, while persons with small hairline fractures, or none at all that can be detected, may sustain more severe intracranial injury, with bleeding. In general, skull films are of little use in the evaluation of traumatic intracranial hemorrhage, and in general need not be obtained except in certain instances of associated facial fracture.

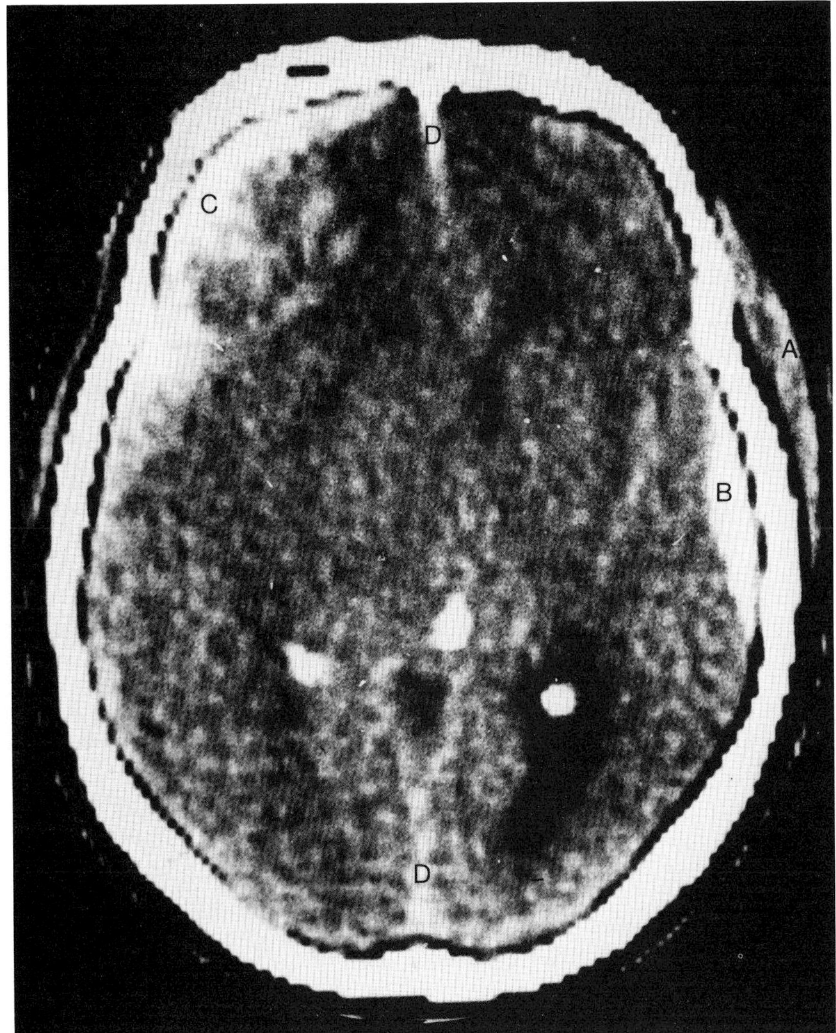

Figure 14-1-1 **Computed Tomography of Multiple Forms of Intracranial Hemorrhage.** Extracranial soft tissue swelling (A) is adjacent to a temporal epidural (biconvex) hematoma (B). A fracture in the temporal bone could be demonstrated using bone window settings. A contrecoup subdural hematoma (C) with underlying cortical contusion is noted in the contralateral frontal lobe. D represents perifalcine subarachnoid hemorrhage. While subdural hematomas usually have the typical curvilinear appearance such as demonstrated by C, and while epidural hematomas have a biconvex appearance as demonstrated by B, surgical exploration may reveal a mixture of lesions. Occasionally, a biconvex lesion of high density may be an old calcified subdural hematoma, and measurement of the densities of such biconvex lesions should be undertaken.

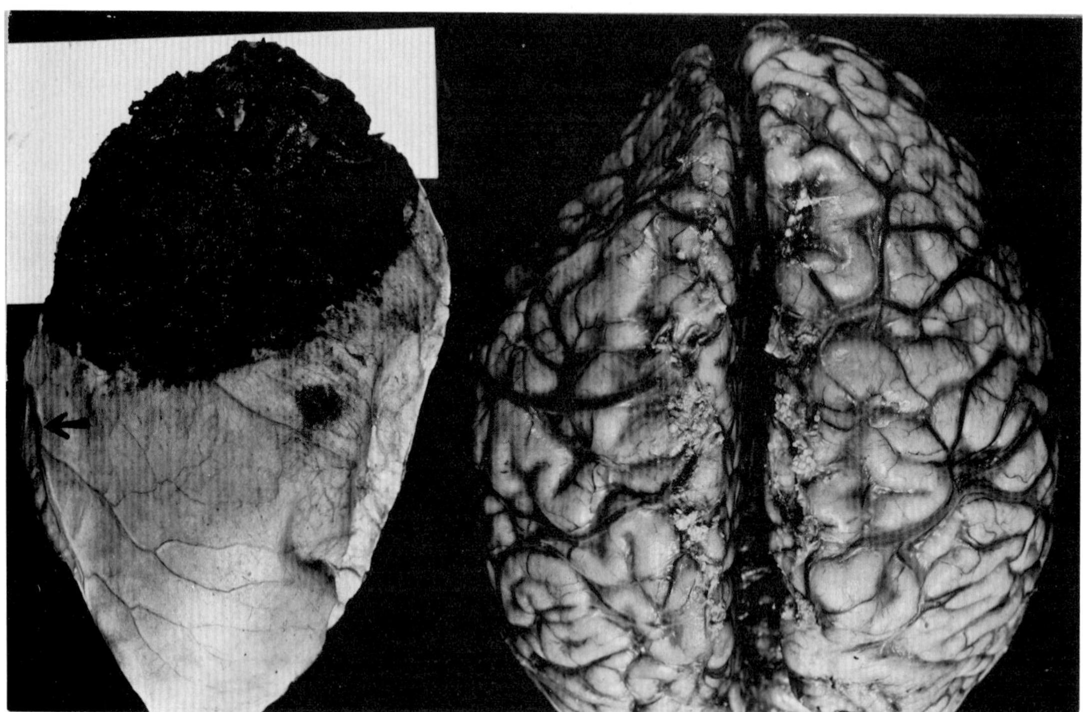

Figure 14-1-2. **Extradural Hematoma.** There is compression of underlying left frontal lobe. Injured middle meningeal arterial branch giving rise to bleeding is buried beneath the clot; a comparable vessel is indicated by arrow. From Dublin, W. B.: *Fundamentals of Neuropathology,* Ed. II, 1967, Charles C Thomas, Springfield, Illinois.

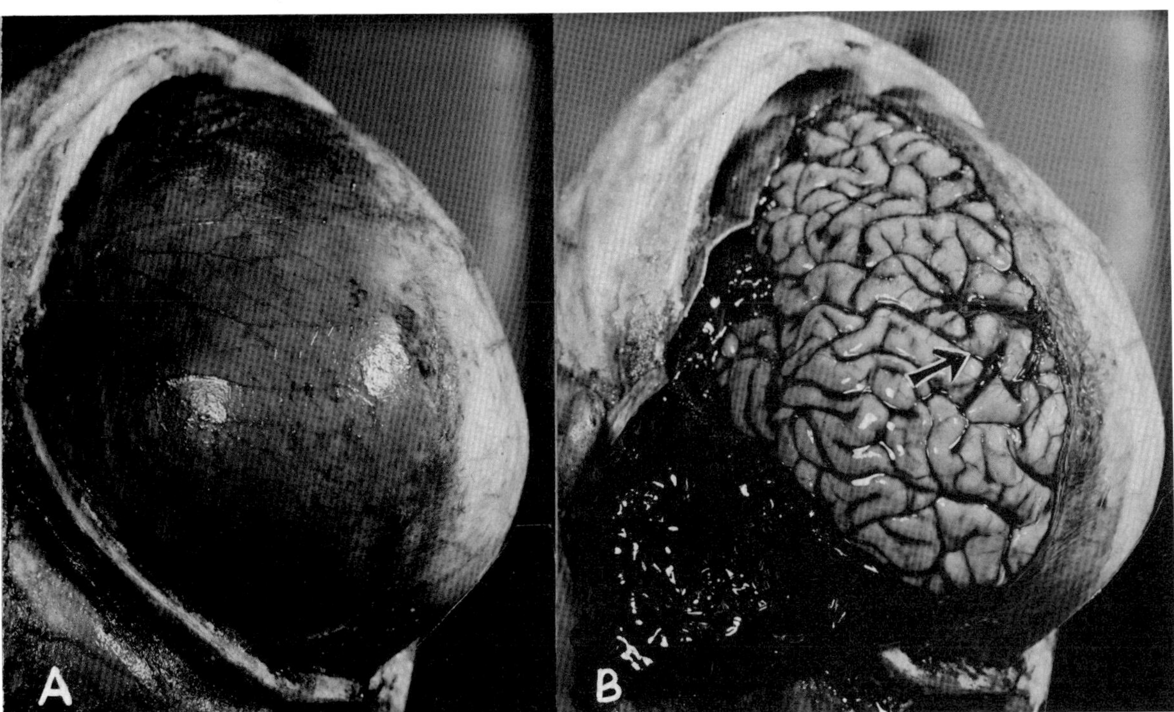

Figure 14-1-3. **Traumatic Subdural Hematoma.**

A. There is dark discoloration of dura on the left, owing to underlying blood.

B. Dura has been reflected, showing layer of blood clot; a large amount of liquid blood
    has escaped. One or more of large veins at vertex (arrow indicates the group)
    appear to have been torn. From Dublin, W.B.: *Fundamentals of Neuropathology,*
    Ed. II, 1967, Charles C. Thomas, Springfield, Illinois.

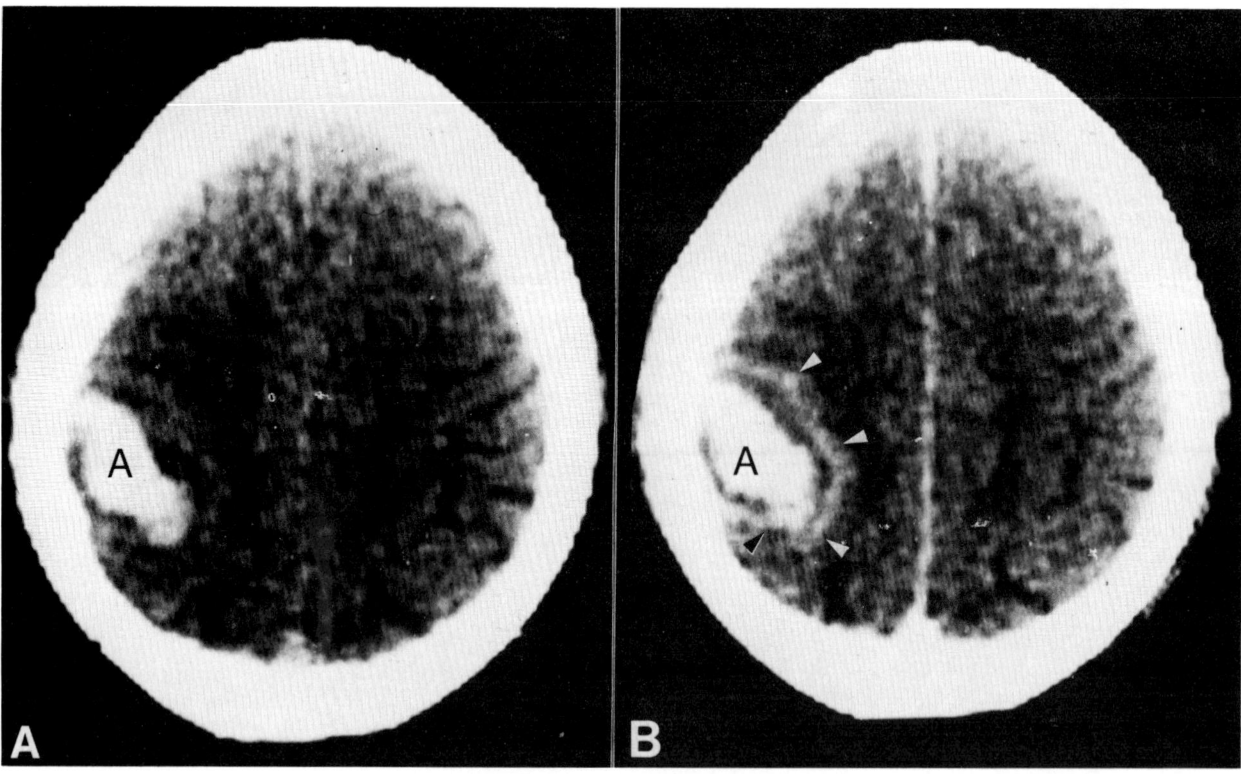

Figure 14-2-1. **Computed Tomography of Acute Intracerebral Hematoma. A.** A hematoma is noted in the parietal lobe posteriorly (A) in this noncontrast scan. **B.** Postcontrast enhancement: ring (arrowheads) surrounds hematoma (A). Usually, the ring is noted more frequently around older (2-3 weeks) hematomas that may have become iso- or hypodense in relationship to normal surrounding brain. However, as this case demonstrates, this phenomenon may be seen acutely. In general, spontaneous (such as hypertensive) hematomas tend to be uniform without satellite lesions, while posttraumatic hematomas tend to have more satellite areas of hemorrhage. However, considerable crossover between these two patterns may be noted, as in this case of traumatic hemorrhage.

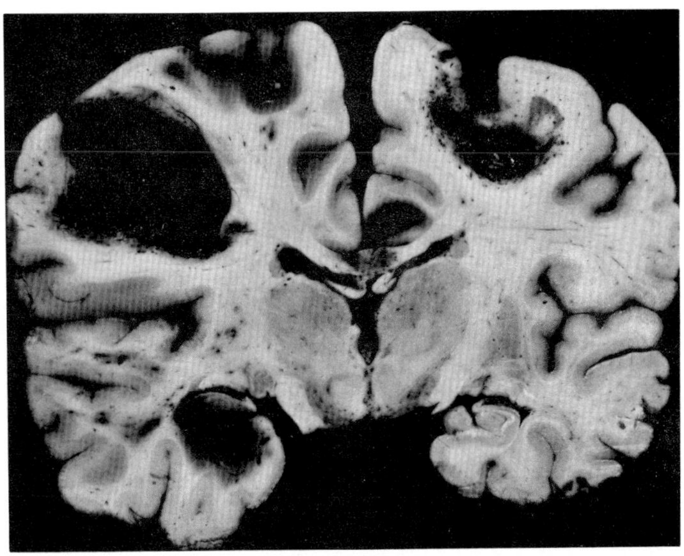

Figure 14-2-2. **Traumatic Intracerebral Hemorrhages.** There is communication of hemorrhagic foci with the subarachnoid space. From Dublin, W.B.: *Fundamentals of Neuropathology,* Ed. II, 1967, Charles C. Thomas, Springfield, Illinois.

Chapter Six

Tumors

Originally, it was thought that an area of "ring-like" contrast enhancement was pathognomic of neoplasm. We now know that this is not the case, since a variety of other lesions including abscess, posttraumatic hemorrhage, and infarct also may present such a pattern. According to recent reports, computed tomography is accurate in 95 per cent of cases in determining the presence or absence of intracranial neoplasm. The use of fourth generation CT scanners has greatly increased the resolution of orbital, pituitary and posterior fossa structures, and in general, the rate of detection of intracranial tumors is now approaching 100 per cent. At UCDMC, computed tomography with and without metrizamide or small amounts of air is the procedure of choice, and often is the only primary tool used in the diagnosis of pituitary neoplasms and/or acoustic neurofibromas.

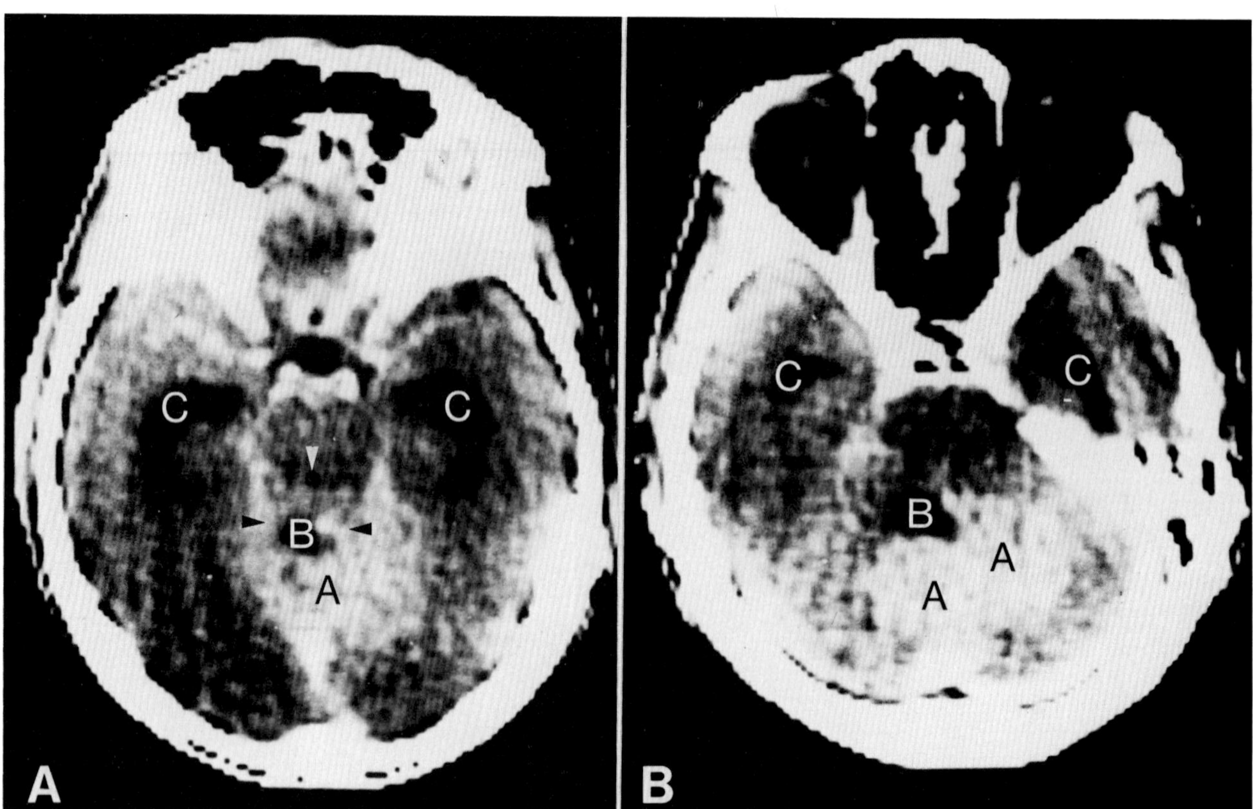

Figure 15-1-1. **Computed Tomography of Neuroglioma, Grade IV, Medulloblastoma Type (Traditionally, Medulloblastoma) Posterior Fossa.** Two levels from a contrast enhanced study demonstrate extensive cerebellar tumor (A) distorting the mid and upper fourth ventricle (B). Tentorial meningeal seeding (*arrowheads*) is identified. Hydrocephalus secondary to fourth ventricular obstruction is evident by dilated inferior horns (C).

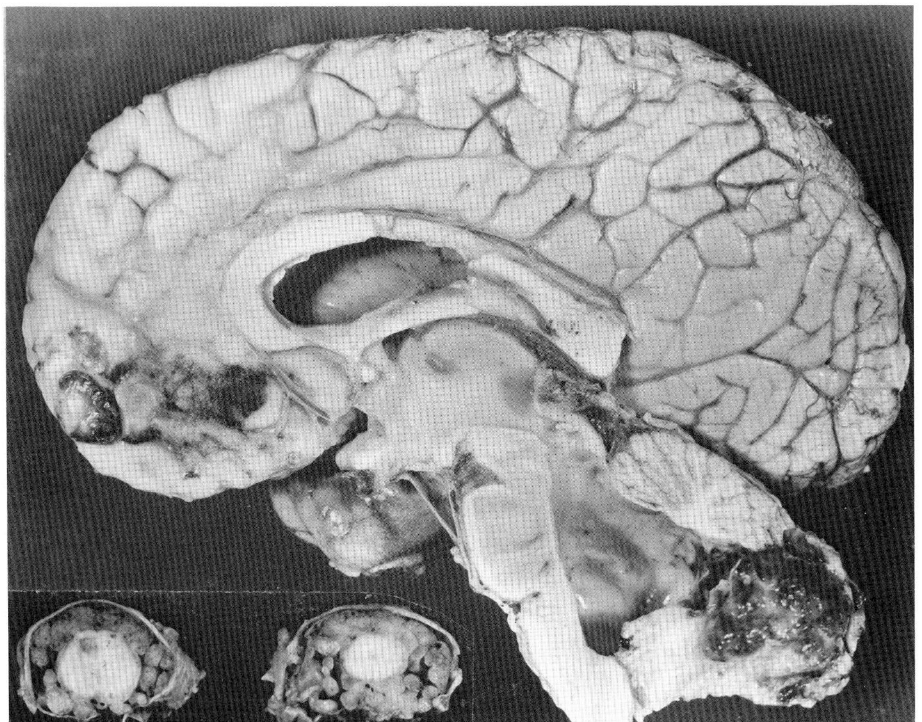

Figure 15-1-2. **Neuroglioma, Grade 4, Medulloblastoma Type (Traditionally, Medulloblastoma) of Midline of Cerebellum.** The ventricular system is greatly enlarged, consequent to obstruction, by tumor, of outflow from the fourth ventricle. Subarachnoid dissemination is shown in the frontal region. Inset shows thick subarachnoid infiltration about lumbar (left) and thoracic (right) spinal cord, with a small focus of intrinsic invasion of the lumbar; the roots of the cauda equina are densely invested by neoplasm. From Dublin, W.B.: *Fundamentals of Neuropathology;* Ed. II, 1967, Charles C. Thomas, Springfield, Illinois.

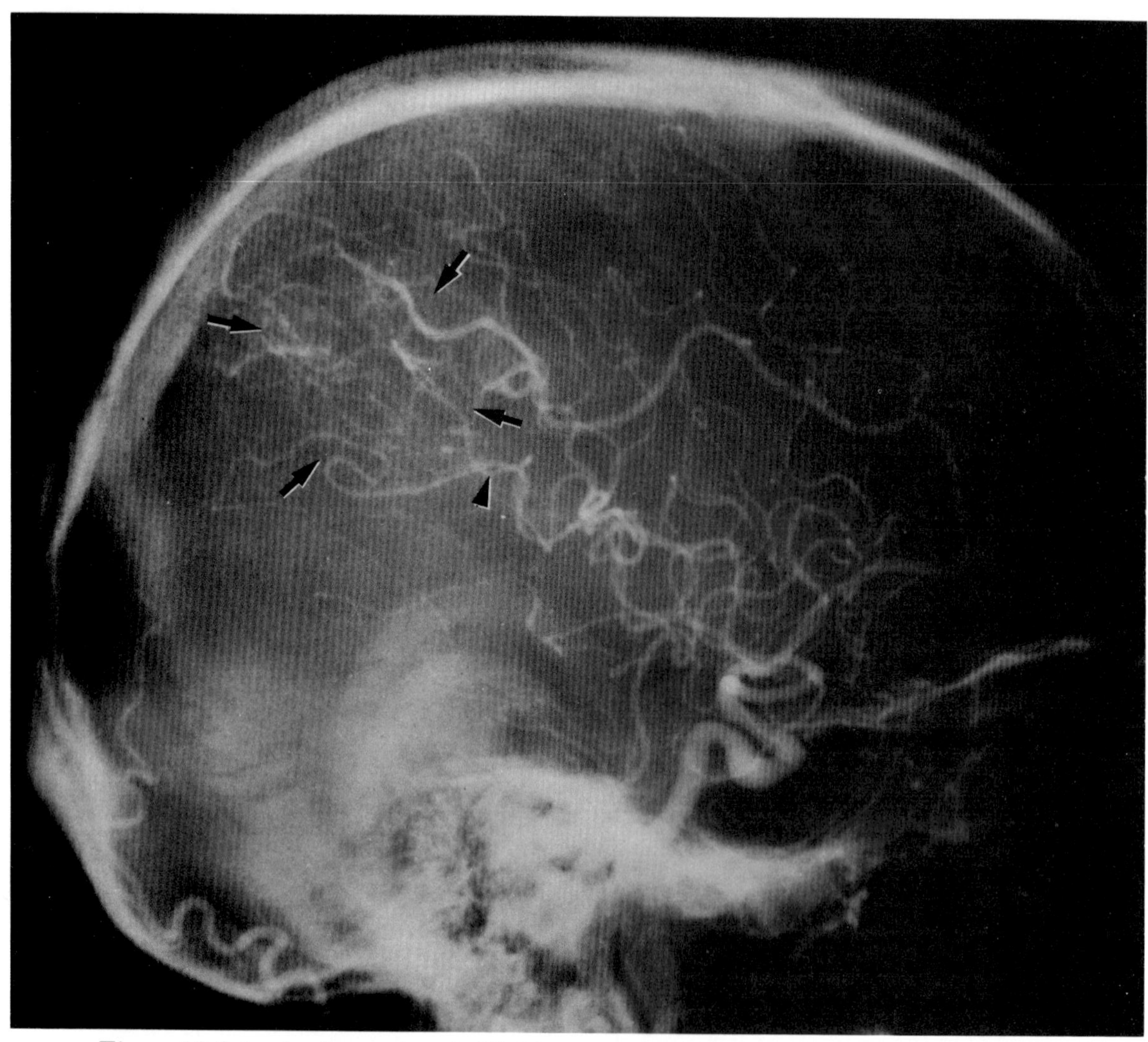

Figure 15-2-1. **Angiography of Glioblastoma Multiforme.** A lateral (late arterial phase) arteriogram demonstrates tumor neovascularity (*arrows*), producing anterior displacement of the sylvian point (*arrowhead*).

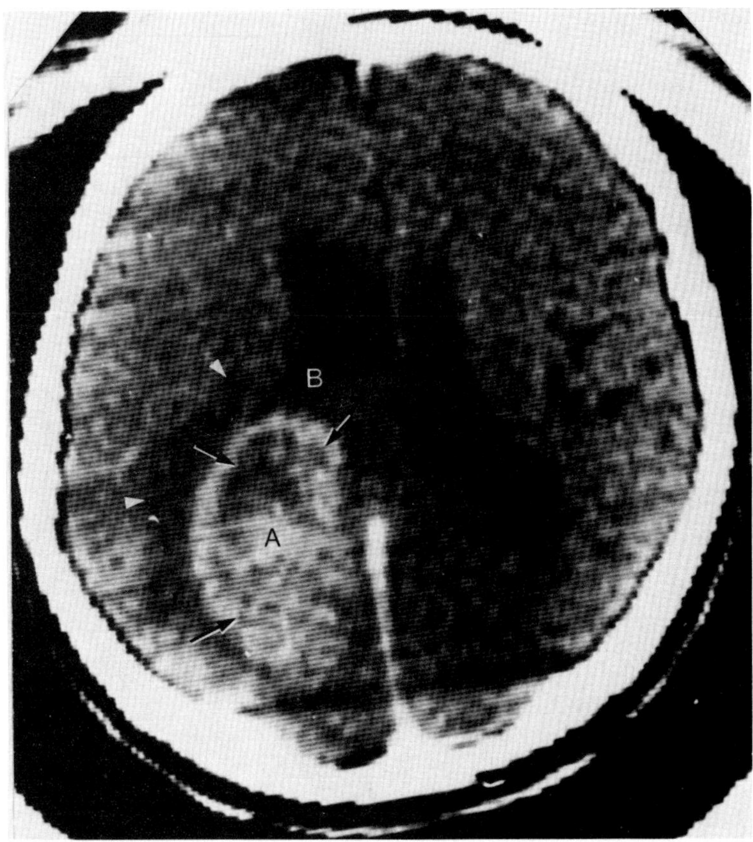

Figure 15-2-2. **Glioblastoma Multiforme.** Same case as 15-2-1. A CT scan demonstrates a hemorrhagic tumor (A) with peripheral contrast enhancement (*arrows*), and adjacent edema (*arrowheads*). Compression and anterior displacement of the ipsilateral lateral ventricle (B) is also identified.

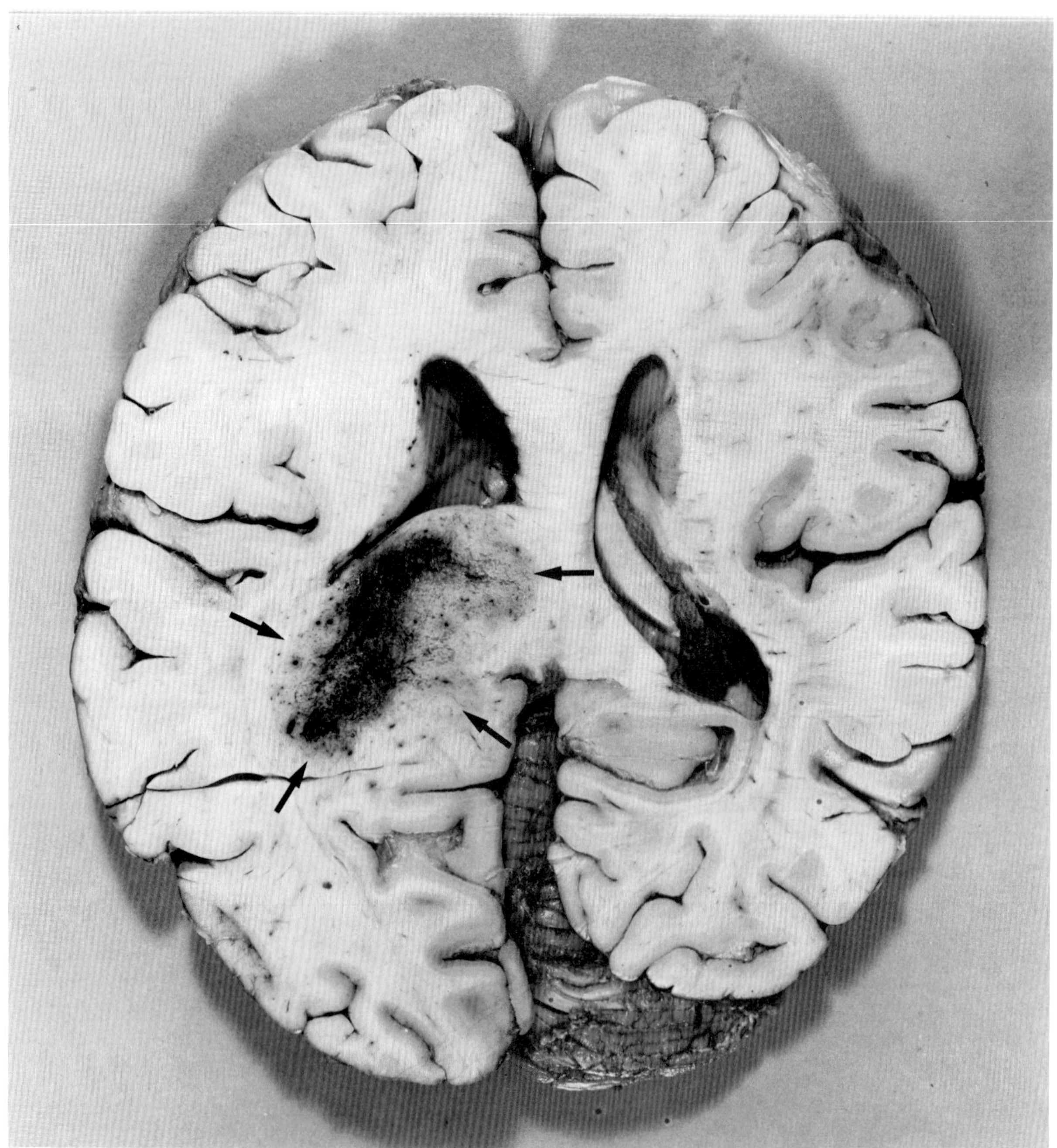

Figure 15-2-3. Continuing from Figure 15-2-2. Axial section corresponding to the CT. Tumor (*arrows*) was pink-gray, and fleshy in consistency. Microscopically, glioblast-oma multiforme.

Figure 15-3-1. **Cavitating Astrocytoma.** (See pages 190 and 191.)

Figure 15-3-1. **Cavitating Astrocytoma.** Postcontrast infusion CT sections (*A-D*), caudal to cephalic, demonstrate a large cavitating frontal lesion (*C-D,* A). A second lesion (*A-B-D,* B), associated with hemorrhage of the corpus striatum and cerebral peduncle, is identified. This multicentric pattern should suggest metastatic disease. However, the tumor proved microscopically to be an astrocytoma (see Figure 15-3-3). The multiple lesions were connected, and this represents extension of a glioma. While the CT scan may be quite helpful in identifying the foci of pathologic alteration, the specific diagnosis can be established more securely by histologic examination. Letters in italics refer to larger letters denoting subdivisions of the illustration. Nonitalicized letters refer to small letters that indicate individual structures in the illustration.

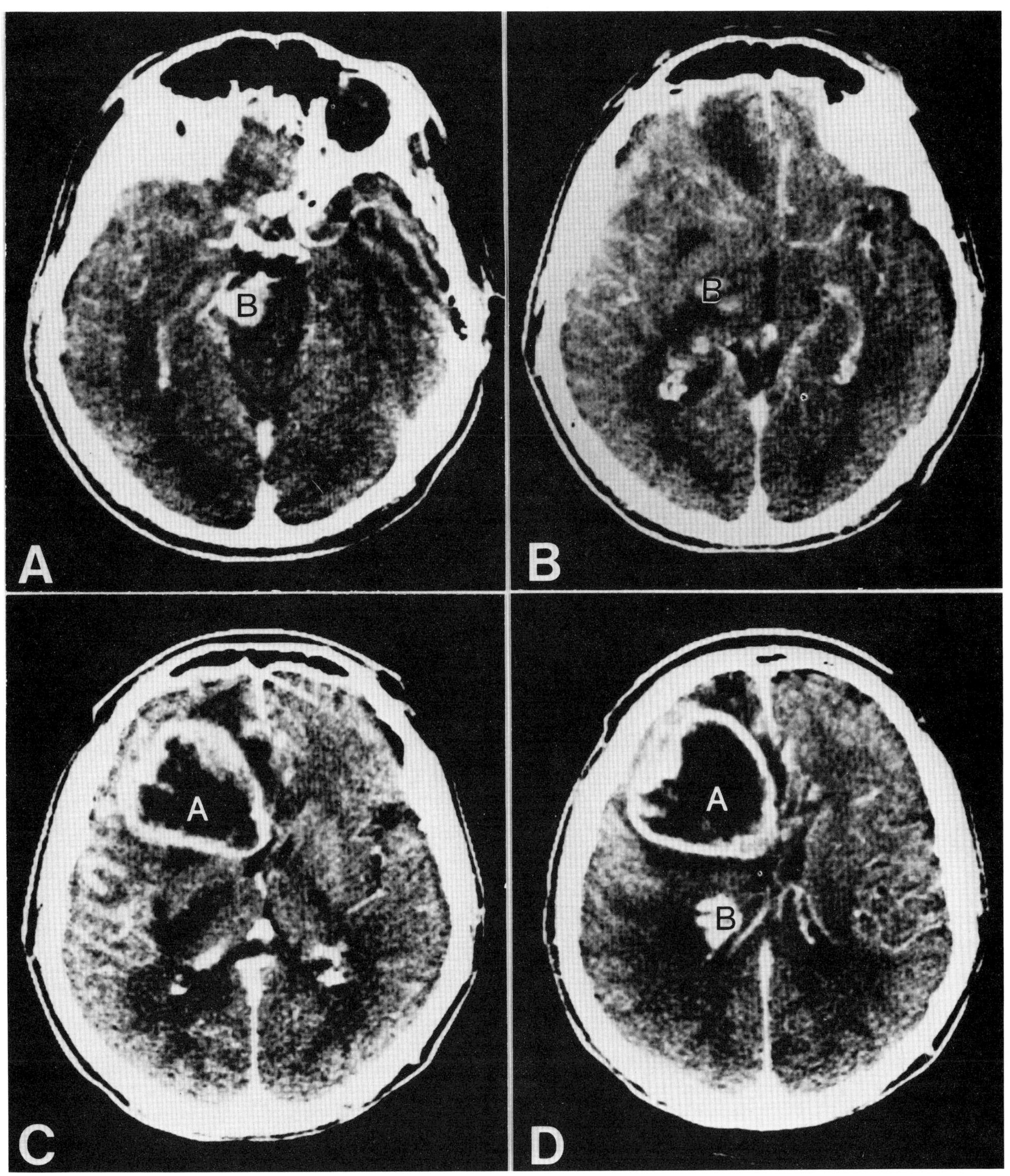
B
B
A
A
B
A
C
D

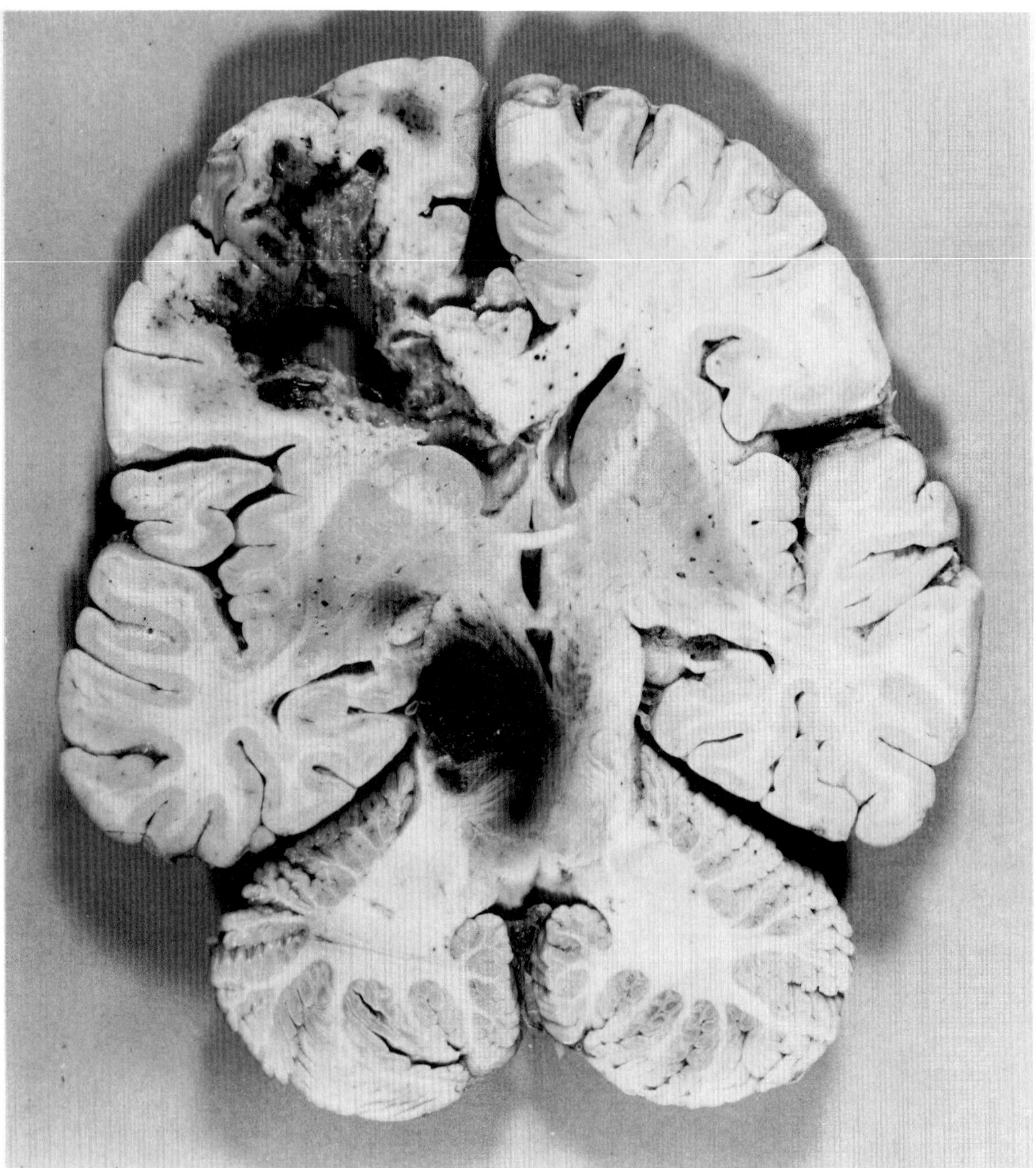

Figure 15-3-2. Continuation of Figure 15-3-1. The cavitating lesion of left frontal lobe is exhibited, corresponding to Figure 15-3-1 *C-D*, A. The corpus callosum is thickened by invading tumor. The left cingulate gyrus is herniated beneath the falx. The hemorrhagic lesion of left cerebral peduncle corresponds to Figure 15-3-1 *A-B-D*, B.

Figure 15-3-3. Continuation of Figure 15-3-2. (See pages 194 and 195.)

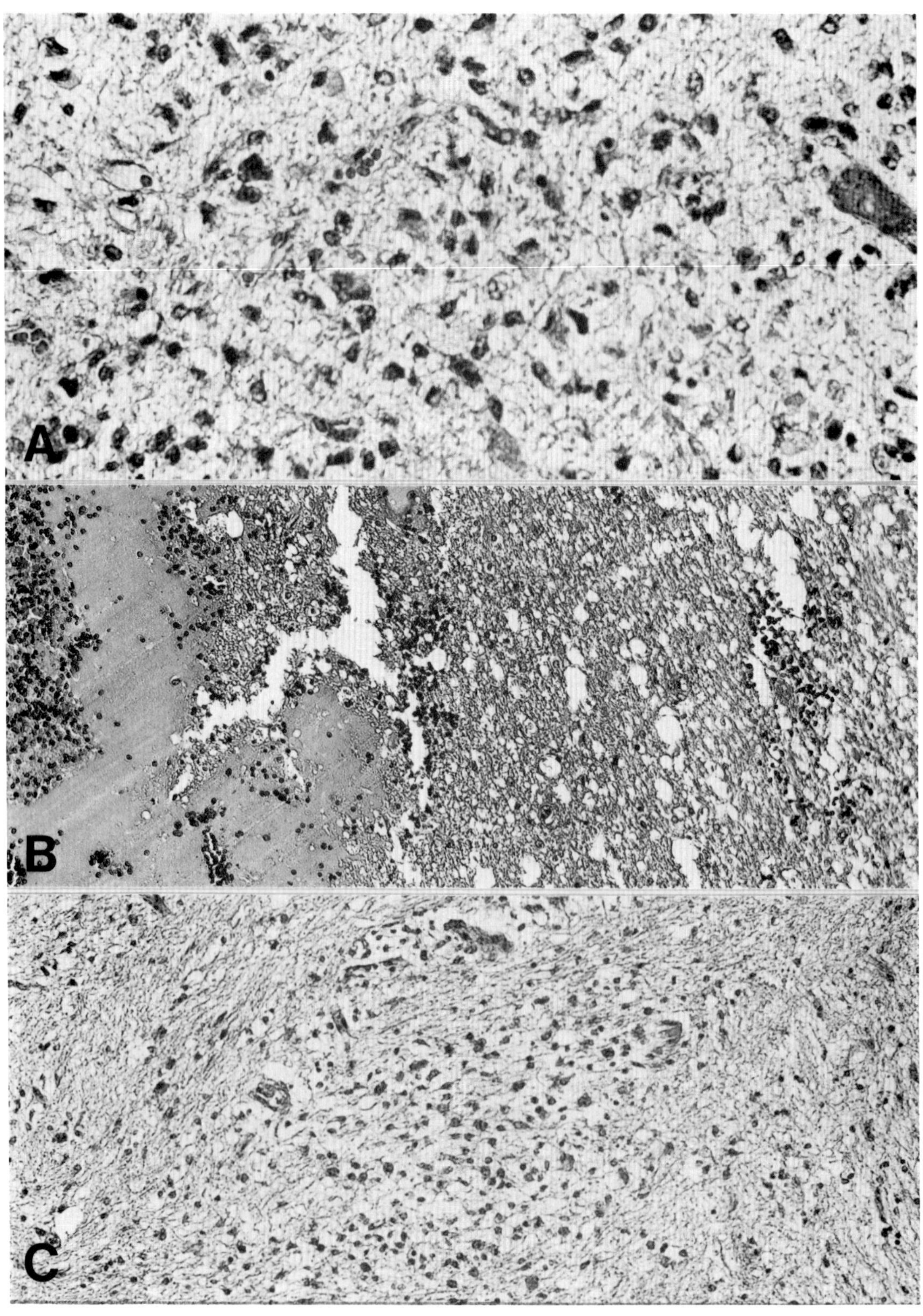

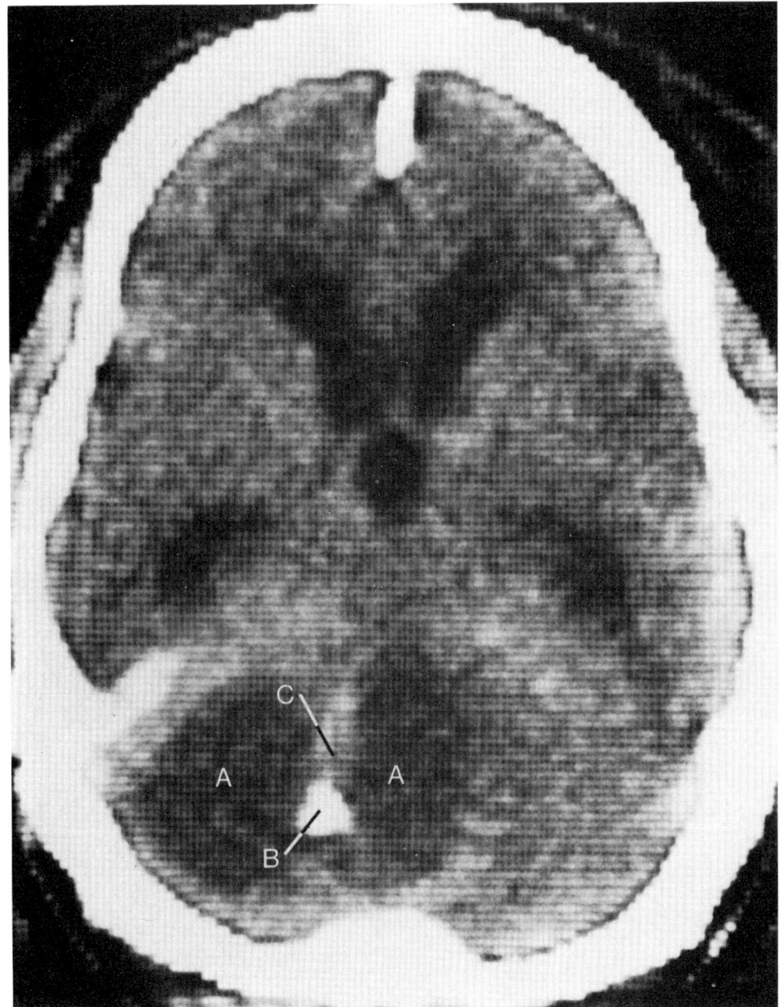

Figure 15-4-1. **Cystic Cerebellar Astrocytoma.** A postcontrast CT shows a low density oval lesion (A) representing the cystic portion of the tumor. Calcification (B) and a small area of tumor enhancement (C) are noted and are typical of this tumor. Note the prominent ventricular structures anterior to the astrocytoma, the former as a result of obstructive hydrocephalus.

←
Figure 15-3-3. Continuation of Figure 15-3-2.
A. Microphotograph of the margin of the tumor cavity shows a well-differentiated astrocytoma.
B. The wall of the hemorrhagic focus shows, for the most part, ecchymosis, edema, and degeneration, with no tumor in the area photographed. Elsewhere, it was scant at most.
C. Section transverse to a line between the cavitating main mass and the hemorrhage showed streams of tumor tissue; one of them is shown in cross section in the photograph (center). The status of the tumor was considered to be one of extension rather than of multicentricity.

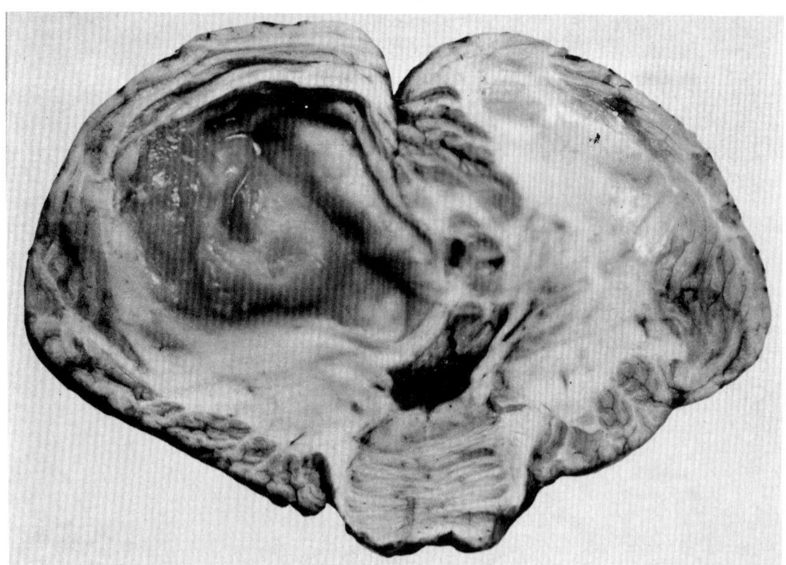

Figure 15-4-2. **Cystic Astrocytoma of Cerebellum.** From Dublin, W. B.: *Fundamentals of Neuropathology,* Ed. II, 1967, Charles C Thomas, Springfield, Illinois.

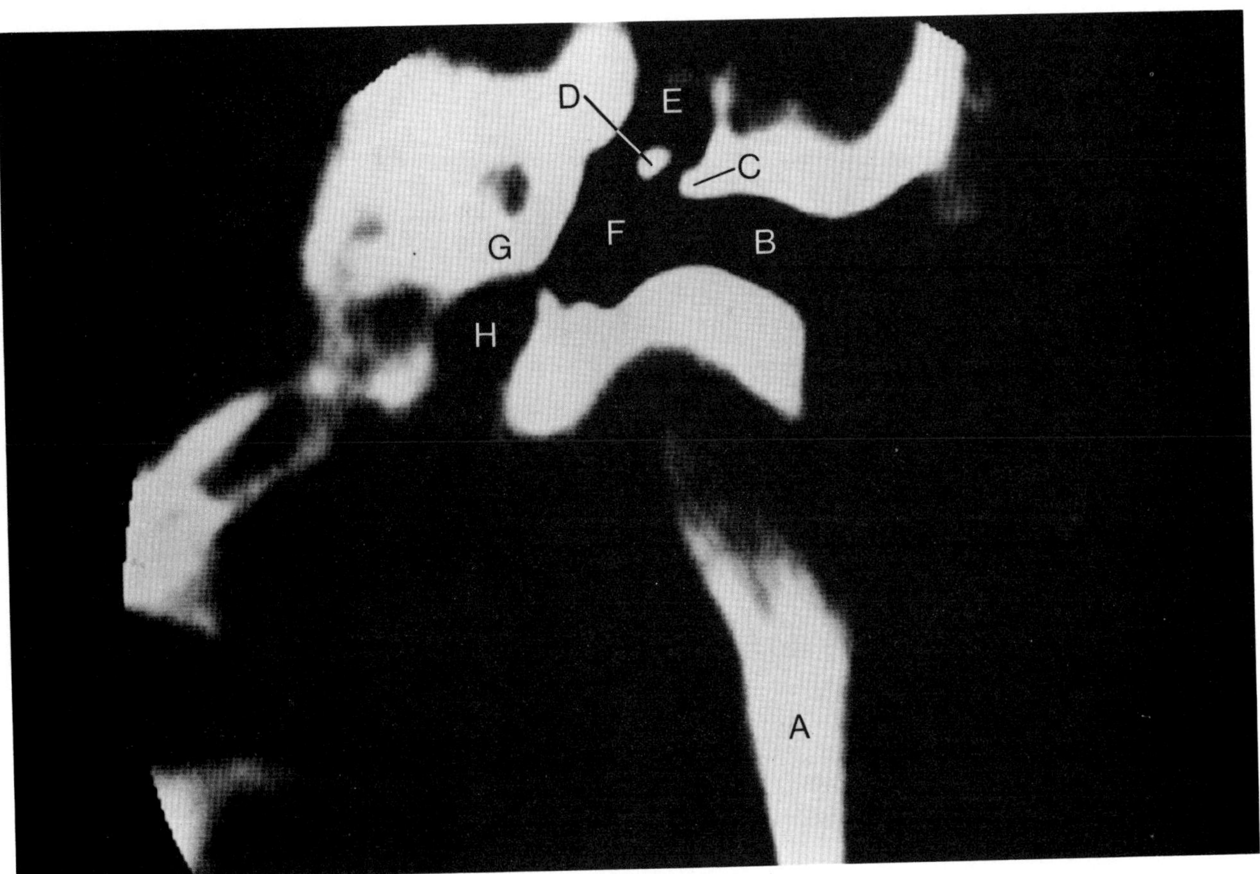

Figure 15-5-1. **Coronal View, Temporal Bone.**
A. Mandible.
B. External auditory canal.
C. Scutum.
D. Head of the malleus.
E. Epitympanic recess.
F. Middle ear.
G. Portion of cochlea.
H. Carotid canal.

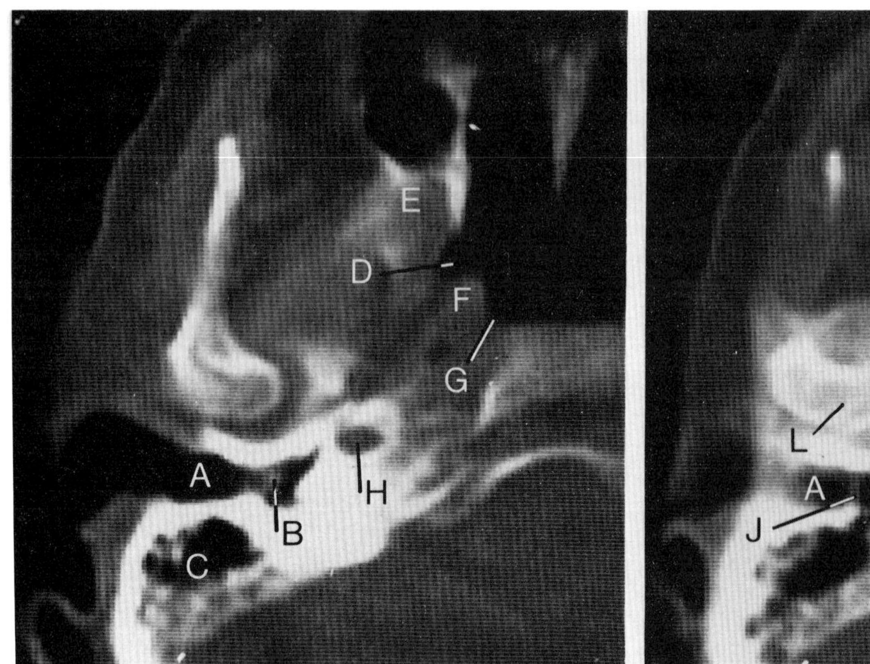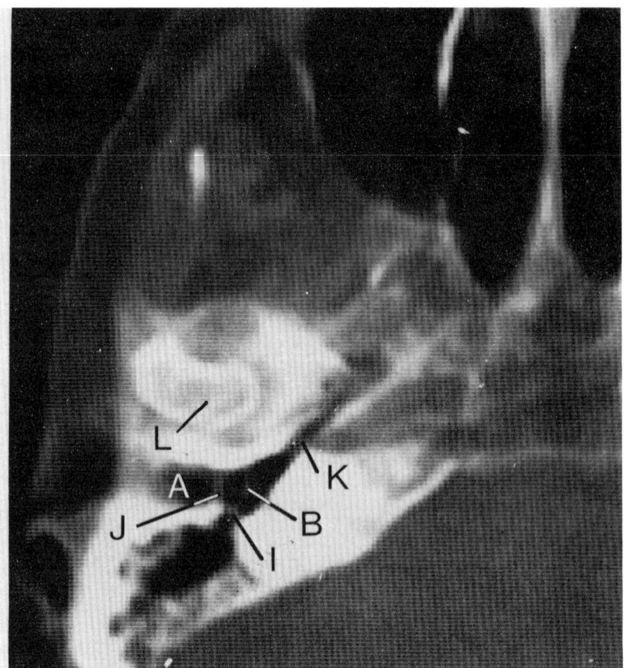

Figure 15-5-2. **Normal Axial Computed Tomographic Section Through the Temporal Bone.**

A. External auditory canal.
B. Middle ear ossicles.
C. Mastoid air cells.
D. Nasopharyngeal eustachian tube orifice.
E. Pterygoid bone.
F. Torus tubarius.
G. Fossa of Rosenmüller.
H. Orifice of carotid canal.
I. Antrum entrance.
J. Tympanic membrane.
K. Eustachian tube.
L. Mandibular condyle.

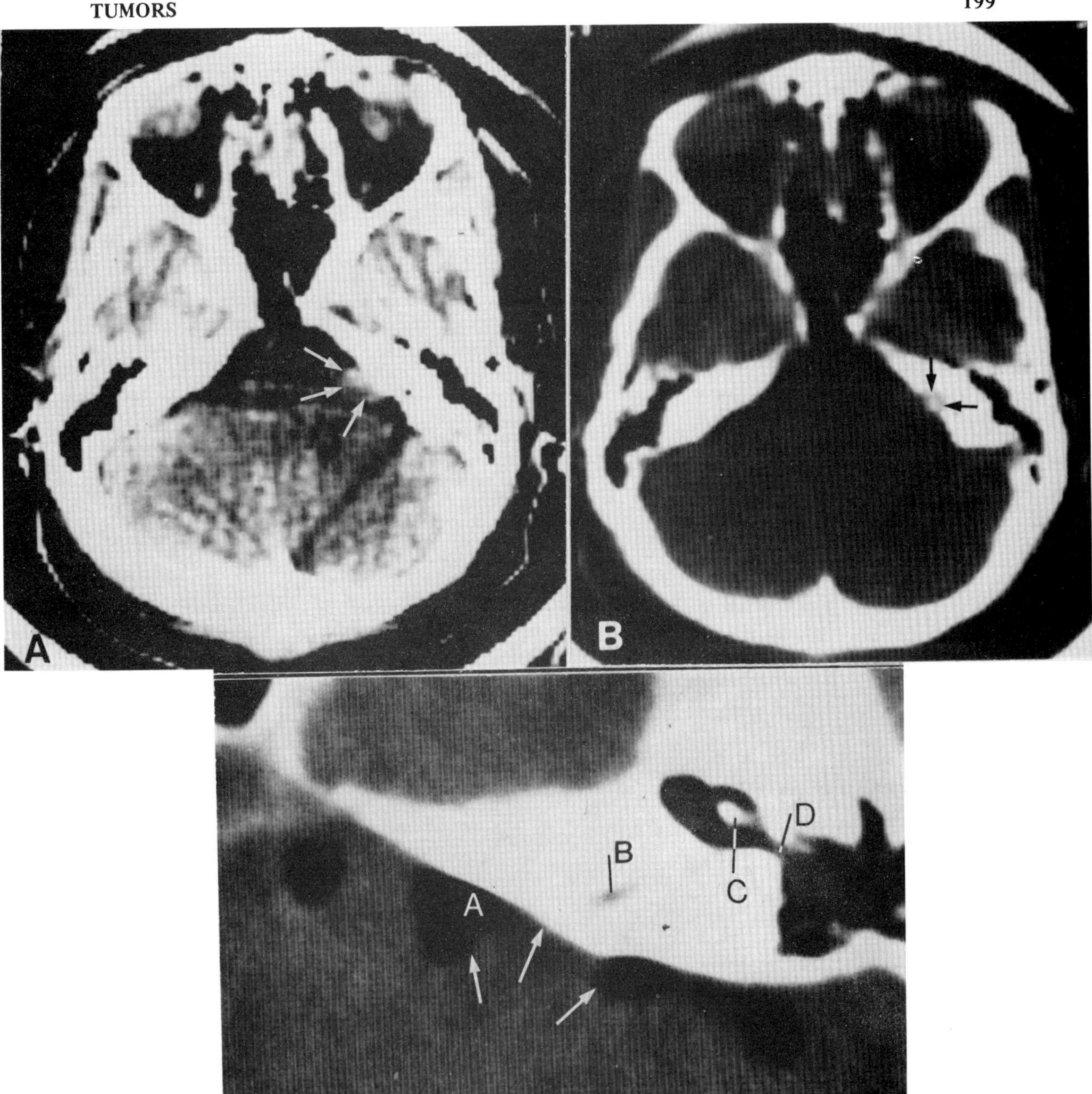

Figure 15-6-1. **CTs of Acoustic Neurofibromas.**

A. A post-contrast CT scan of an individual with unilateral hearing loss shows a small area of tumor enhancement (*arrows*) adjacent to the porus acousticus, in the acoustic recess cistern.

B. Same section as **A**, with window settings to emphasize bone structures. Enlargement of the porus acousticus with extension of contrast enhancing tumor into the latter structure, is demonstrated (*arrows*).

C. Air CT cisternogram performed in patient different from **A, B.** The patient is postioned in a lateral decubitus manner, with the patient's nose to the viewer's left, occiput to the viewer's right. Air (A) is seen within the CP angle cistern surrounding a 13 mm tumor (*arrows*), the latter of which prevents the entrance of air into the internal auditory canal (B). Incidental note is made of ossicles within the middle ear hamber (C), anterior to the additus of the mastoid air cells (D).

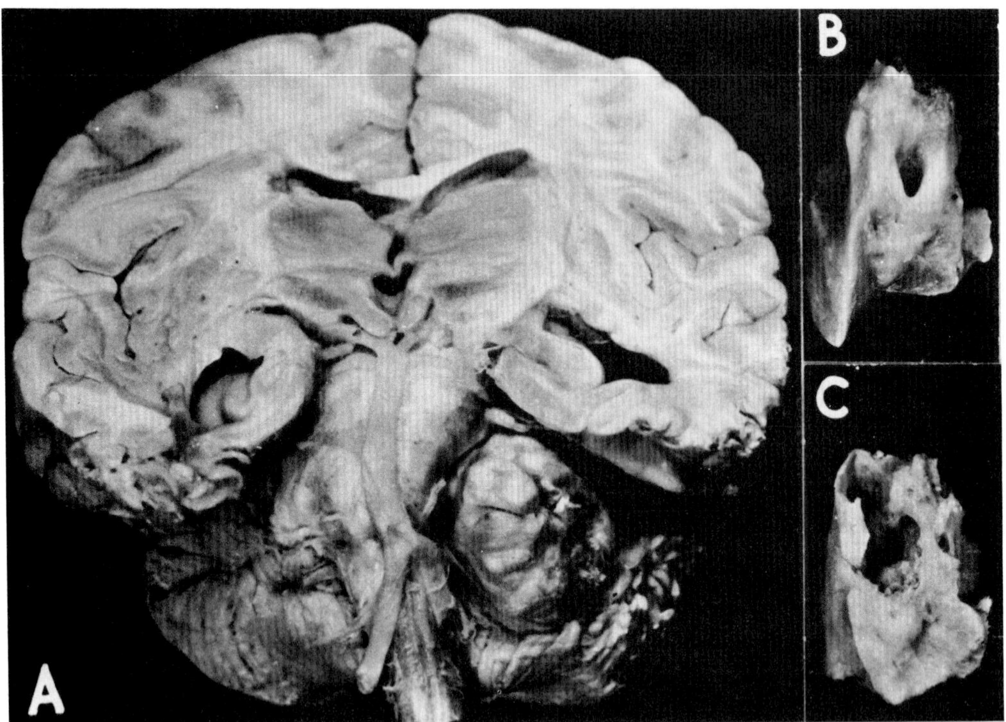

Figure 15-6-2. **Acoustic Neurofibroma.**
A. The tumor is growing in the acoustic recess, margined by cerebellum, pons, and medulla. Considerable destruction of contiguous tissue has occurred.
B. Right petrous bone, showing normal internal auditory meatus, for comparison.
C. Enlargement of left internal auditory meatus by the growing neoplasm. This, as well as the considerable destruction of adjoining brain tissue, as seen in A, is a comparatively late manifestation.
From Dublin, W. B.: *Fundamentals of Sensorineural Auditory Pathology,* 1976, Charles C Thomas, Springfield, Illinois.

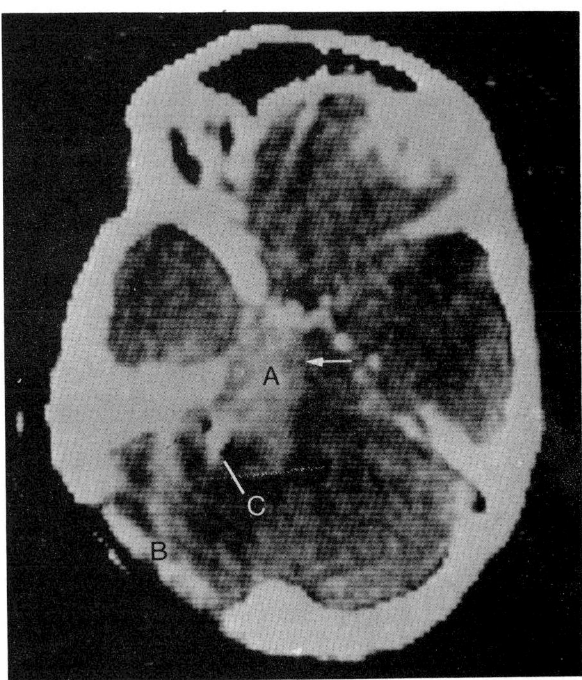

Figure 15-7-1. **Acoustic Recess Meningioma.** A post-contrast scan from the same case as Figure 15-7-2 shows the enhancing tumor (A) which has extended anterior to the edge of the brain stem (arrow). A craniotomy defect (B) is identified from the previous subtotal removal of this lesion. On the base scan, acoustic neuromas tend to be slightly hypodense or isodense, as compared to normal cerebellar tissue. Meningiomas tend to be slightly hyperdense, occasionally with areas of calcification (C). Both types of neoplasms enhance greatly and rather homogeneously. Statistically, acoustic neuromas account for 80%, and meningiomas 10%, of acoustic recess lesions.

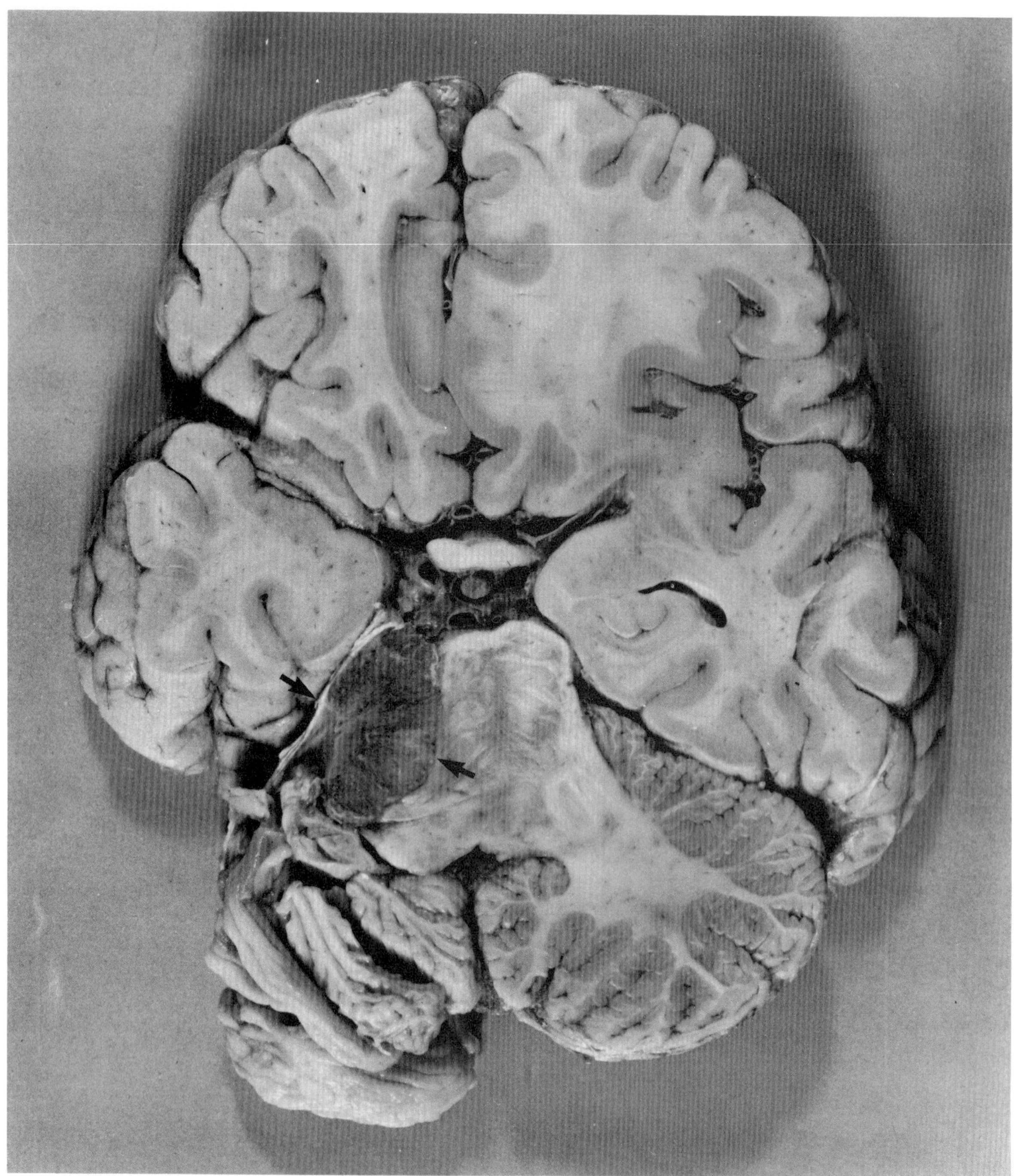

Figure 15-7-2. **Meningioma of Acoustic Recess (*Arrows*), Inferior View.** The histologic type was not suspected until microscopic study had been performed.

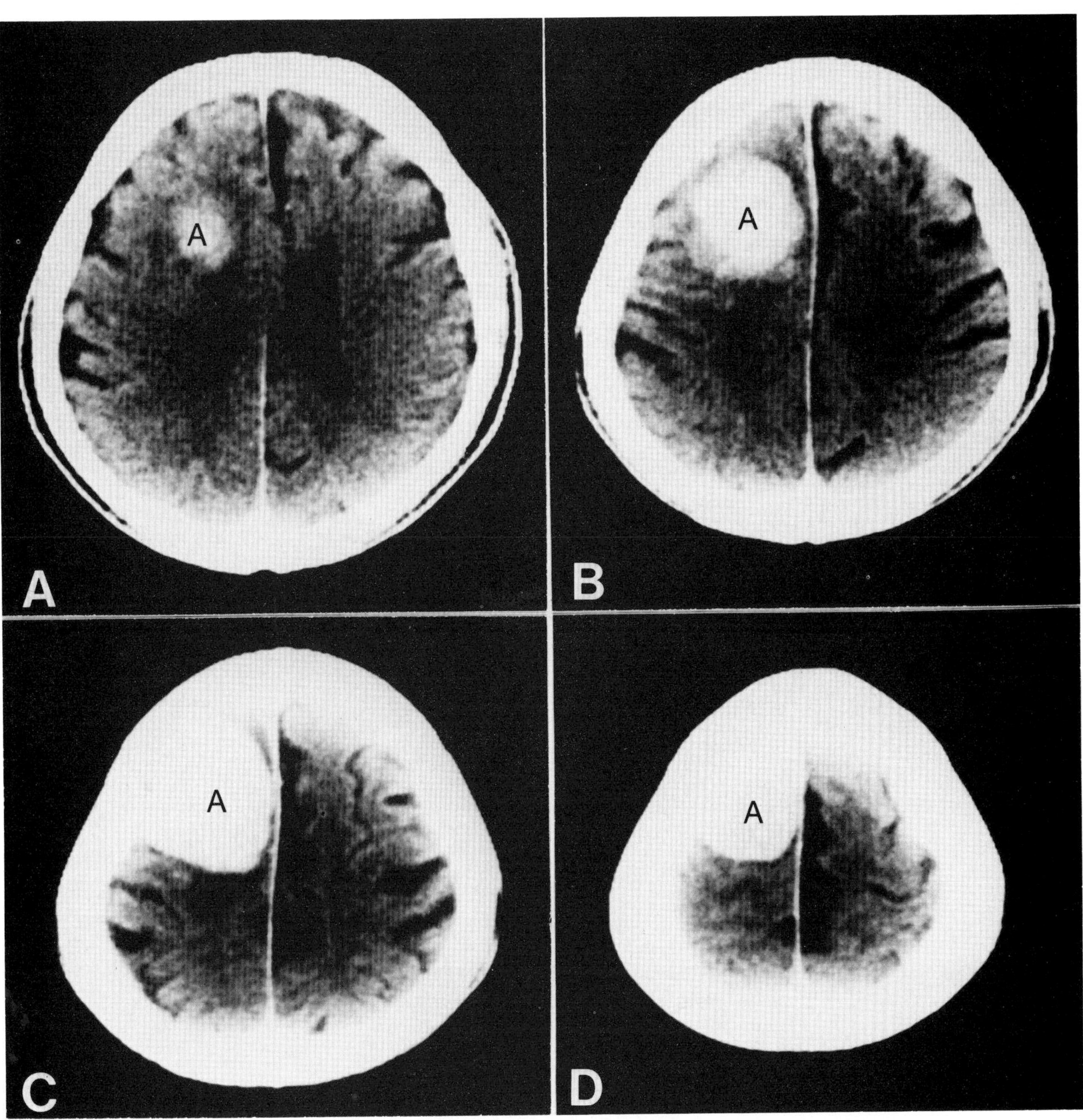

Figure 15-8-1. **Computed Tomography of Meningioma.** Same case as Figures 15-8-2, 3. **A-D** represent caudal to cephalic sections through a homogeneously enhancing neoplasm (A). In **A**, the neoplasm shows some mass effect upon the left lateral ventricle, and compression of the left ipsilateral longitudinal fissure against the falx cerebri. This lesion based on this single section could represent a variety of pathologic conditions including a primary brain tumor. However, the lack of significant edema, and the homogeneity of enhancement seen on this level and subsequent higher levels, coupled with the juxtaposition of this tumor to the bony calvarium (**C, D**) in higher levels suggest the diagnosis of meningioma.

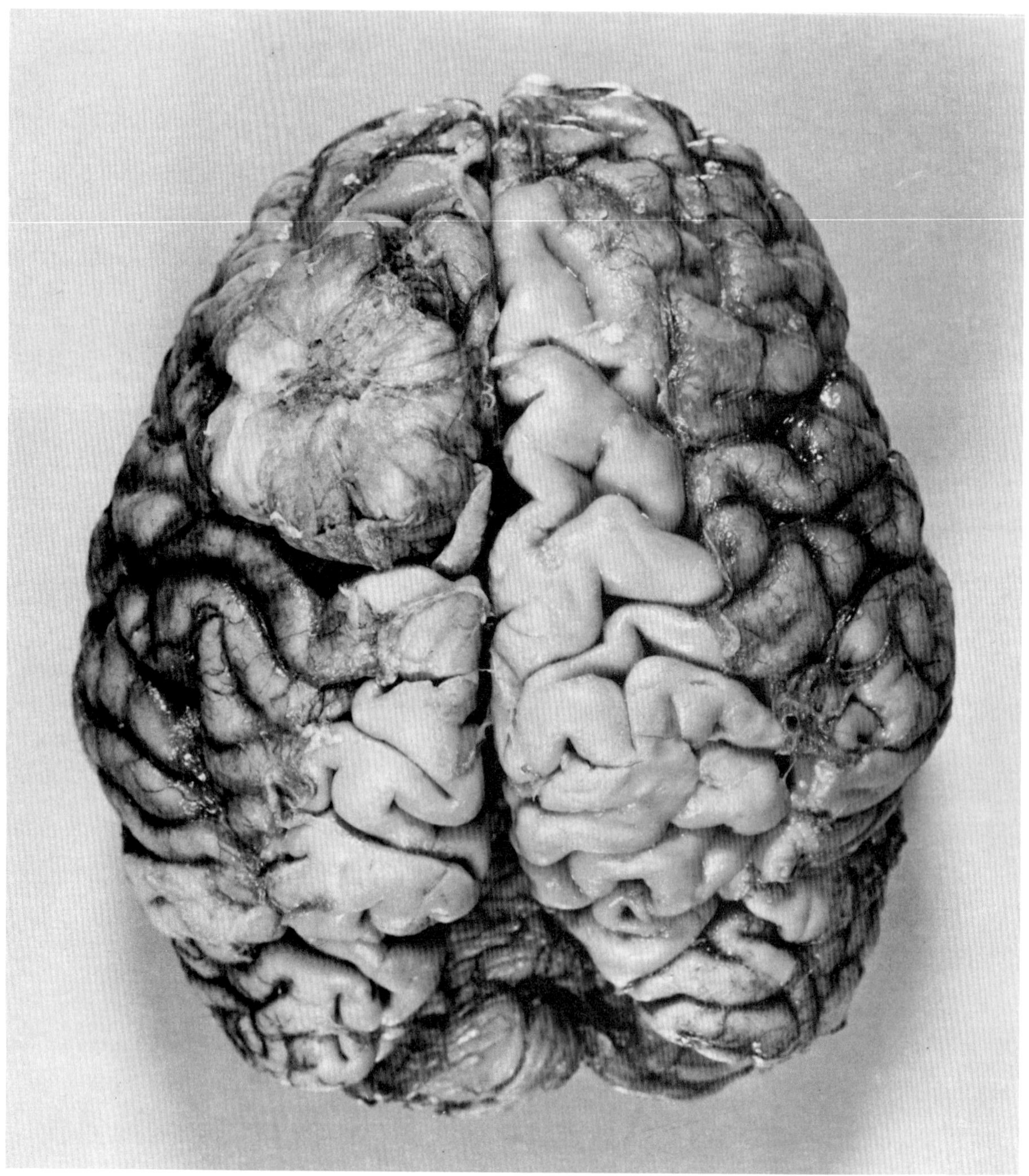

Figure 15-8-2. **Meningioma.** See also Figures 15-8-3 and 15-8-4, to follow. View of vertex of brain, showing the tumor.

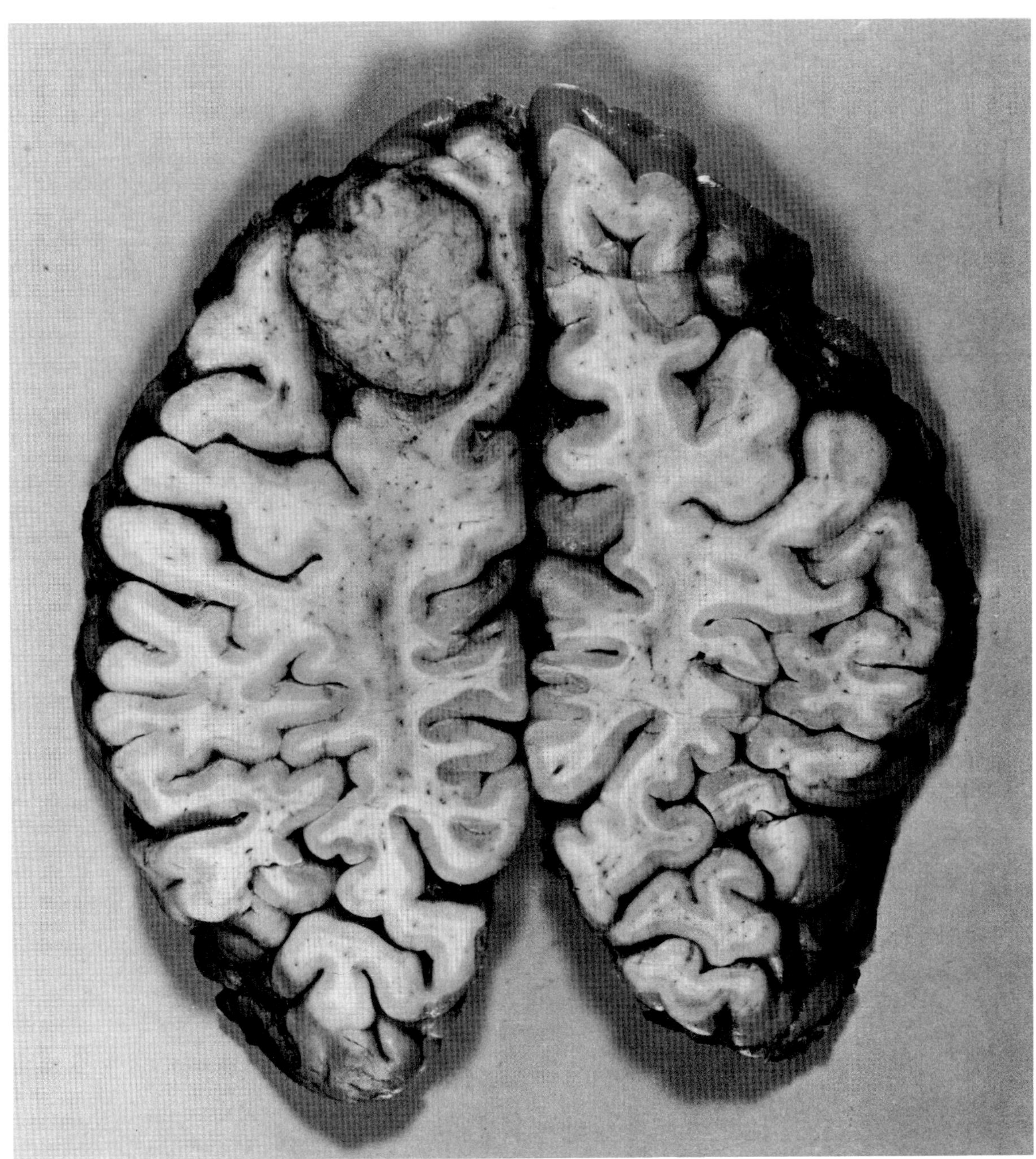

Figure 15-8-3. **Meningioma.** 15° Axial section showing the tumor.

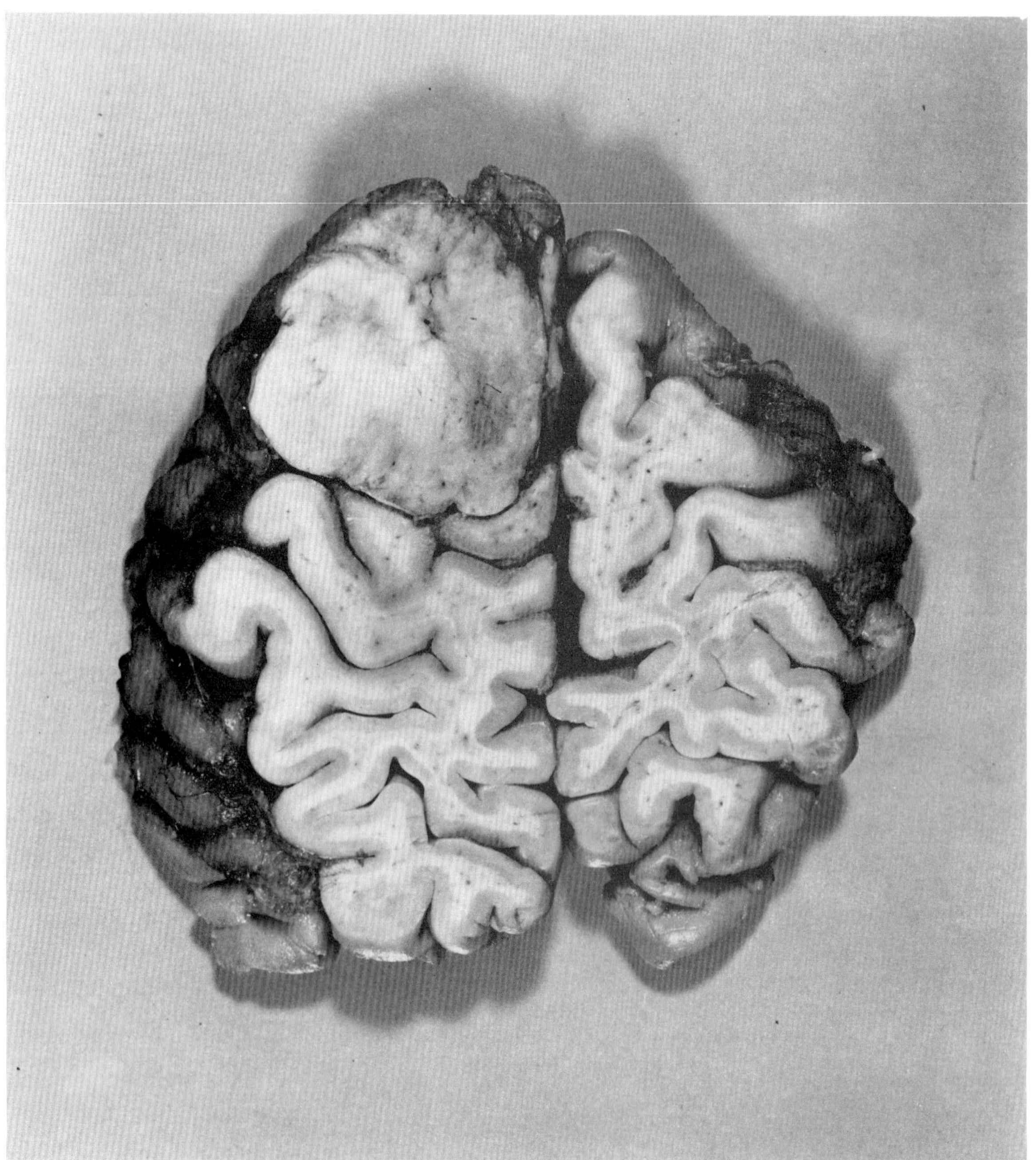

Figure 15-8-4. **Meningioma.** 15° Axial section, nearer the vertex than in the preceding.

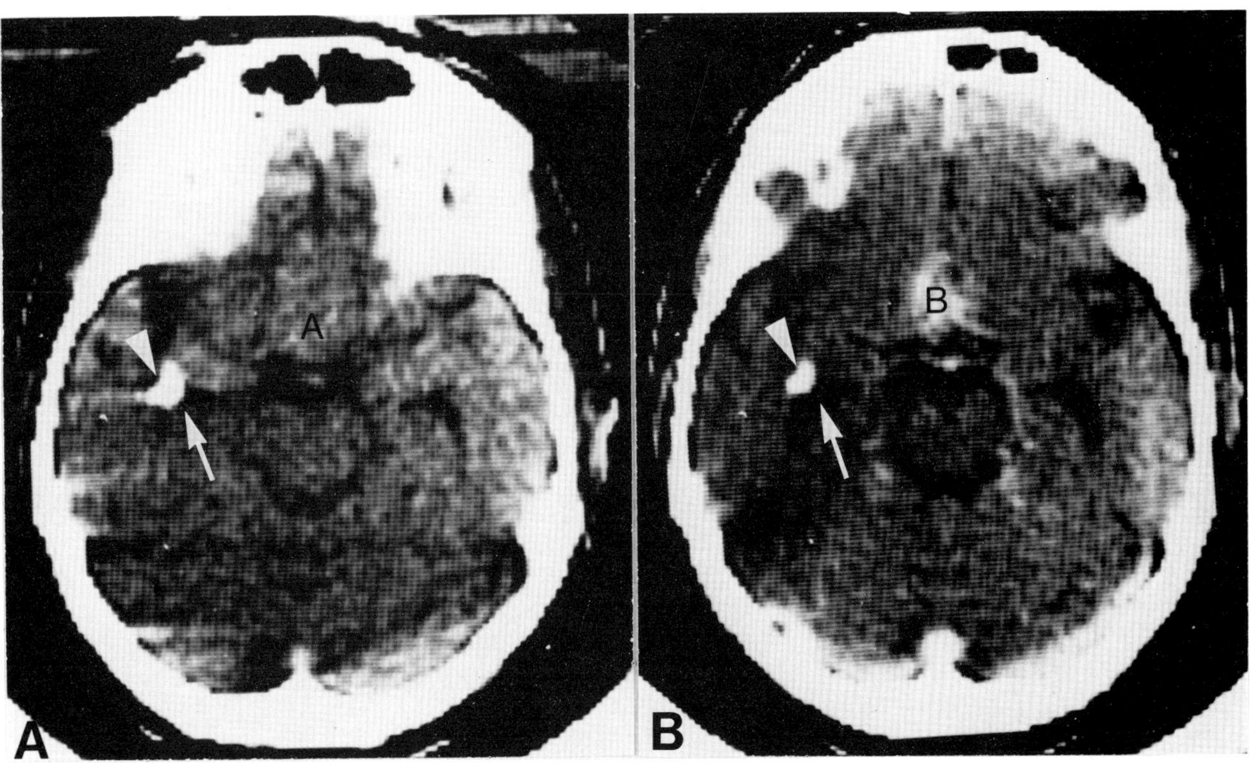

Figure 15-9-1. **Computed Tomography of Suprasellar Meningioma, with Temporal Lobe Calcification.** Same case as Figures 15-9-2, 3. Noncontrast (**A**) and postcontrast (**B**) CT scans demonstrate an area of calcification (*arrowhead*) adjacent to the temporal horn of the lateral ventricle (*arrow*). The noncontrast study also shows a suprasellar mass (A) obliterating the anterior suprasellar cistern, with contrast enhancement (B) of the tumor following iodine infusion.

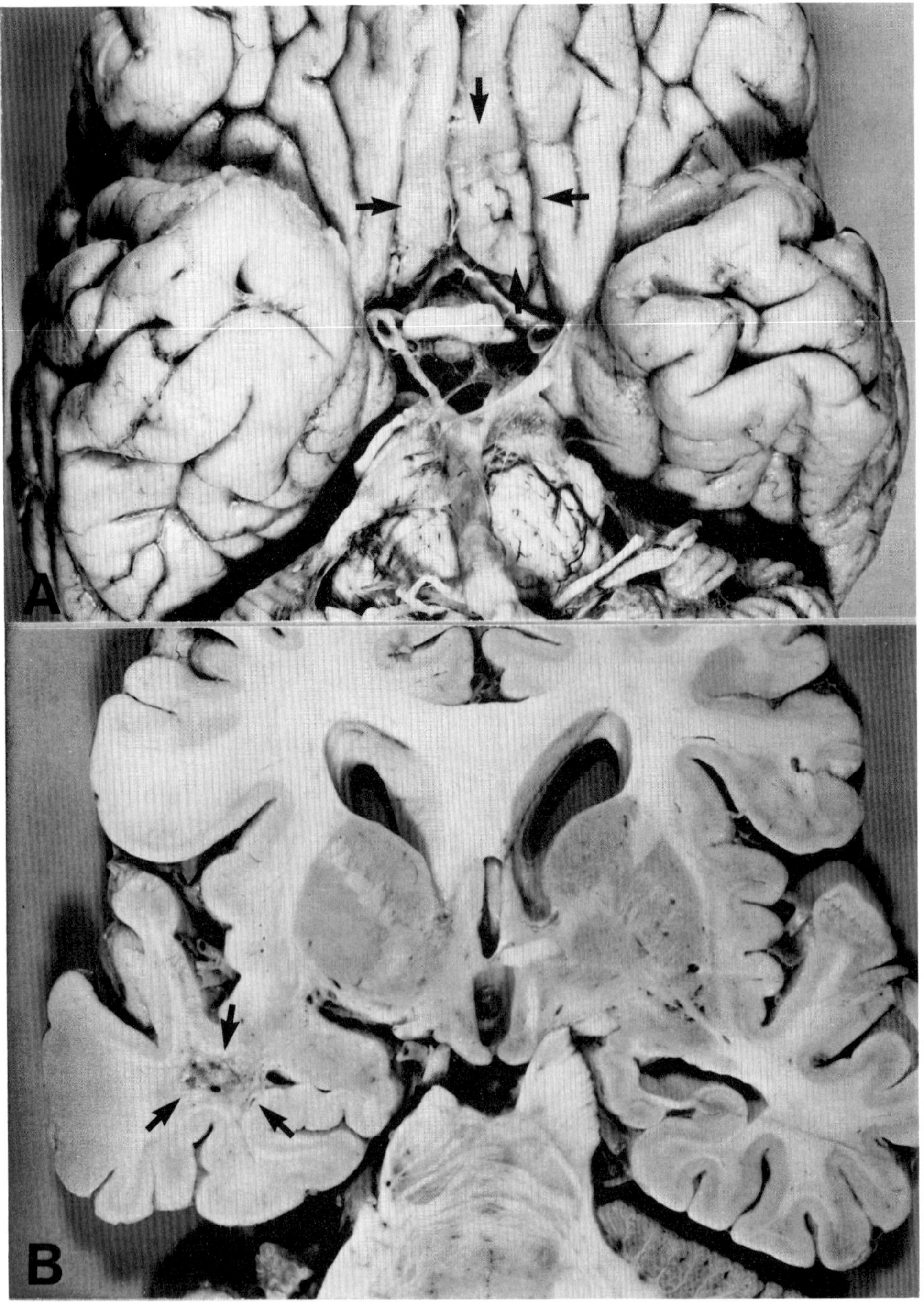

Figure 15-9-2. **Meningioma:** gross corresponding to CT of Figure 15-9-1.
A. Ventral surface of brain. The suprasellar density seen in the CT scan proved to be a meningioma. The tumor made a very shallow saucer-like impression in the orbital surfaces of the frontal lobes, more on the left (on reader's right) (*arrows*).
B. 15° axial section. The density shown in the CT scan, marked with arrows, proved in the microscopic section to be a focus of calcification adjoining the inferior horn of the lateral ventricle (*arrows*).

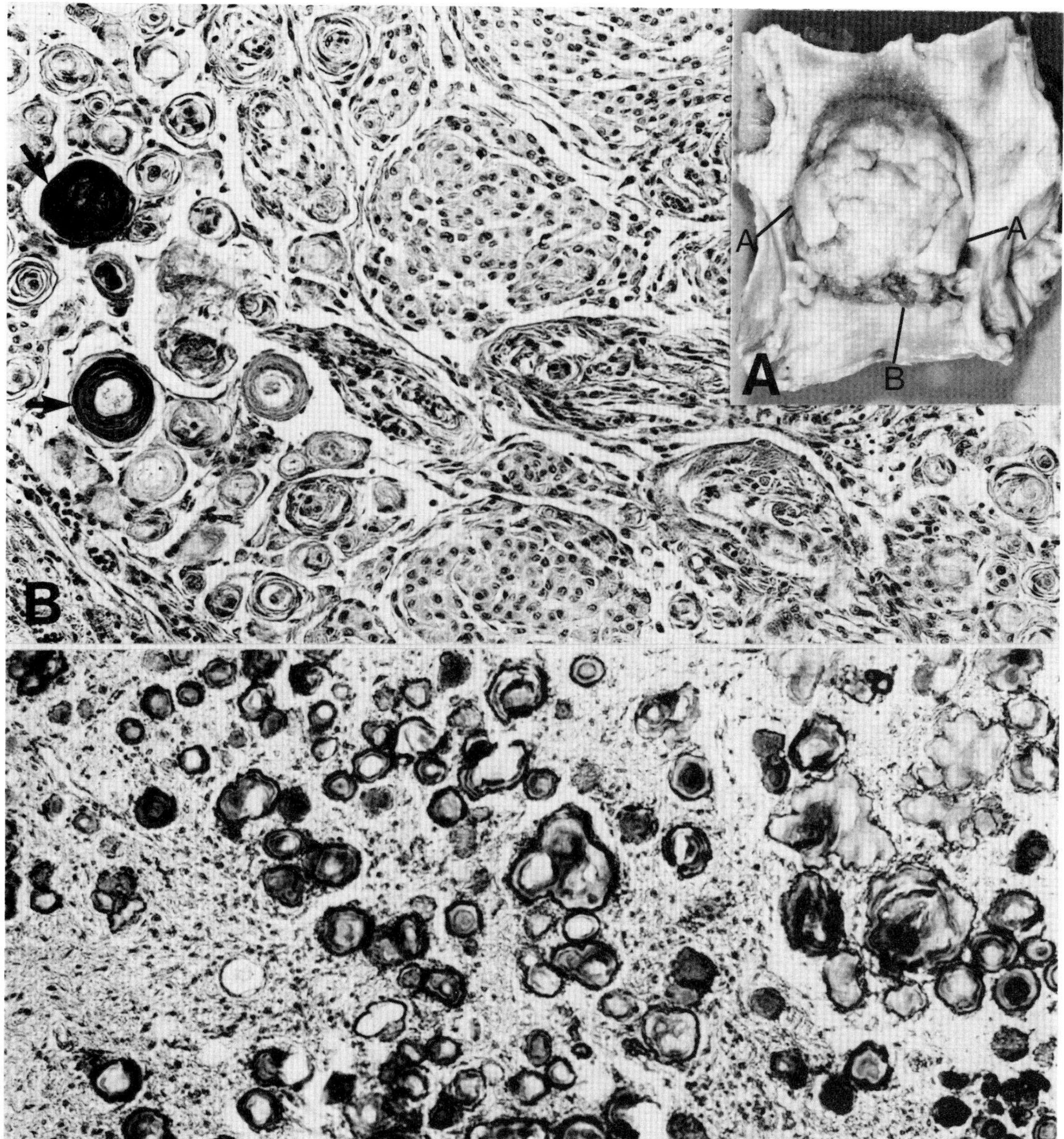

Fig. 15-9-3. **Meningioma.** Continuation of Fig. 15-9-2.

A. Gross view of tumor in situ.
   A. Displaced and compressed optic nerves.
   B. Displaced and engulfed pituitary stalk.
B. Microphotograph of tumor. The whorled pattern of an arachnoidal villoma (mesothelial: "meningiotheliomatous") is seen. There is focal calcification (arrows).
C. More extensive calcification is seen ("psammomoa bodies.").

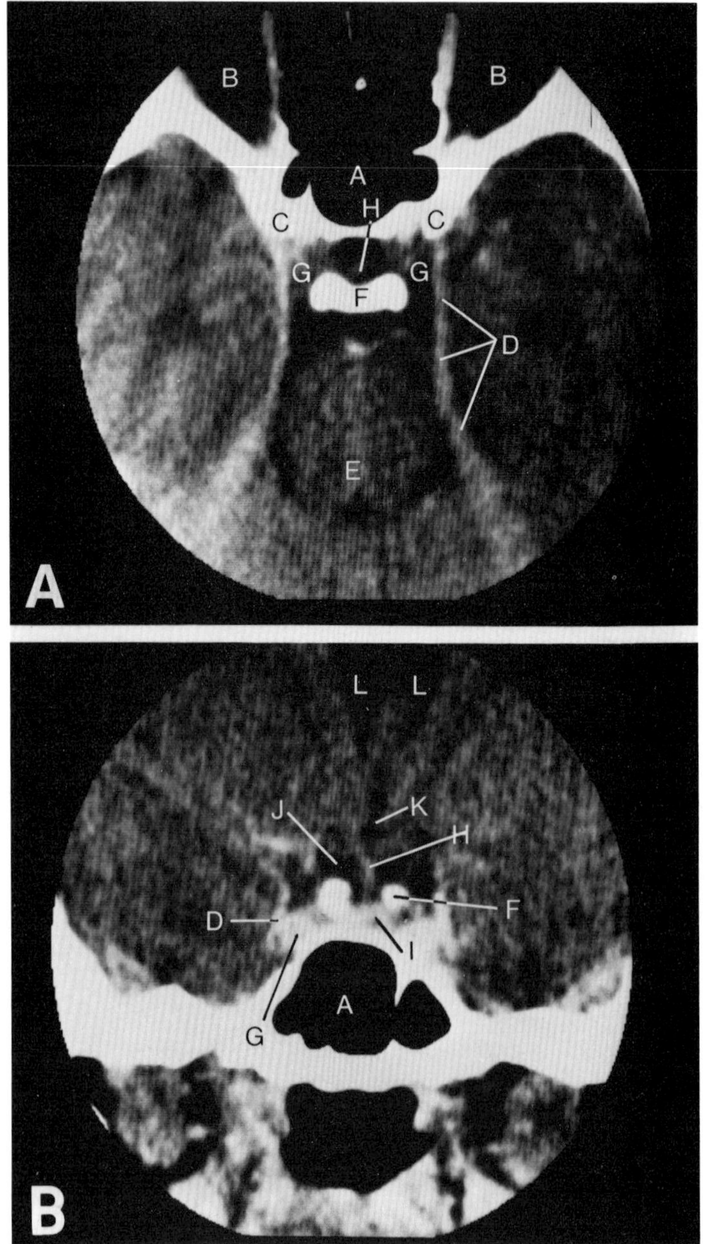
B
B
A
H
C
C
G
G
F
D
E
A
L
L
J
K
H
D
F
I
A
G
B

←
Figure 15-10. **Normal Pituitary. A** (axial) and **B** (coronal), post-contrast, demonstrate the following structures:

A. Sphenoid sinus.
B. Orbits.
C. Anterior clinoid.
D. Enhancing dura lateral to the sella and more posteriorly along the tentorial edge.
E. Brain stem.
F. Dorsum sella with posterior clinoids.
G. Cavernous sinus.
H. Pituitary stalk surrounded by cerebrospinal fluid.
I. Pituitary gland.
J. Suprasellar cistern.
K. Third ventricle.
L. Lateral ventricle.

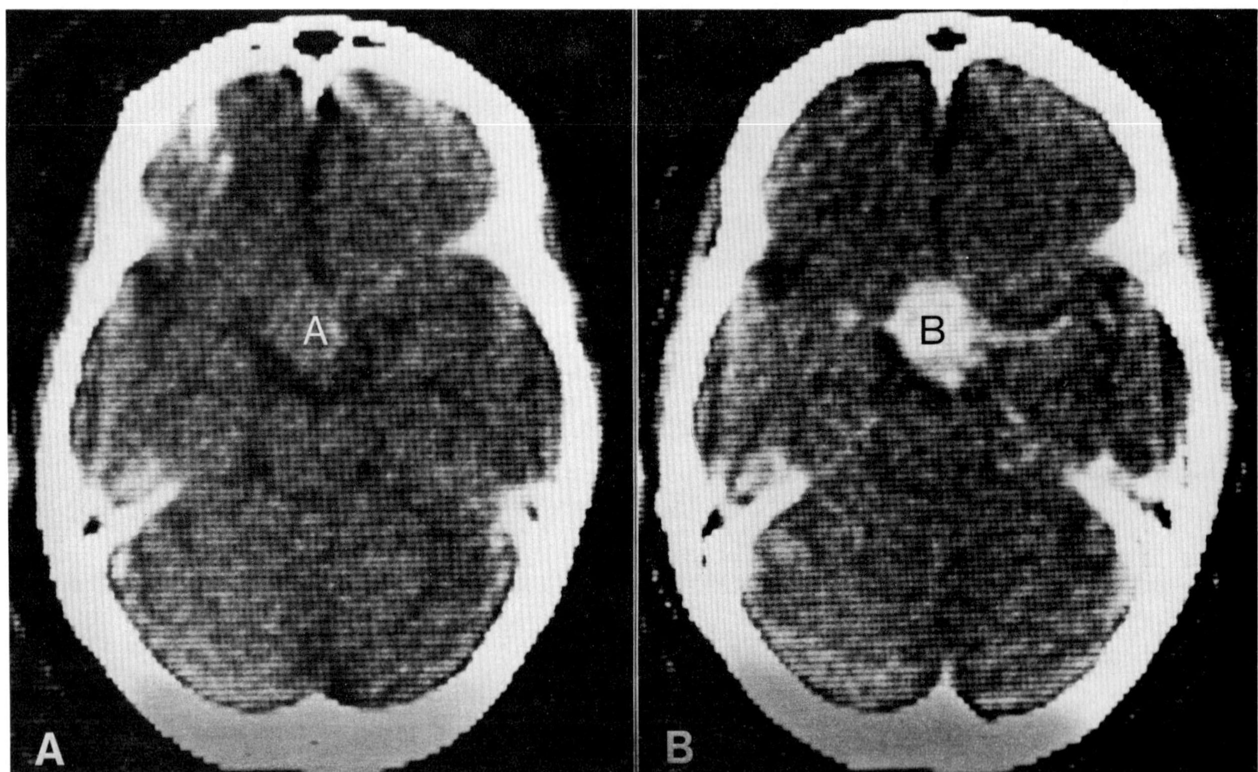

Figure 15-11-1. **Pituitary Adenoma.** *A, C* (precontrast) and *B, D* (postcontrast) demonstrate obliteration of the suprasellar cistern (which should be normally identified in all cases) by an ovoid enhancing mass (A, B). While this type of lesion is compatible with a pituitary adenoma, an extensive differential diagnosis would include among others; meningioma, suprasellar germinoma, metastasis, and aneurysm. *C* and *D* are pre- and postcontrast respectively, taken at a slightly more caudal level through the sella turcica, and show a large tumor with some erosion of the left anterior clinoid (C) and destruction of the dorsum sella (D). Since most of the tumor is within the sella turcica, pituitary adenoma is more likely than other tumor types. Letters in italics refer to larger letters denoting subdivisions of the illustration. Nonitalicized letters refer to small letters that indicate individual structures in the illustration.

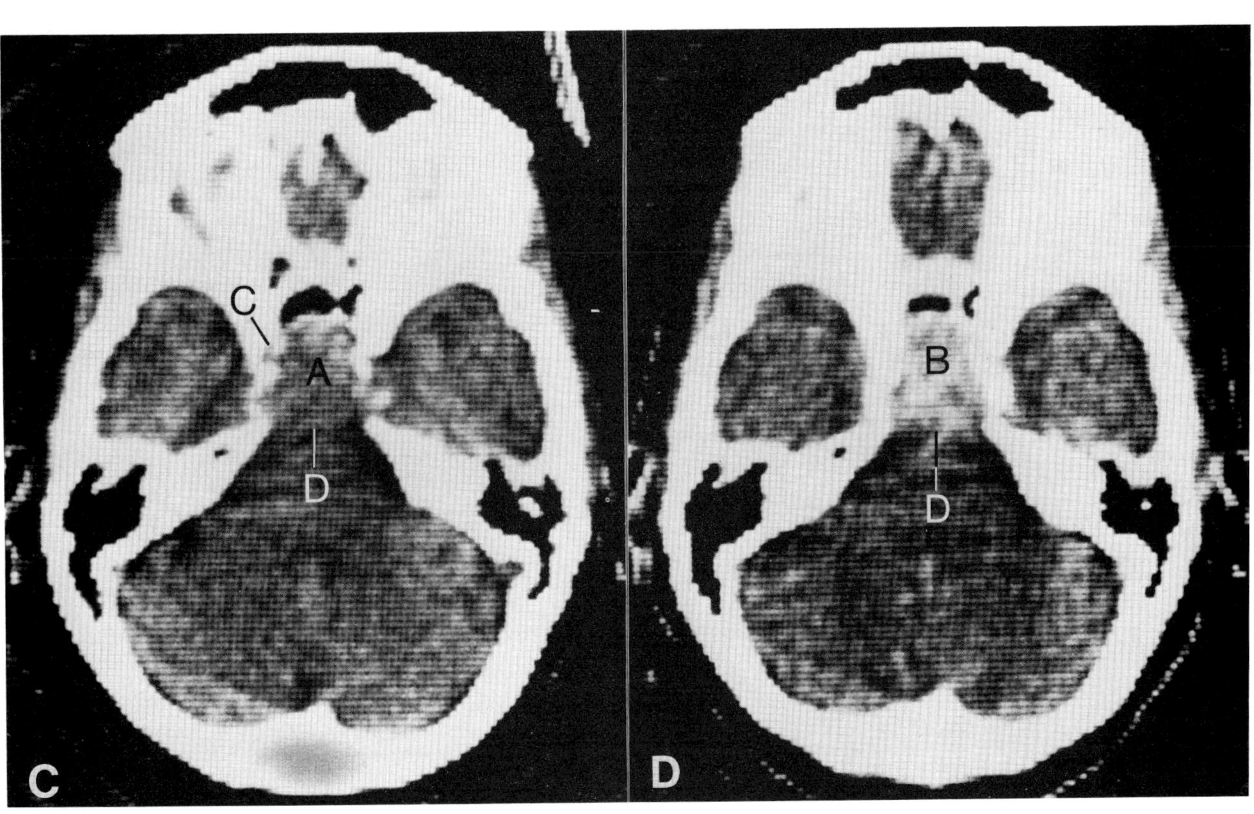
C
C
A
D
B
D

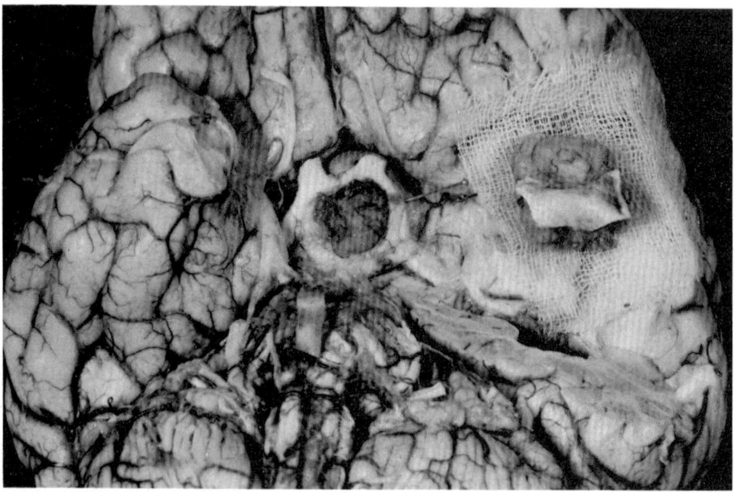

Figure 15-11-2. **Pituitary Adenoma (Chromophobe).** The intrasellar portion of the tumor has been removed, and has been placed on a gauze square, to the reader's right. A portion of dura remains attached. The suprasellar portion of the tumor is seen invading the optic chiasm and extending upward into the base of the brain. A point of compression of the margin of the chiasm by the pulsating internal carotid artery is seen as a thin dark band, marked by a pin. From Dublin, W. B.: *Fundamentals of Neuropathology,* Ed. II, 1967, Charles C Thomas, Springfield, Illinois.

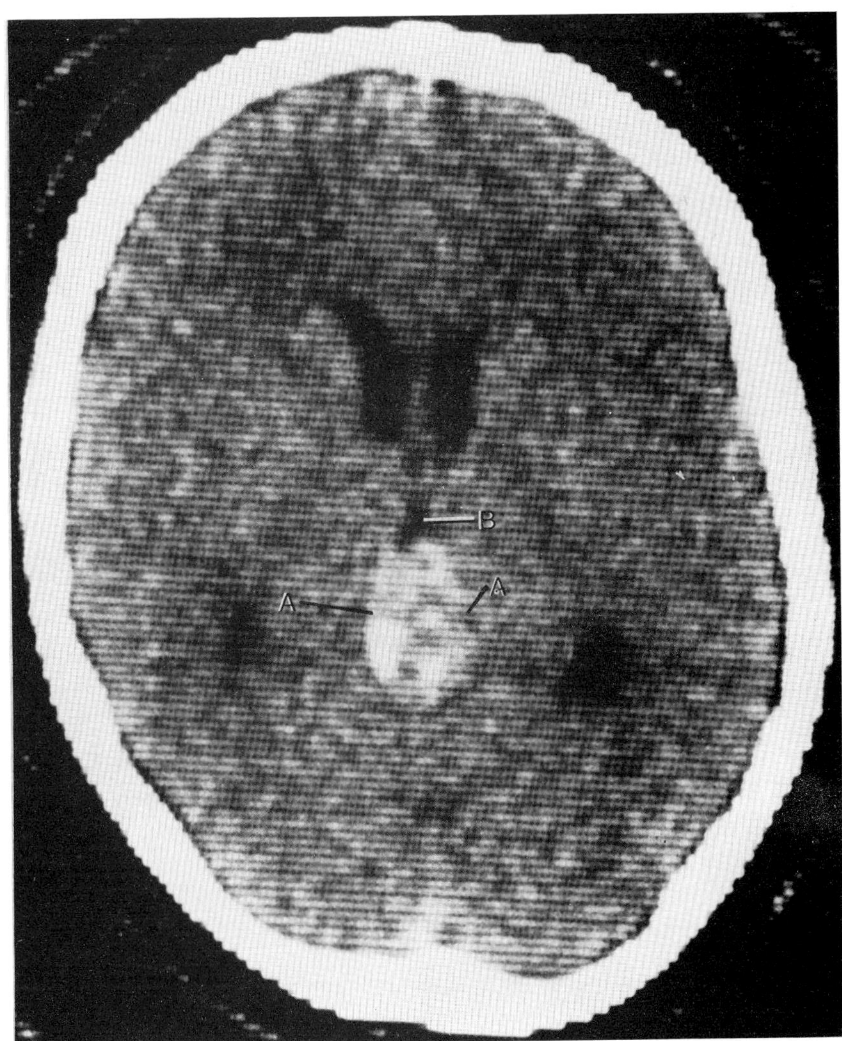

Figure 15-12-1. **Pinealoma.** A precontrast CT study shows a partially calcified oval high density tumor (A) encroaching upon the anterior third ventricle (B), producing mild obstructive hydrocephalus. Metastatic seeding to the inferior third ventricular and hypothalamic structures is not uncommon with pineal tumors, particularly with germinomas. Such extension may be very difficult to ascertain by CT alone, even with sagittal reconstruction, and negative or positive plain tomographic contrast studies of the inferior third ventricular recesses may be necessary.

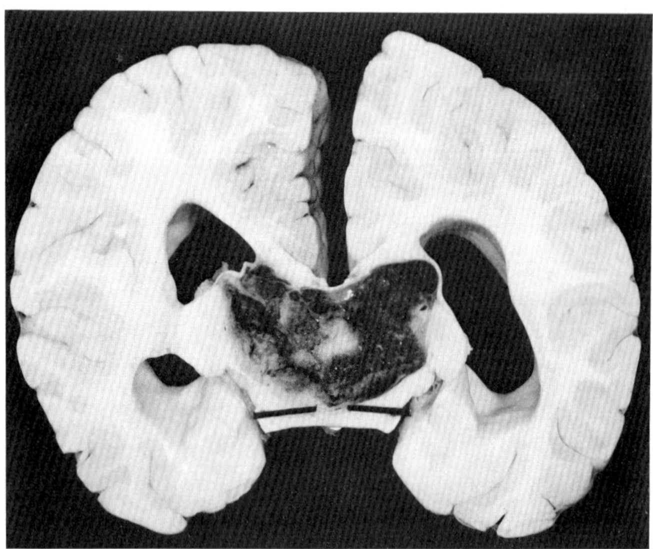

Figure 15-12-2. **Pinealoma.** The tumor has destroyed portions of the corpus callosum and of the roof of the midbrain. Markers indicate compressed and scarcely visible aqueduct. The tumor proved to be a glioma of ependymal type. From Dublin, W. B.: *Fundamentals of Neuropathology,* Ed. II, 1967, Charles C Thomas, Springfield, Illinois.

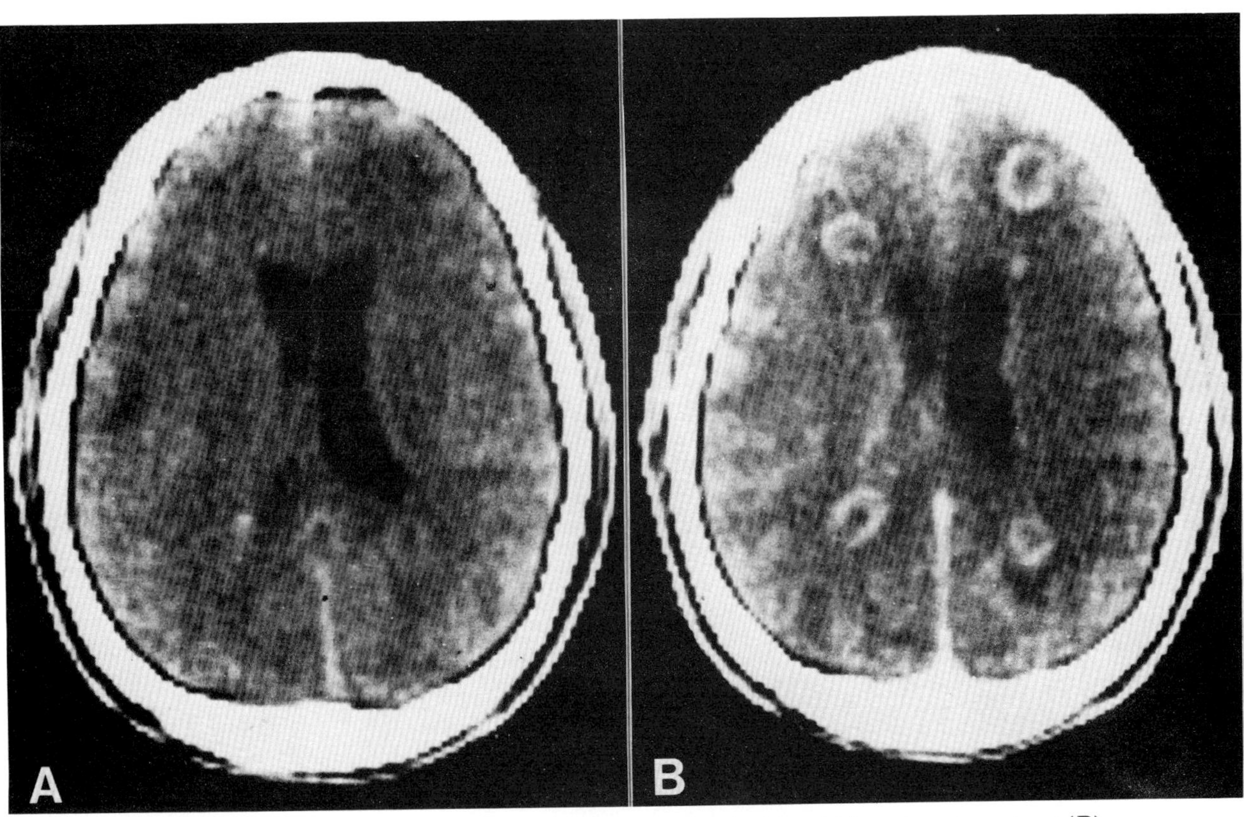

Figure 15-13. **Lung Tumor Metastatic to the Brain.** Pre- (A) and post-contrast (B) sections from the same patient demonstrate multiple areas of circular enhancement, with surrounding areas of edema, typical of metastatic deposits, particularly of a **squamous**-cell origin.

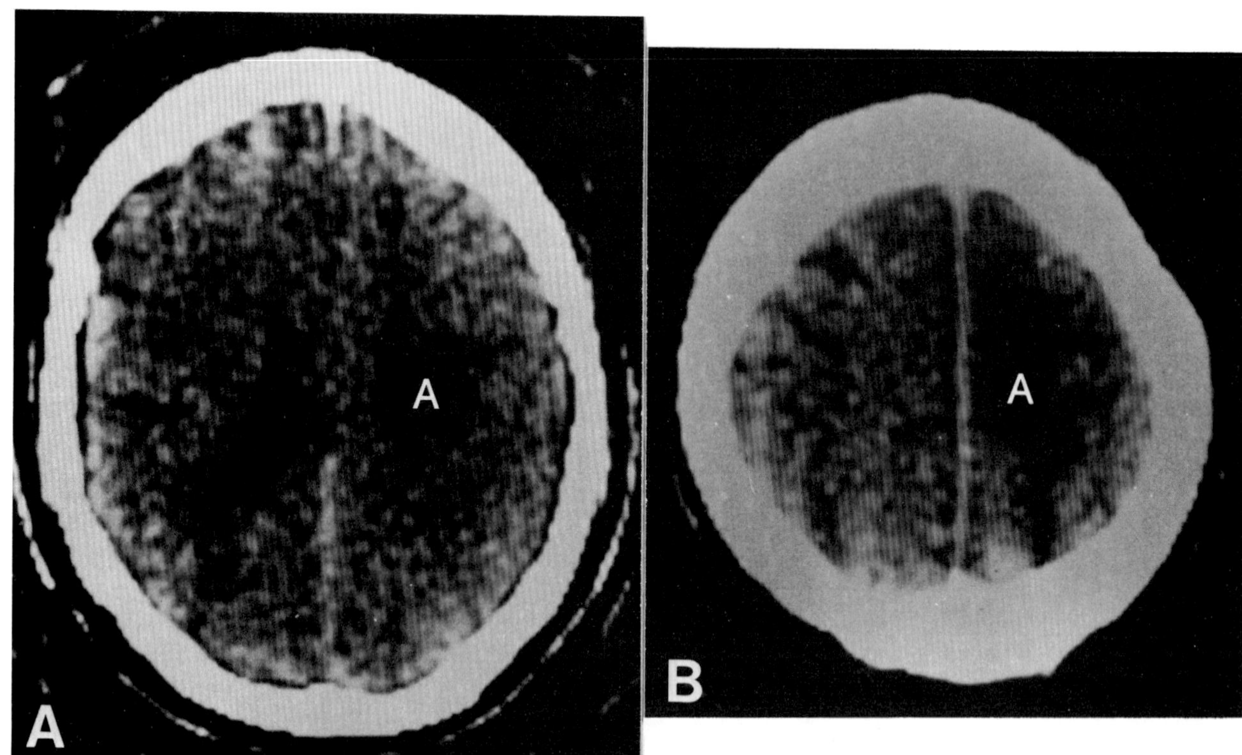

Figure 15-14-1. **Cerebral Metastasis.** Same case as Figure 15-14-2. Two postcontrast CT scans show a considerable amount of white matter hypodensity representing edema (A). No enhancing tumor nodule is identified. This sequence of scans demonstrates the importance of obtaining high vertex levels to search for tumor presence, so as not to mislead the investigator. Coronal scans may be necessary for proper identification. This pattern might be confused with embolic infarction, but the latter, especially of this size, almost always involves cortical structures as well.

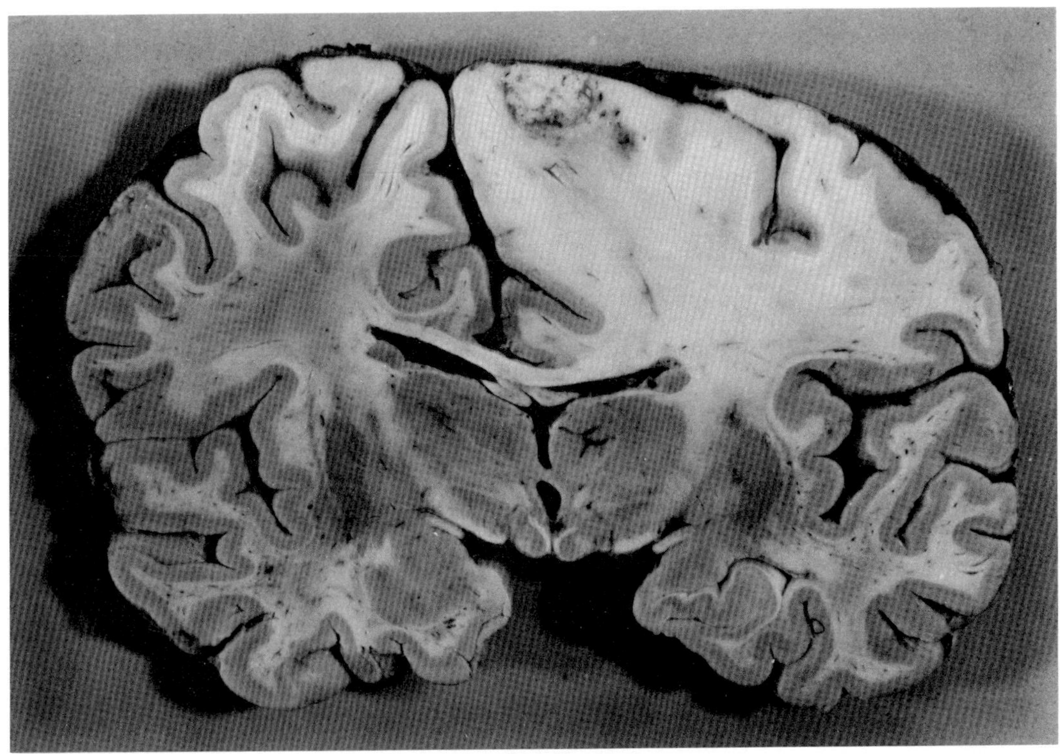

Figure 15-14-2. **Metastasis to Brain from Carcinoma of Lung.** Same case as Figure 15-14-1. A solitary metastasis was found in the precentral (motor) area. The location of the tumor correlated well with clinical manifestation in that there was paresis of the contralateral upper extremity. Marked edema has developed about the tumor nodule.

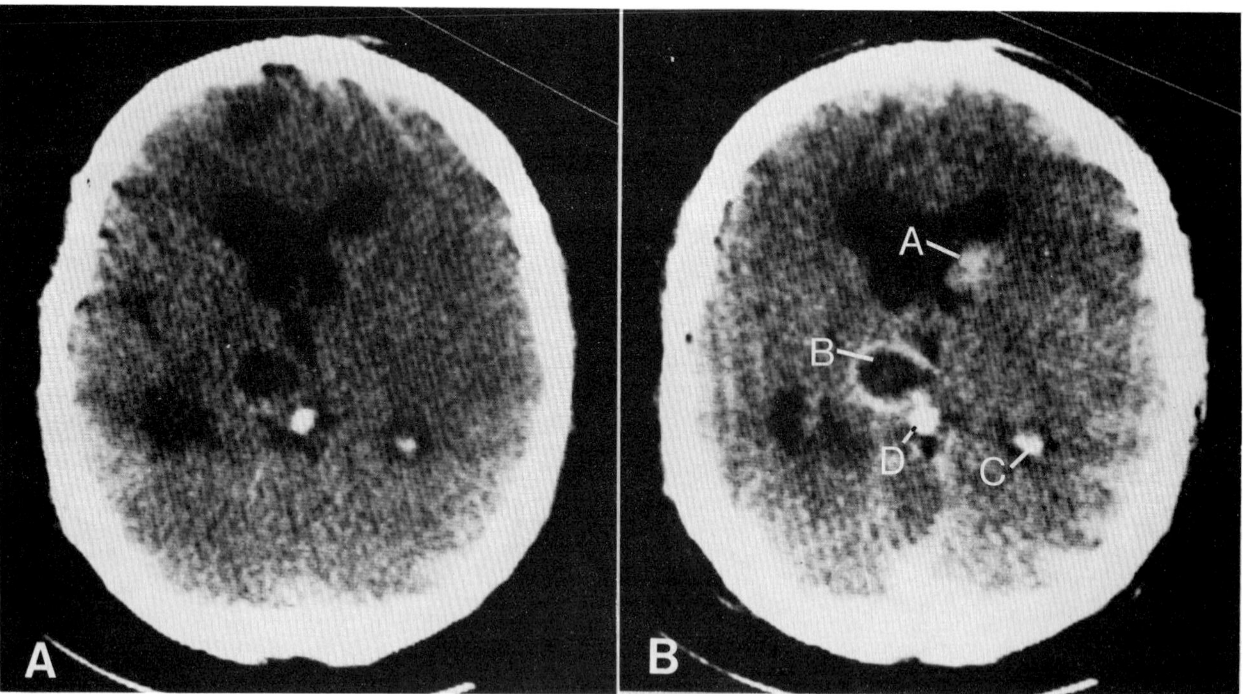

Figure 15-15-1. **Computed Tomography of Multiple Metastases.** Same Case as Figure 15-15-2. **A** (precontrast) and **B** (postcontrast) demonstrate two areas of metastasis. One is located in the head of the caudate nucleus (A), and the second within the thalamus (B). Normal choroid calcification with slight enhancement is represented by C, and pineal by D. This case demonstrates the different pattern of metastatic enhancement from solid nodular (A) to "ring-like" (B). Some authors suggest that smooth, thin "ring-like" enhancement may vary considerably between abscess and primary and secondary tumor.

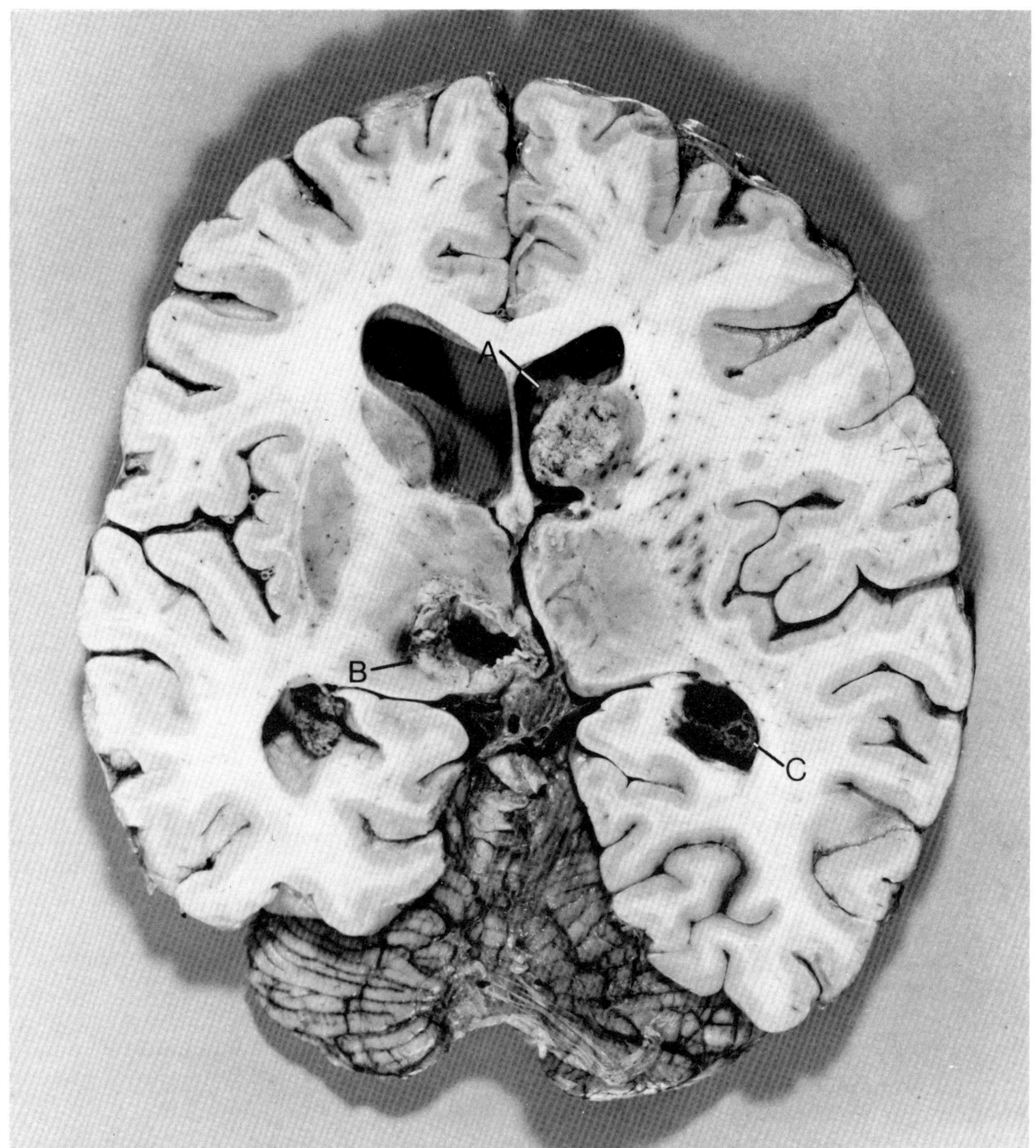

Figure 15-15-2. **Multiple Metastases to Brain from Carcinoma of Lung.**

A. Metastasis to head of right caudate nucleus. Edema of adjacent tissue has effected swelling to a degree that the right cerebral hemisphere at this point is considerably wider than the left.

B. Metastasis to left thalamus.

C. Cystic choroid plexus in first part of inferior horn, lateral ventricle. Appreciable calcium was not found, and there was no evidence of metastasis to this structure.

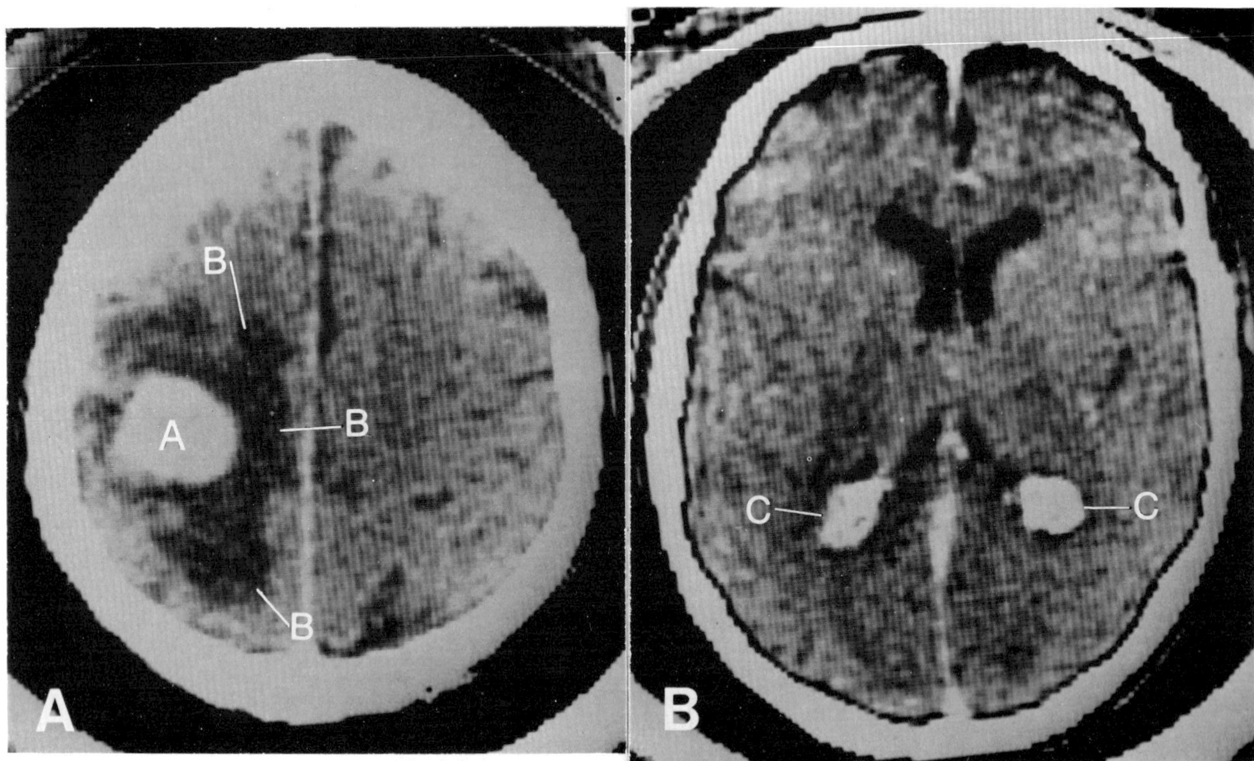

Figure 15-16-1. **Metastatic Large Bowel Carcinoma to Brain.** Same case as Figures 15-16-2 through 5. *A* demonstrates an enhancing tumor (A) surrounded by a large zone of decreased density (B). The CT pattern might suggest meningioma. However, higher sections (not demonstrated) did not show continuity of the tumor mass with the bony calvarium. Coronal cuts may be necessary at times to demonstrate such relationships. In addition, the large amount of surrounding edema (B) is unusual for a neoplasm, especially secondary. *B* shows incidental heavy calcification (C) in the choroid plexuses of the atria of the lateral ventricles. Letters in italics refer to larger letters denoting subdivisions of the illustration. Nonitalicized letters refer to small letters that indicate individual structures in the illustration.

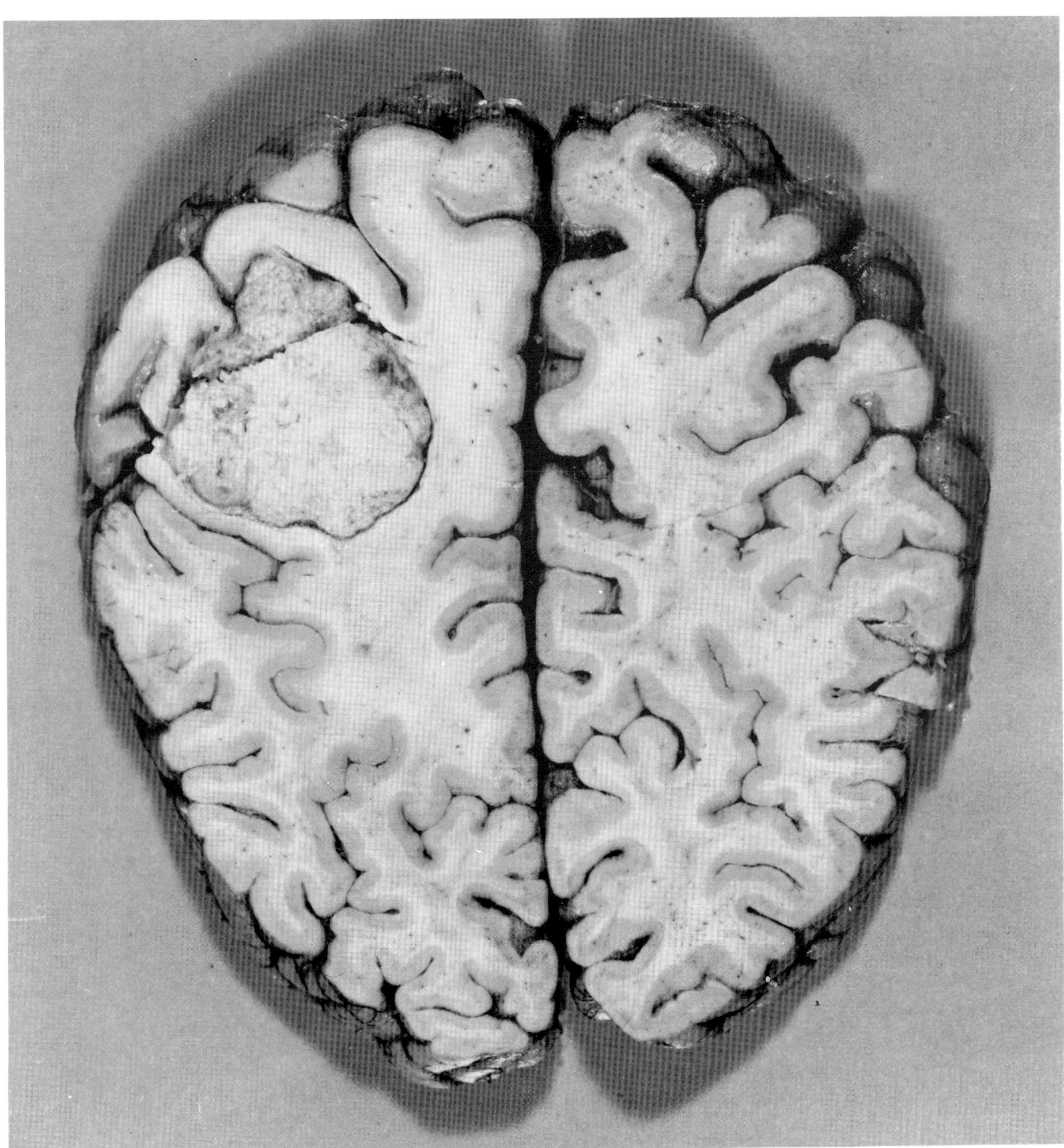

Figure 15-16-2. **Metastasis to Brain from Carcinoma of Colon.** 15° Axial section. The lesion demonstrated in the CT, Figure 15-16-1 *A* A, is a tumor nodule. On a basis of gross features of distinct demarcation, continuity of tumor with meninges, and fine nodularity, metastasis and meningioma were considered possibilities.

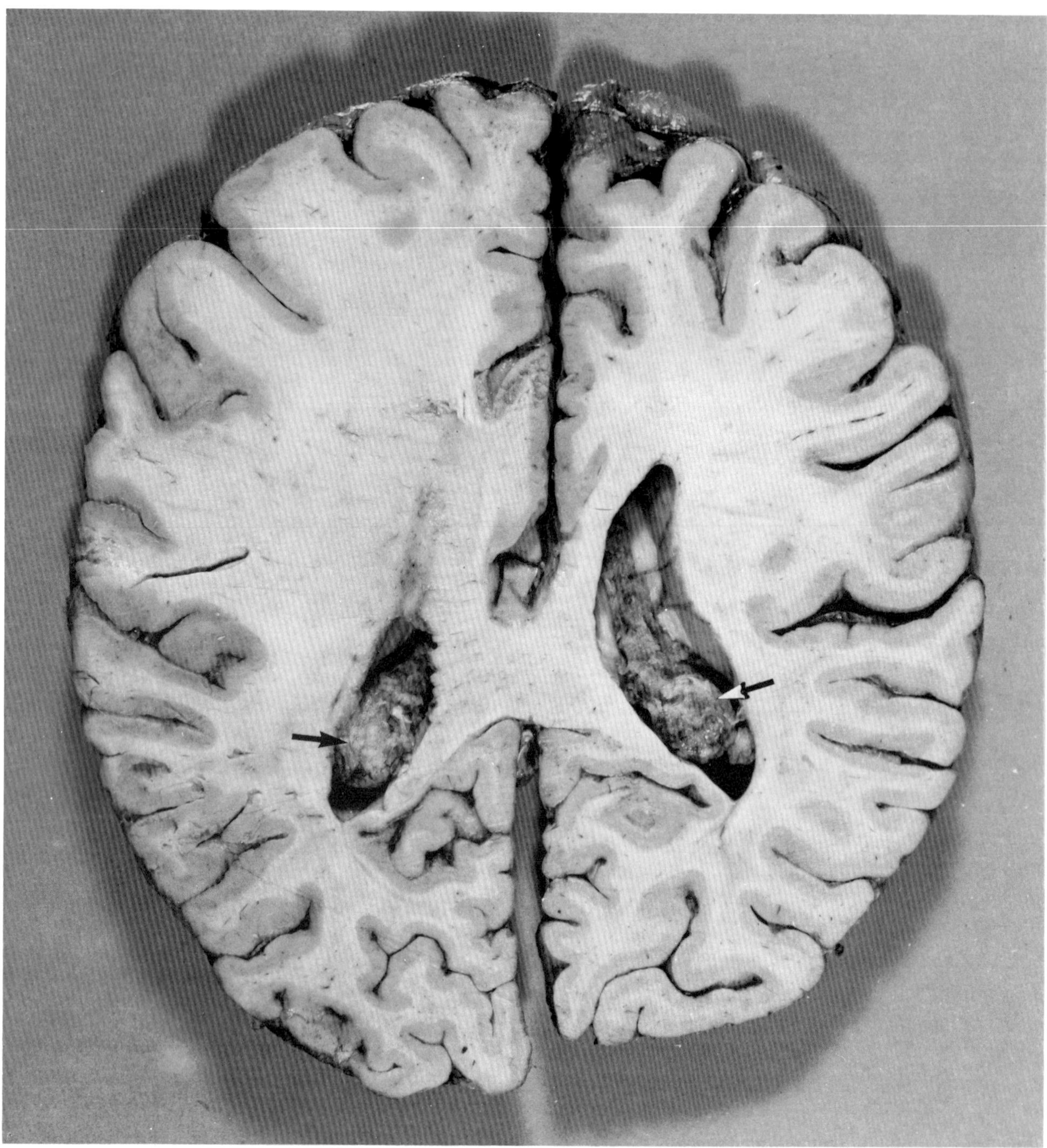

Figure 15-16-3. **Metastasis to Brain from Carcinoma of Colon; Calcification of Choroid Plexus.** In addition to the tumor nodule, a 15° axial section, nearer the base, shows bilateral nodular hypertrophy of choroid plexuses of inferior horns of lateral ventricles (*arrows*), with calcium deposit.

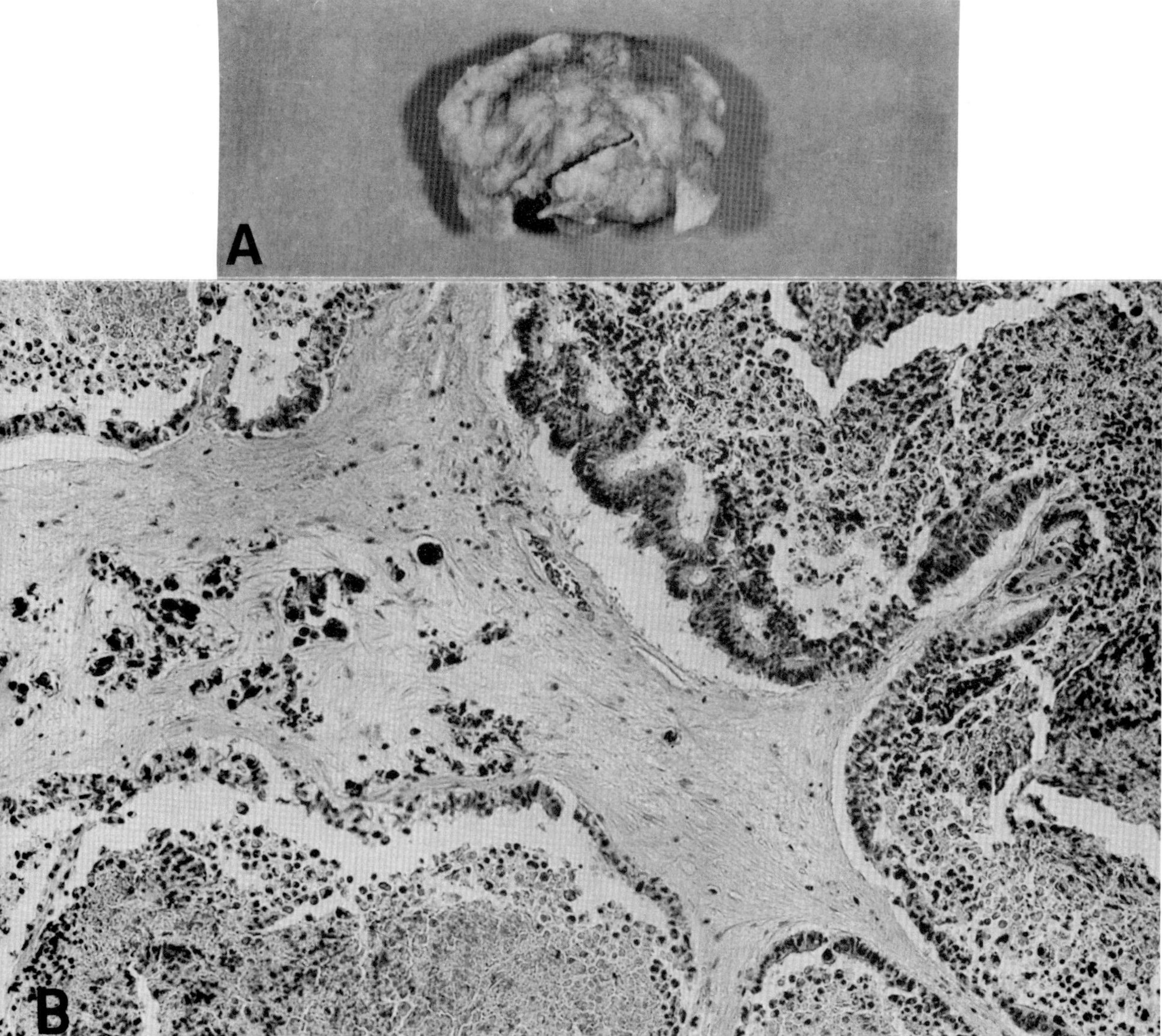

Figure 15-16-4. **Metastasis to Brain from Carcinoma of Colon.** Continuation.
A. A portion of the tumor shown in Figure 15-16-2, exhibiting some of the surface margin, with nodular texture.
B. Microphotograph of the tumor, showing lobular pattern of carcinoma metastatic from colon, correlating with the nodular gross texture.

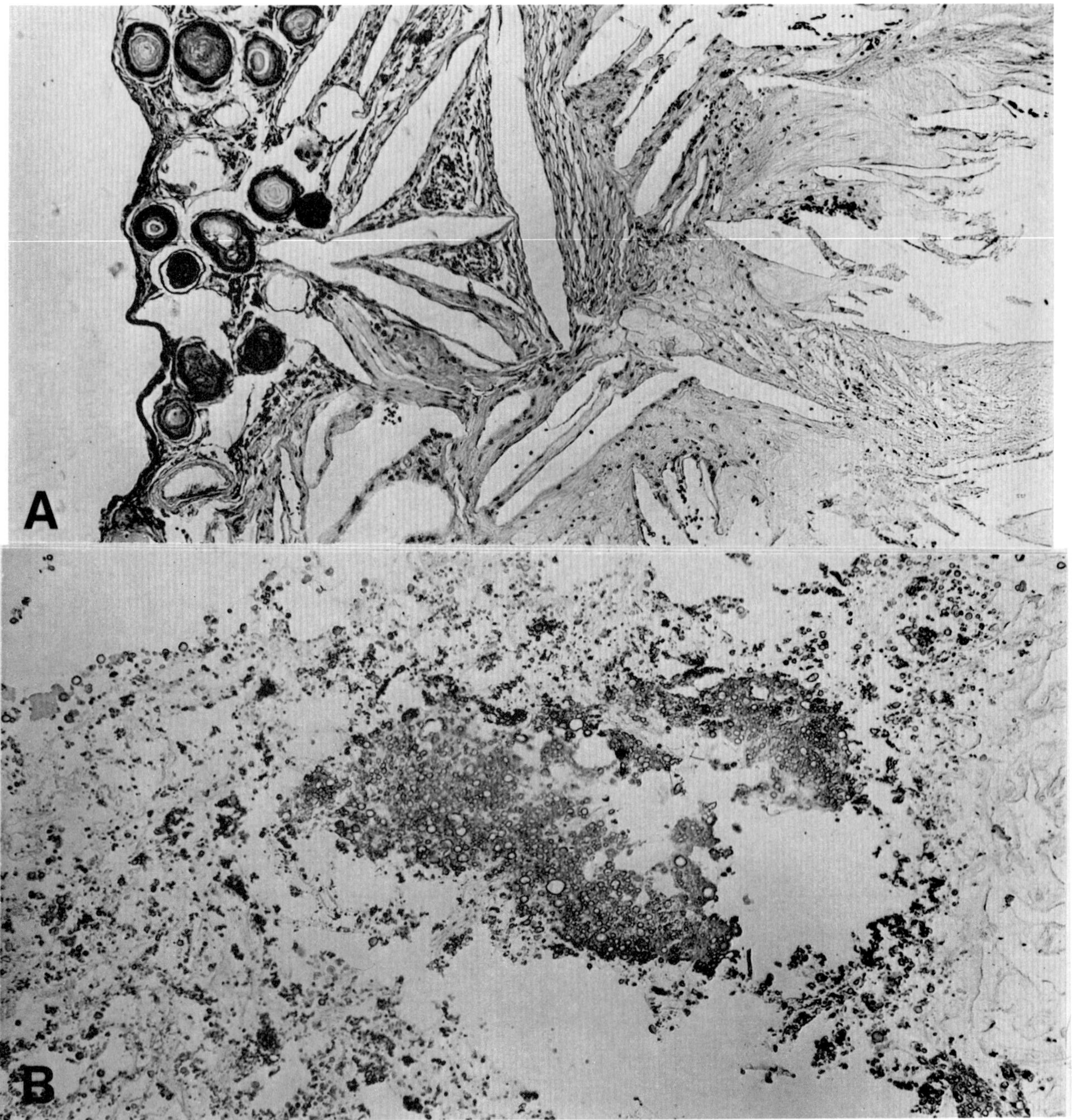

Figure 15-16-5. **Metastasis to Brain from Carcinoma of Colon; Calcification of Choroid Plexuses.** Continuation.
A. Microphotograph of choroid plexus, showing cholesterol clefts (center), with formation of psammoma bodies (on left), and with cystic degeneration and hyalinization (on right).
B. Microphotograph of choroid plexus, showing an area of granular calcium deposit.

Chapter Seven

Metabolic Disturbances—Vascular Lesions

An infarct can be detected with radionuclide scanning and/or computed tomography. In general, the CT mass effect (which tends to be minimal) from a non-hemorrhagic infarct usually is at maximum 2 to 3 days after the initial insult. The ideal time for observation of contrast enhancement in infarcts is approximately 2 weeks after the initial episode. Massive amounts of contrast enhancement within an area of infarction may be indicative of a high risk of hemorrhage; heparin treatment may be reserved in such cases. CT can also demonstrate the presence or absence of intracranial hemorrhage, hydrocephalus, or large arteriovenous malformation, and often may exclude the possibility of neoplasm as a source of infarction. Angiography, however, remains the diagnostic procedure of choice for the evaluation of vascular disorders.

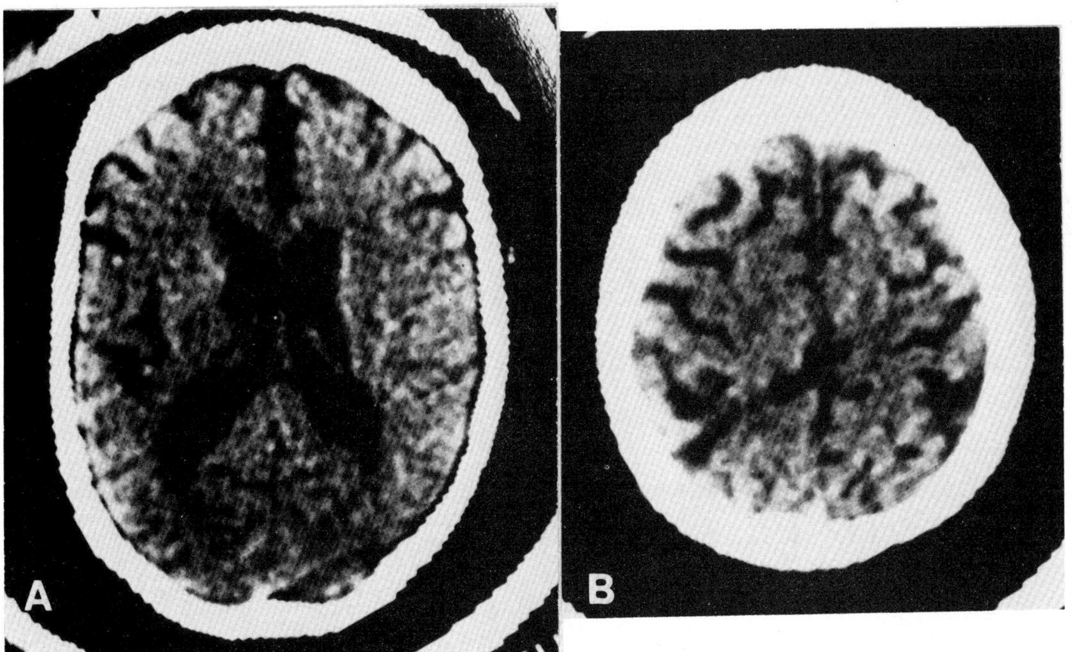

Figure 16-1-1. **Computed Tomography of Cerebral Atrophy. A** and **B** demonstrate enlargement of the lateral ventricles which is consistant with the degree of severe sulcal prominence. These findings are typical of cerebral atrophy, in this case related to normal aging processes.

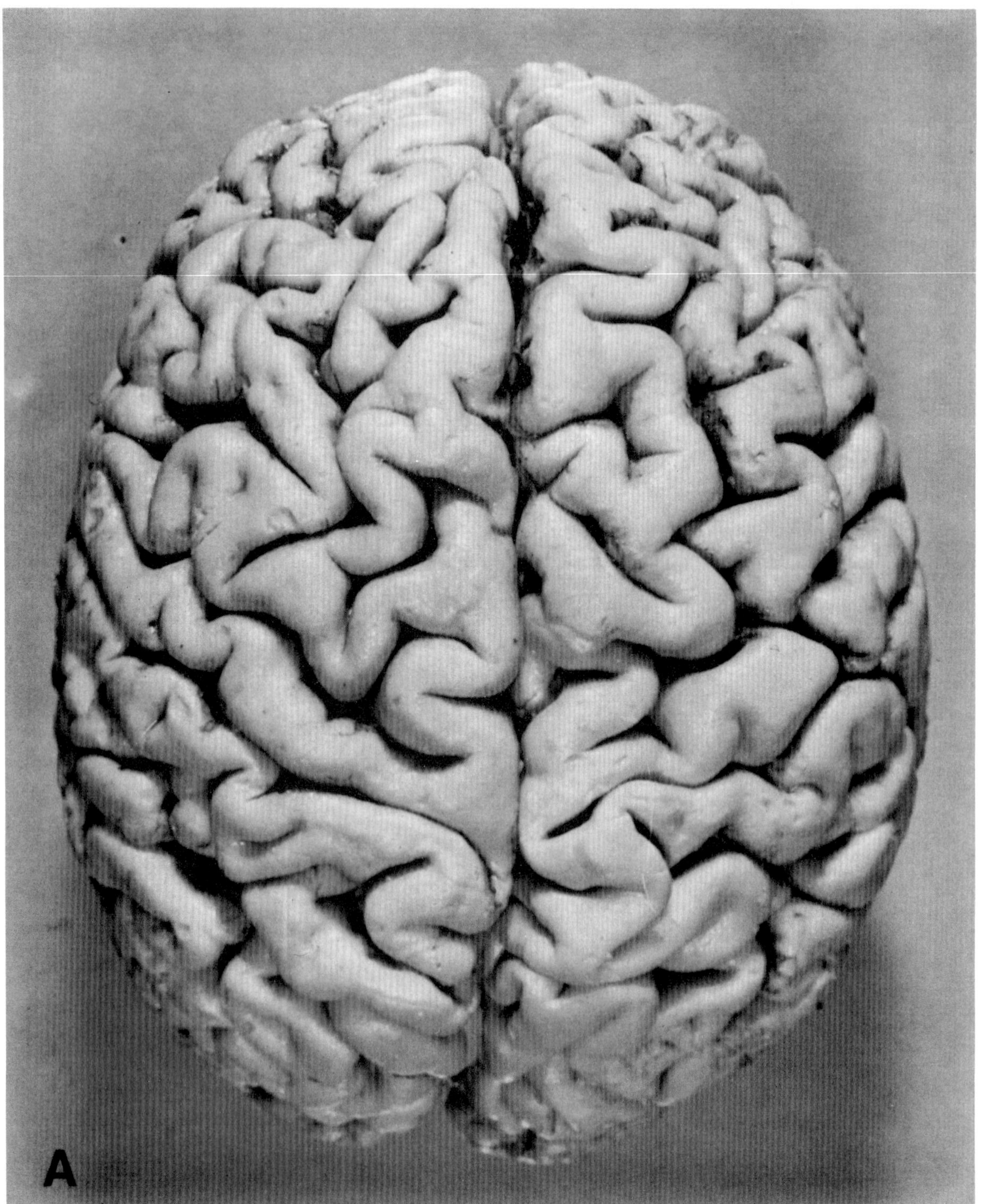

Figure 16-1-2A. **Cerebral Atrophy, Moderate (Aging Process).** Corresponds to CT of Figure 16-1-1. View of vertex of brain. There is moderate atrophy, with commensurate widening of sulci.

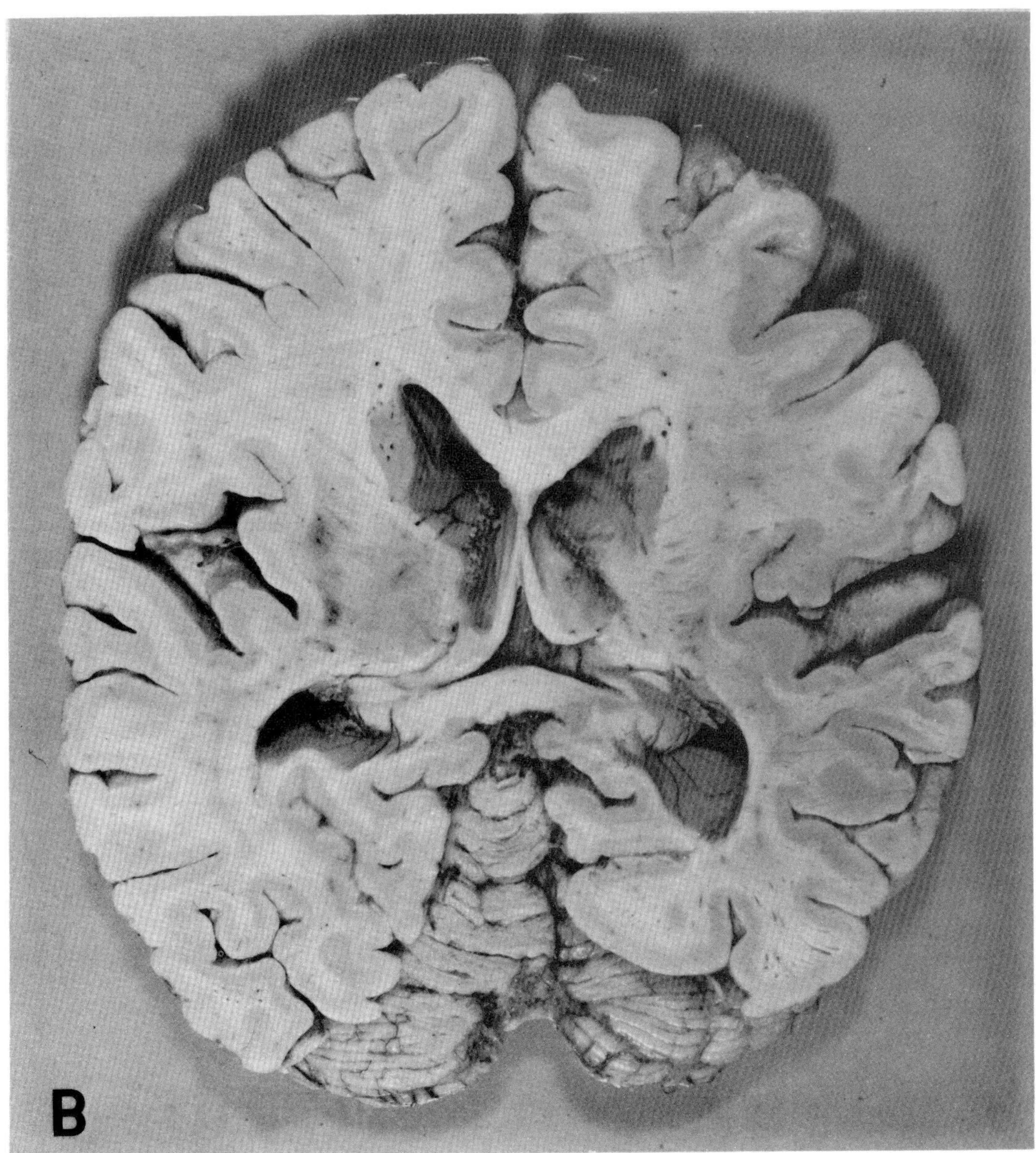

Figure 16-1-2B. **Cerebral Atrophy, Moderate (Aging Process).** 15° Axial section corresponding to CT of Figure 16-1-1 A. There is moderate narrowing of convolutions, with widening of sulci, and the ventricles are enlarged.

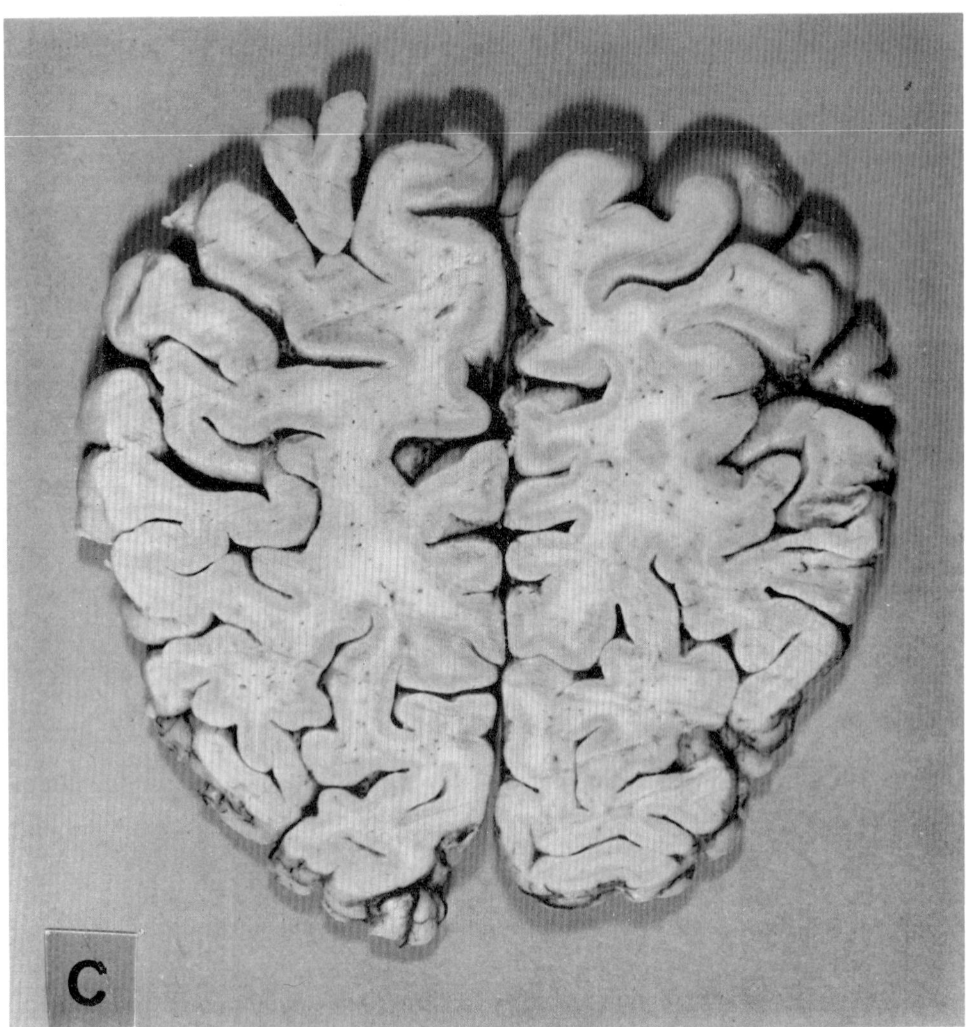

Figure 16-1-2C. **Cerebral Atrophy, Moderate (Aging Process).** 15° Axial section corresponding to CT of Figure 16-1-1 B. There is narrowing of convolutions, especially in frontal region (at top), with widening of sulci.

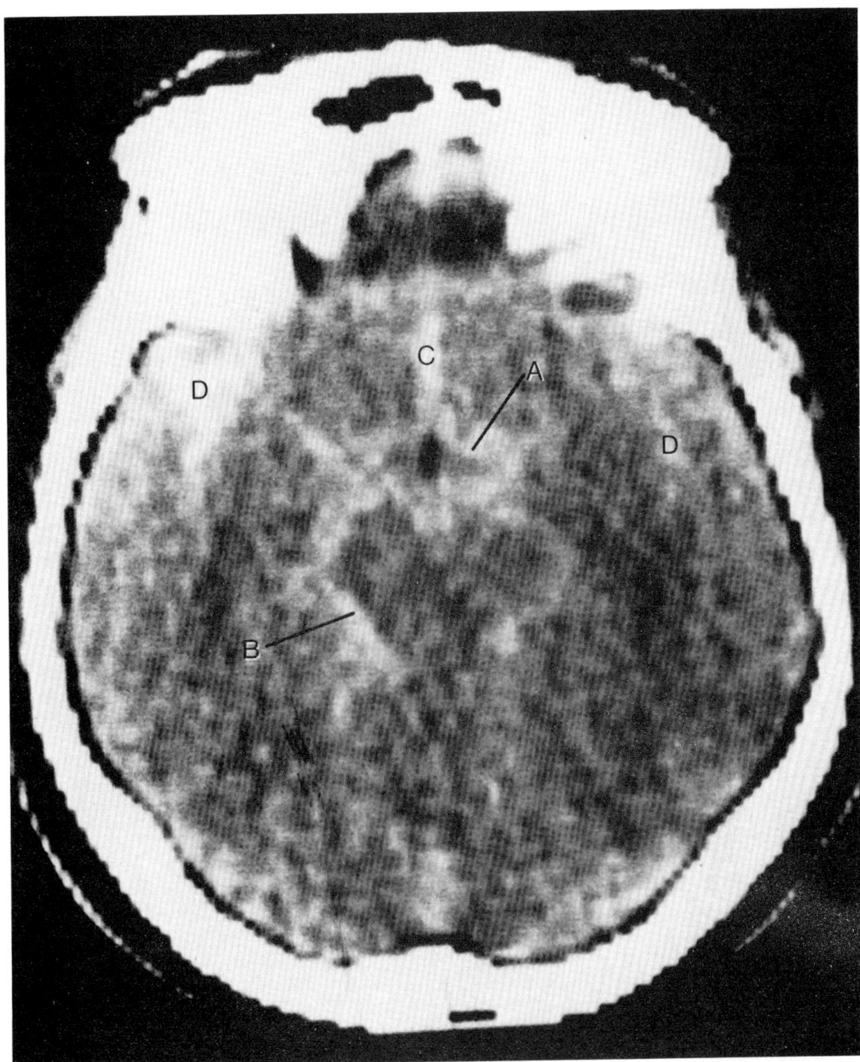

Figure 16-2-1. **Subarachnoid Hemorrhage, Computed Tomography.** Diffuse subarachnoid blood is identified in the chiasmatic cistern (A), around the brain stem (B), in the cistern of the lamina terminalis (C), and in the sylvian cisterns anteriorly (D). The presence of subarachnoid hemorrhage in ruptured aneurysms can be detected in approximately 80 to 85% of cases examined by computed tomography. On occasion, the area of possible aneurysmal rupture can be determined from the scan as follows: blood primarily within the cistern of the lamina terminalis, particularly associated with frontal lobe edema or hematoma is most likely the result of an anterior communicating artery aneurysm. Blood within the cistern of the middle cerebral artery or lateral sulcus is most likely the result of rupture of a middle cerebral artery aneurysm. Blood within the interpeduncular fossa results from basilar tip artery aneurysms and blood collected primarily around the brain stem and in the superior cerebellar cistern may result from basilar tip aneurysms, posterior communicating artery aneurysms, or posterior cerebral artery aneurysms.

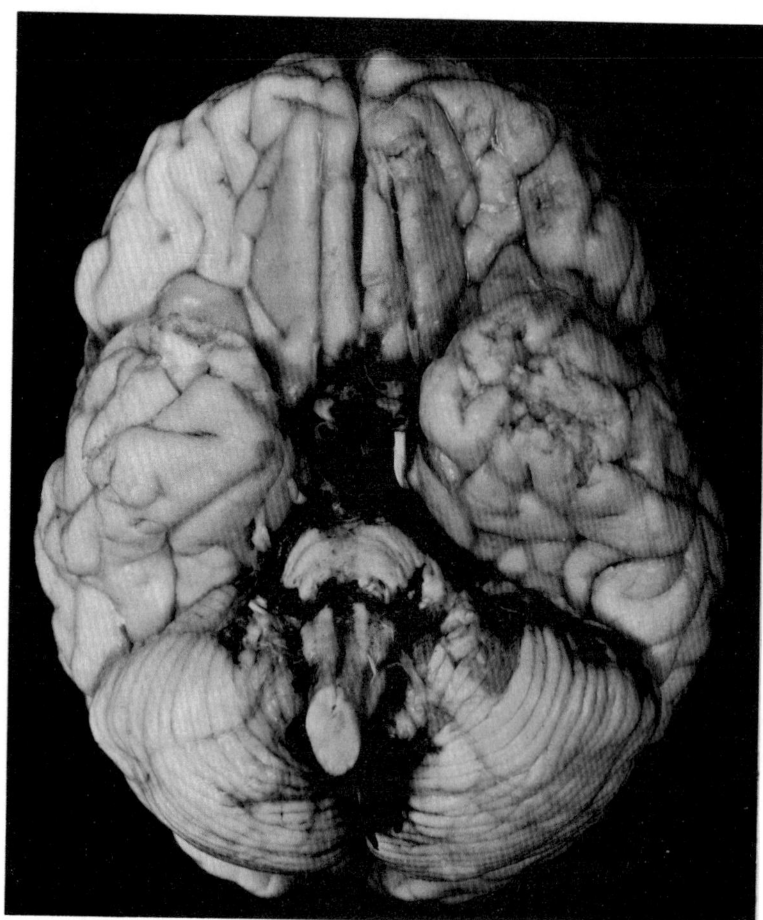

Figure 16-2-2. **Subarachnoid Hemorrhage.** From Dublin, W. B.: *Fundamentals of Neuropathology,* Ed. II, 1967, Charles C Thomas, Springfield, Illinois.

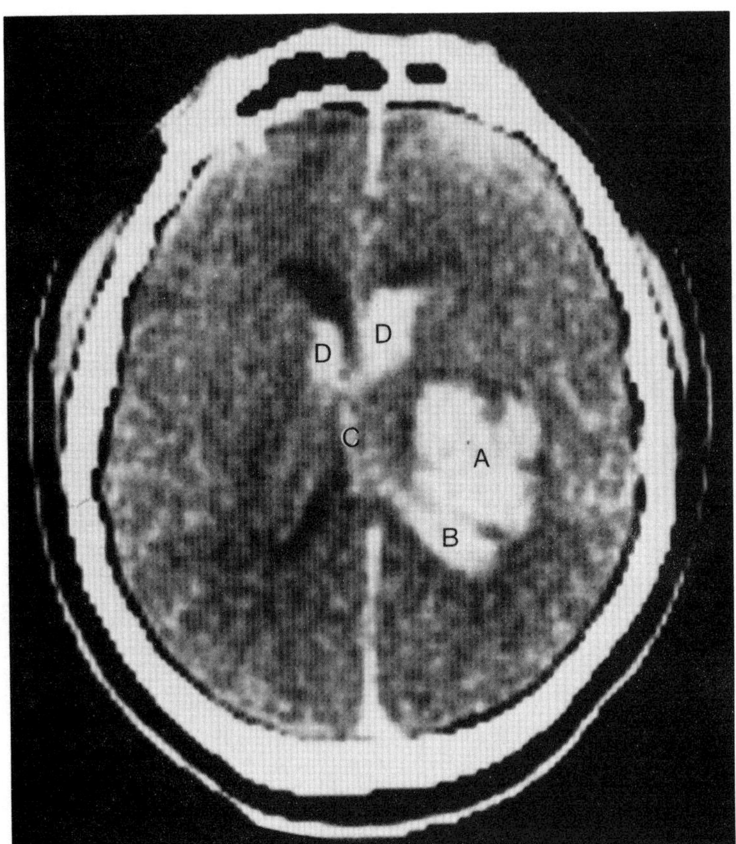

Figure 16-3-1. **Hypertensive Intra-axial Hemorrhage.** A noncontrast CT scan demonstrates a hematoma in the superior basal ganglia and associated white matter (B) which has ruptured into the adjacent atrium of the lateral ventricle. Blood is also seen in the displaced third ventricle (C) and in the anterior bodies of the lateral ventricles (D). This pattern is typical of a hypertensive hemorrhage, in that the hematoma (A) is fairly "clean," without significant satellite hemorrhages. The location of the lesion (basal ganglia structures) and rupture into the ventricular structures is also characteristic of the hypertensive hemorrhage.

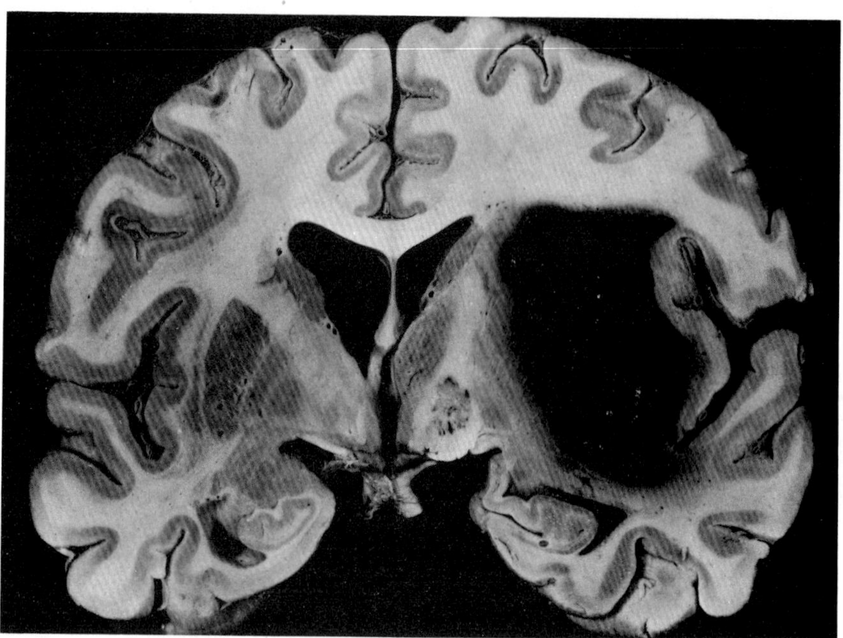

Figure 16-3-2. **Hypertensive Encephalopathy.** There is a hemorrhage arising in the lenticular nucleus (lenticulostriate), with destruction of contiguous tissues, and with swelling of the hemisphere, and of the brain generally, with commensurate flattening of gyri, and with ventricular distortion. From Dublin, W. B.: *Fundamentals of Neuropathology,* Ed. II, 1967, Charles C Thomas, Springfield, Illinois.

Figure 16-4. **Computed Tomographic Appearance of Massive Infarction with Contrast Enhancement. A.** A noncontrast scan demonstrates an ill-defined lucency in the right temporal lobe (A), without mass effect. **B.** A contrast scan of the same level, demonstrates massive enhancement without mass effect in a "sheet-like manner" is typical of cerebral infarction. Involvement of the parahippocampal gyrus adjacent to the tentorium and temporal cortical areas is typical of a posterior cerebral distribution.

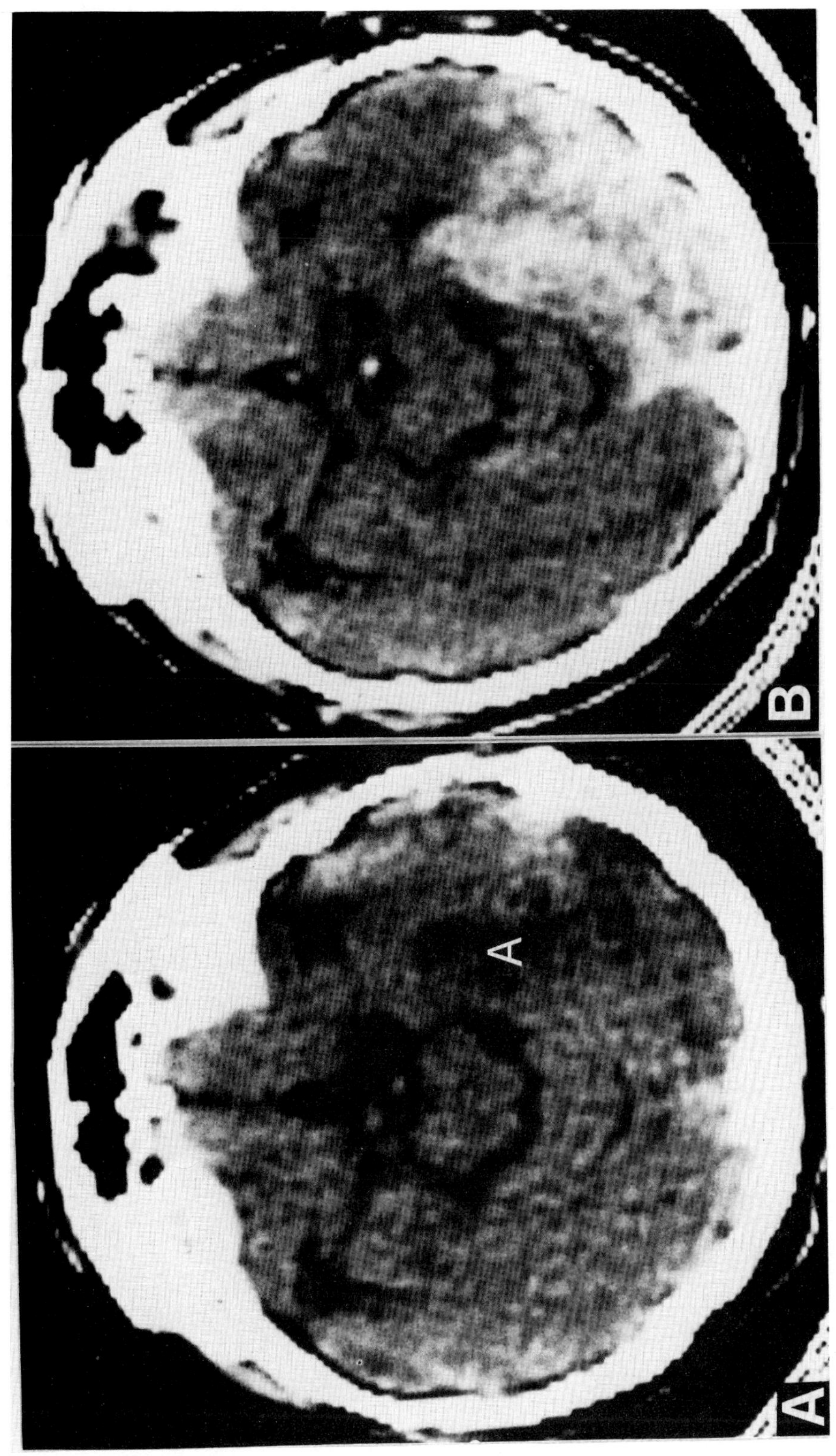

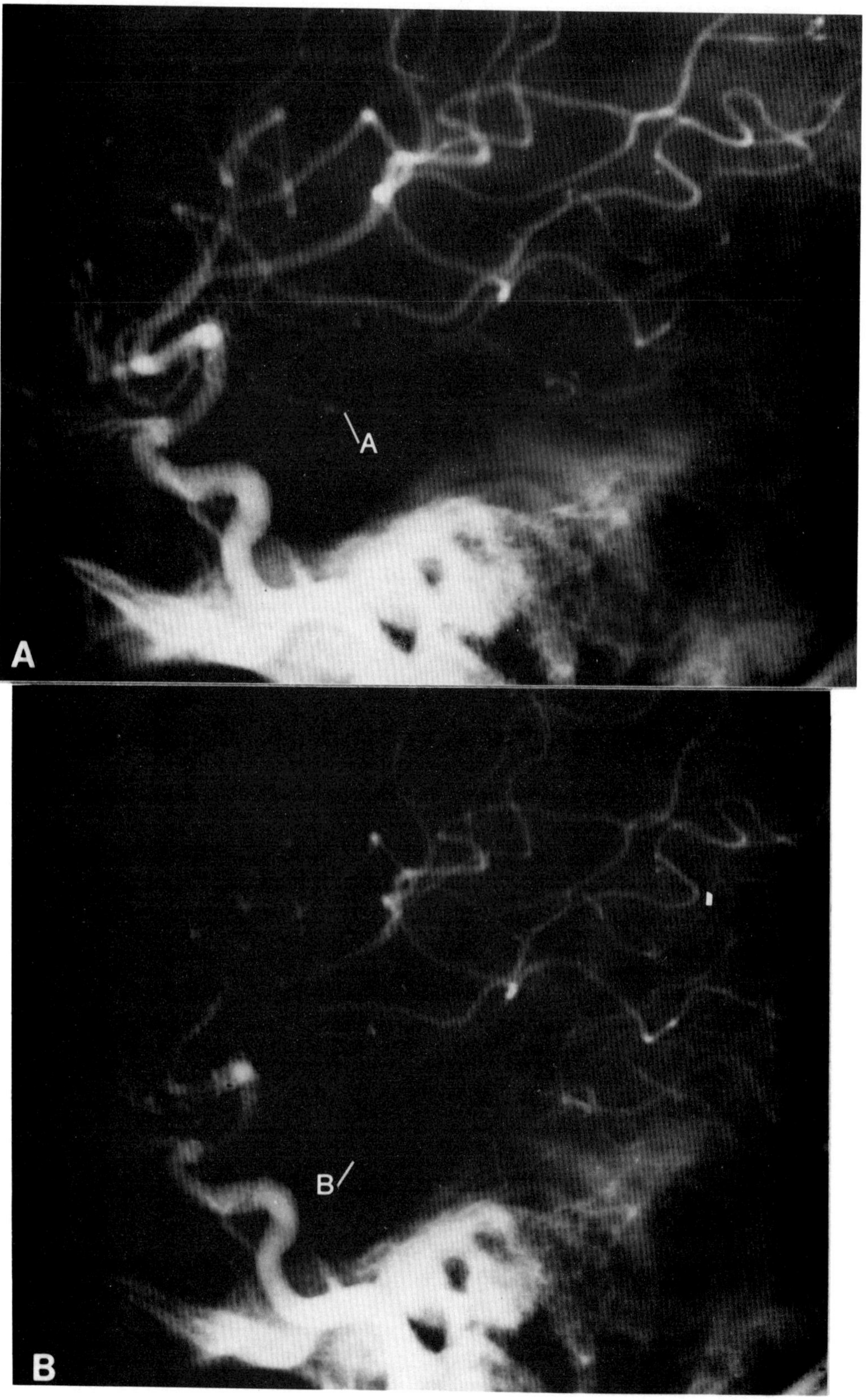

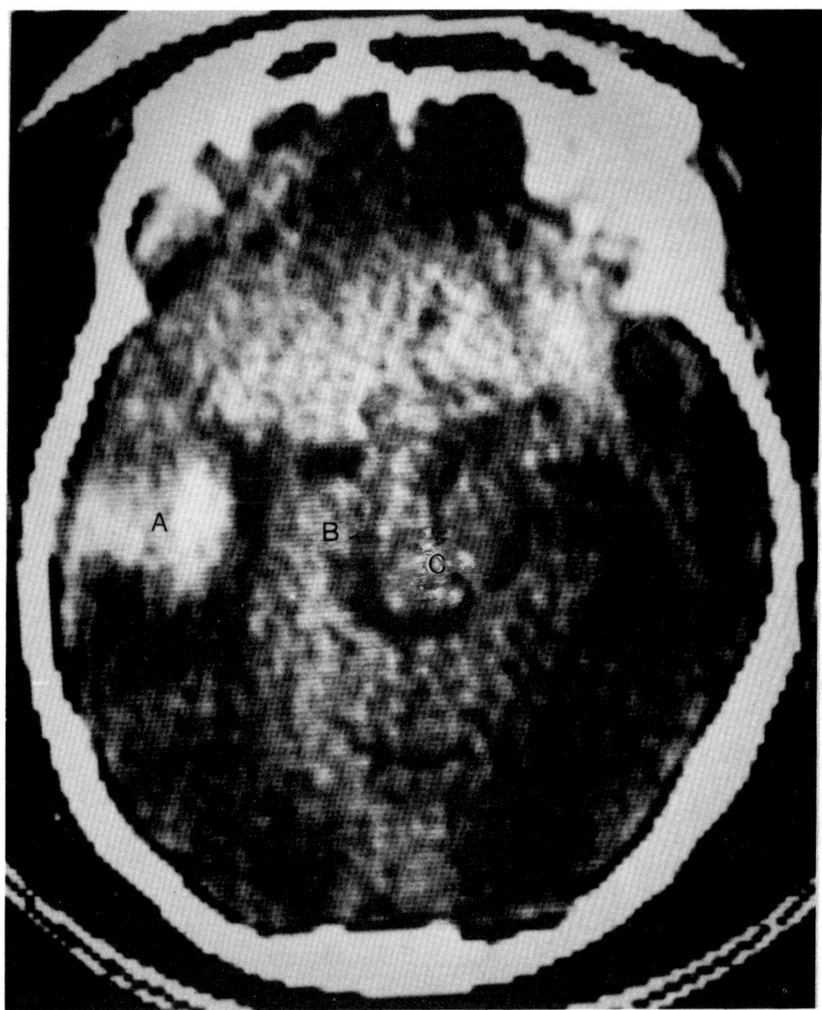

Figure 16-5-2. **Uncal Herniation.** The CT scan shows an area of contusion (A) which has produced uncal herniation (B) with encroachment upon, and displacement of, the brain stem (C).

←

Figure 16-5-1. **Lateral Angiographic Demonstration of Uncal Herniation. A** represents an angiogram performed in a young individual who suffered cerebral anoxia. A points to the normal course of the posterior cerebral artery and posterior communicating artery. **B** was taken several days later after clinical evidence of uncal herniation. Note the downward migration of the posterior communicating artery and proximal posterior cerebral artery (**B**), which have been inferiorly displaced due to uncal herniation and notching.

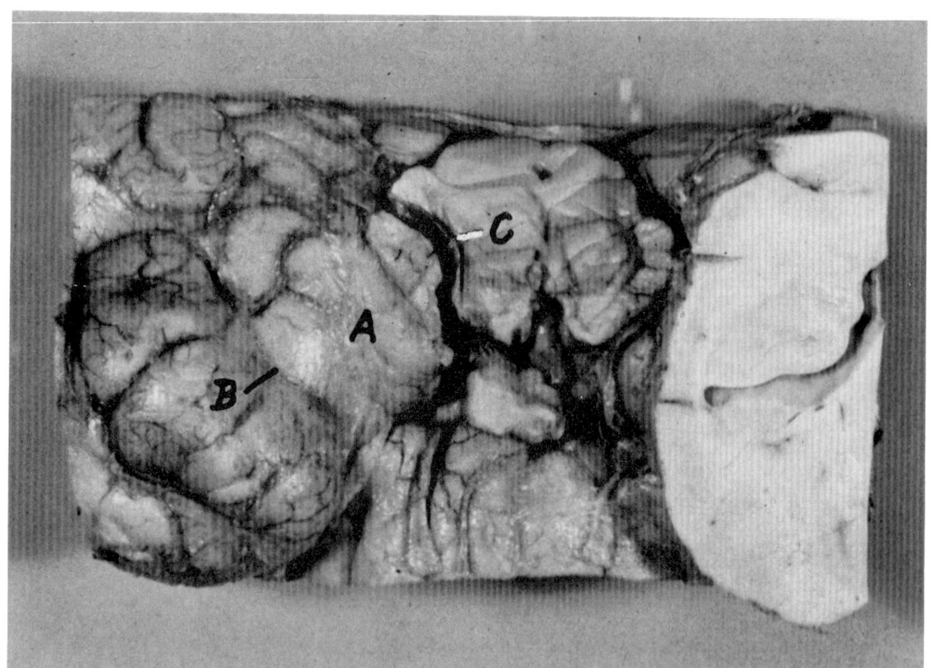

Figure 16-5-3. **Uncal Herniation.** this may result in the presence of brain swelling from any cause. In the present case, there was a hemorrhagic infarct. The attendant swelling resulted in severe herniation of the uncus over the edge of the tentorium, with deep grooving and with indentation of the midbrain (the latter being unusual).

A. Uncus.

B. Line of grooving.

C. Margin of Indentation of brainstem.

From Dublin, W. B.: *Fundamentals of Neuropathology,* Ed. II, 1967, Charles C Thomas, Springfield, Illinois.

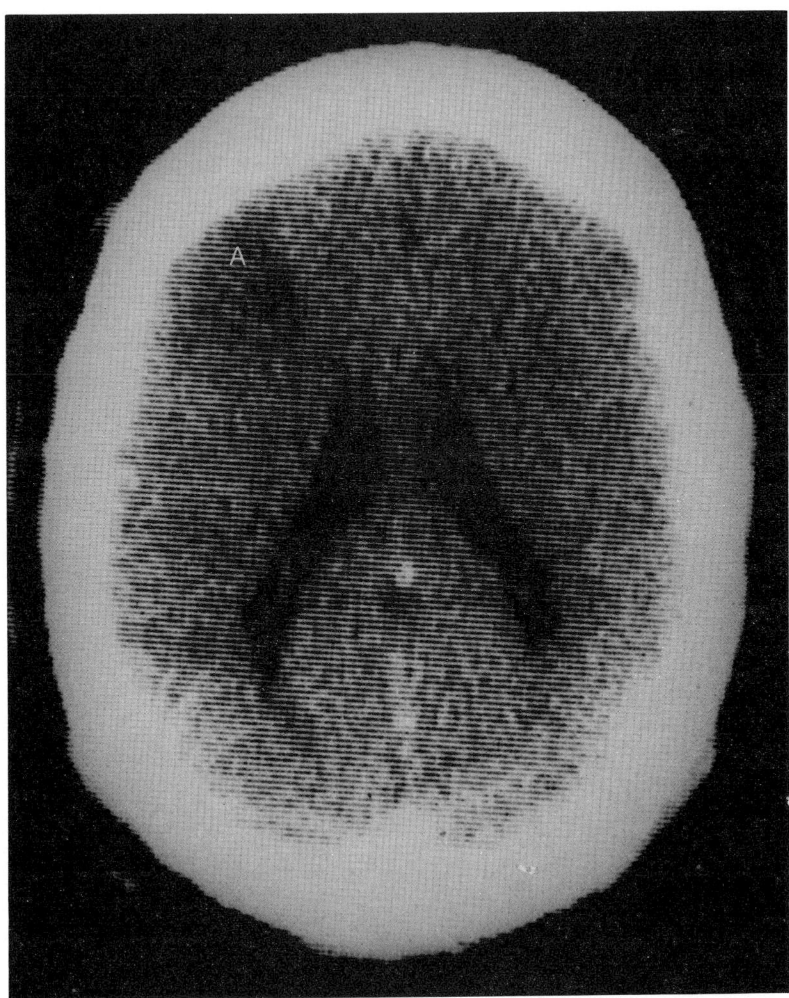

Figure 16-6-1. **Recent Infarct.** A noncontrast CT section of the same case as Figure 16-6-2 demonstrates a wedge-shaped hypodensity (A) with essentially no mass effect, typical of an infarctive process.

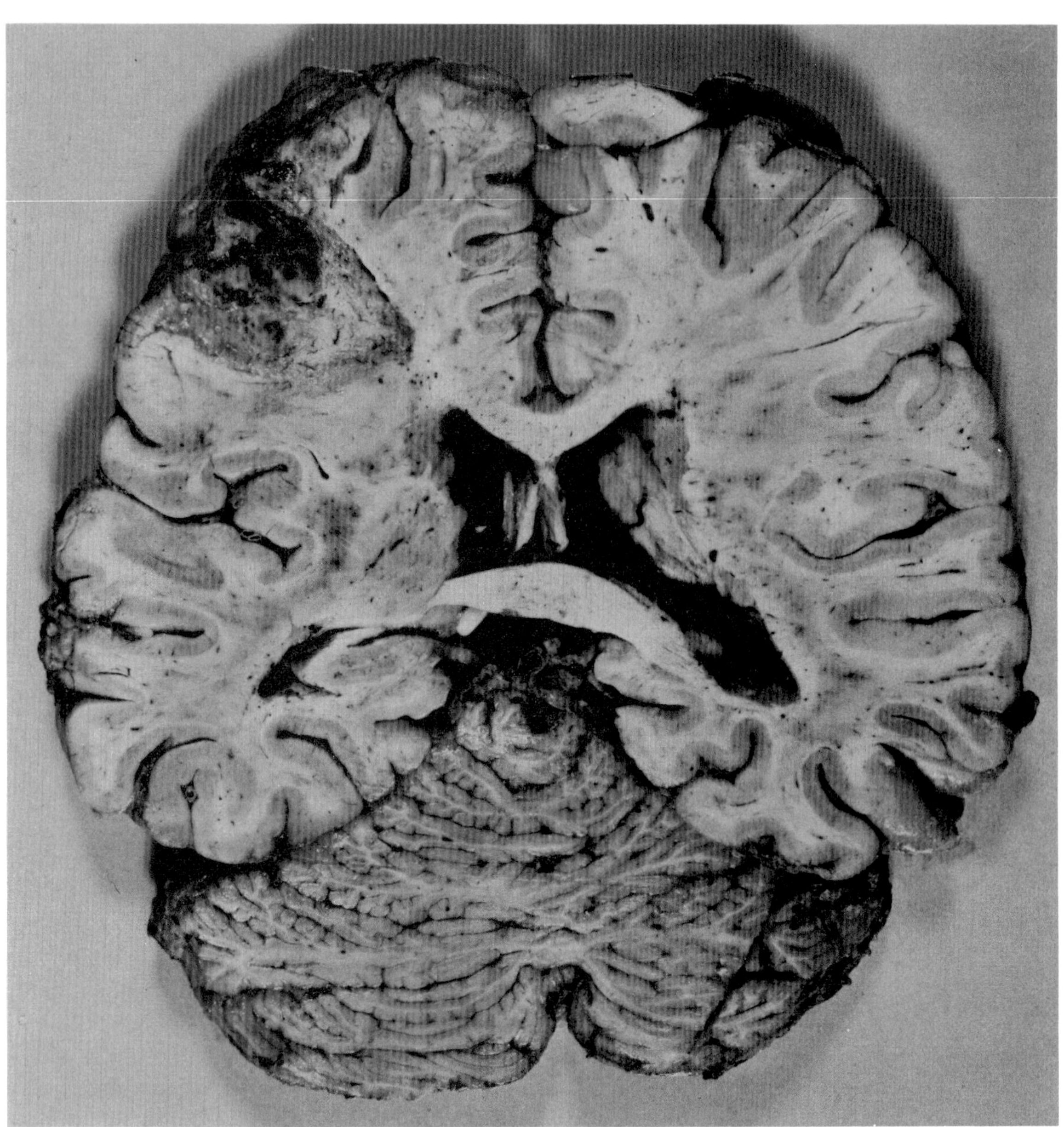

Figure 16-6-2. **Recent Infarct.** 15° Axial section corresponding to the CT in Figure 16-1-1. An infarct is seen in the left frontal lobe. It has reached a stage of necrosis, and there is focal ecchymosis (the darker portion). The lesion occurred in hypertensive vascular disease.

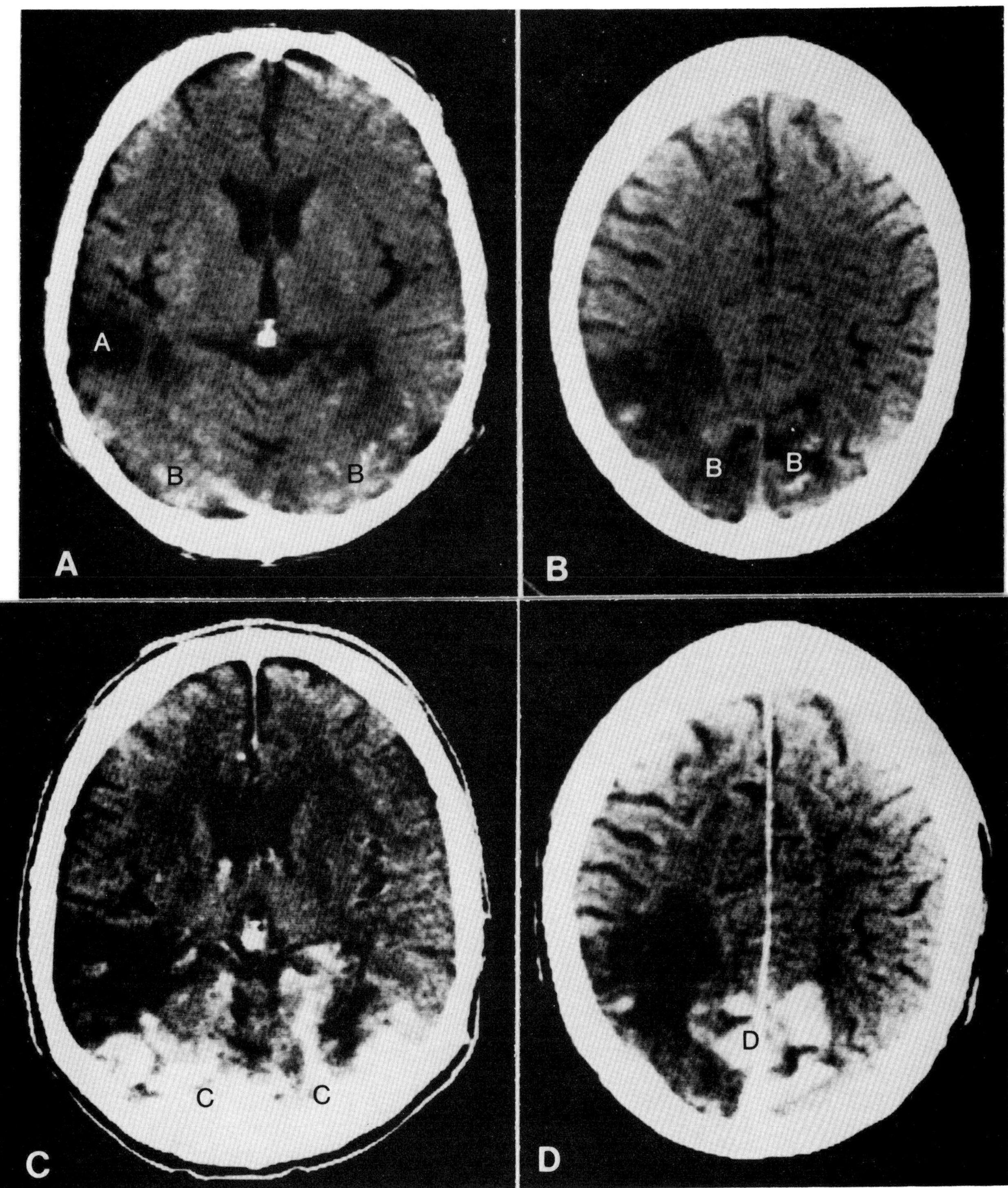

Figure 16-7-1. **Massive Occipital and Temporal Infarction.** Same case as Figure 16-7-2. Two precontrast (**A, B**) scans demonstrate areas of infarction (hypodensity) in the temporal lobe (A), with similar areas of hypodensity and mottled hemorrhage in the occipital lobes (B) as well. Comparable post contrast levels (**C, D**) show areas of massive enhancement in the occipital lobes (C), particularly in the region of the calcarine cortex (D). This pattern of massive CT enhancement, with minimal mass effect, is typical of infarction. Occasionally, it may be difficult or impossible to exclude underlying arterio-venous malformations.

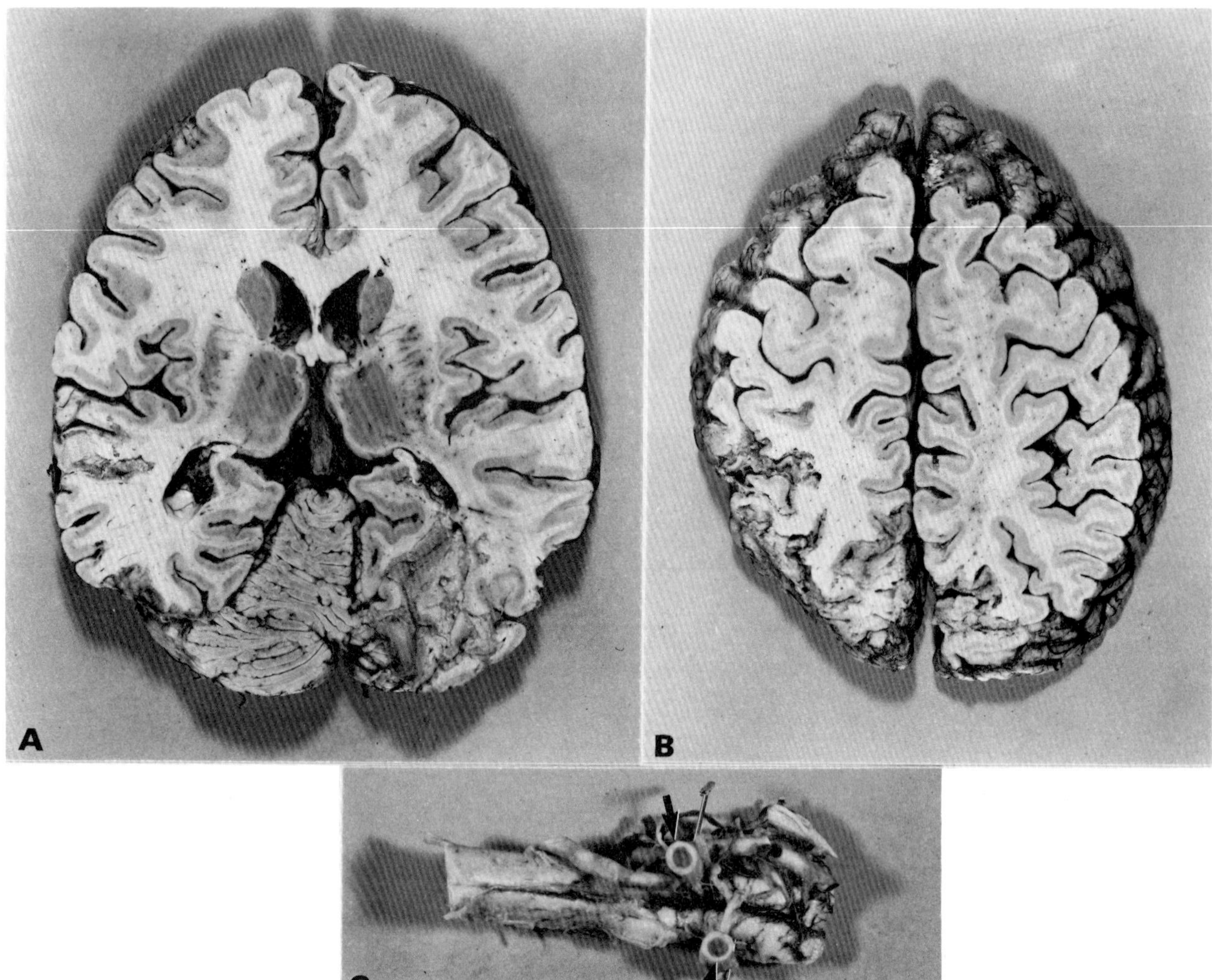

Figure 16-7-2. **Bilateral Occipital Lobe Infarction, with Basilar Artery Thrombosis.**
A and **B** show 15° axial sections of brain corresponding to the CT scans of Figure 16-7-1. Much of the infarcted tissue was stained green (the patient was jaundiced); the implication of breakdown of blood-brain barrier, in relation to strong enhancement of the infarcted regions in the CT, is manifest.

C. The brain stem is seen, with basilar artery; the latter is thrombosed, as shown in cross section. The thrombus was stained green. The brain stem does not appear infarcted; it must have been served by collateral circulation, independent of the basilar artery. The mechanism of the occipital infarction is not explained. The patient inevitably experienced bilateral blindness. This at one time was thought to be hysterical.

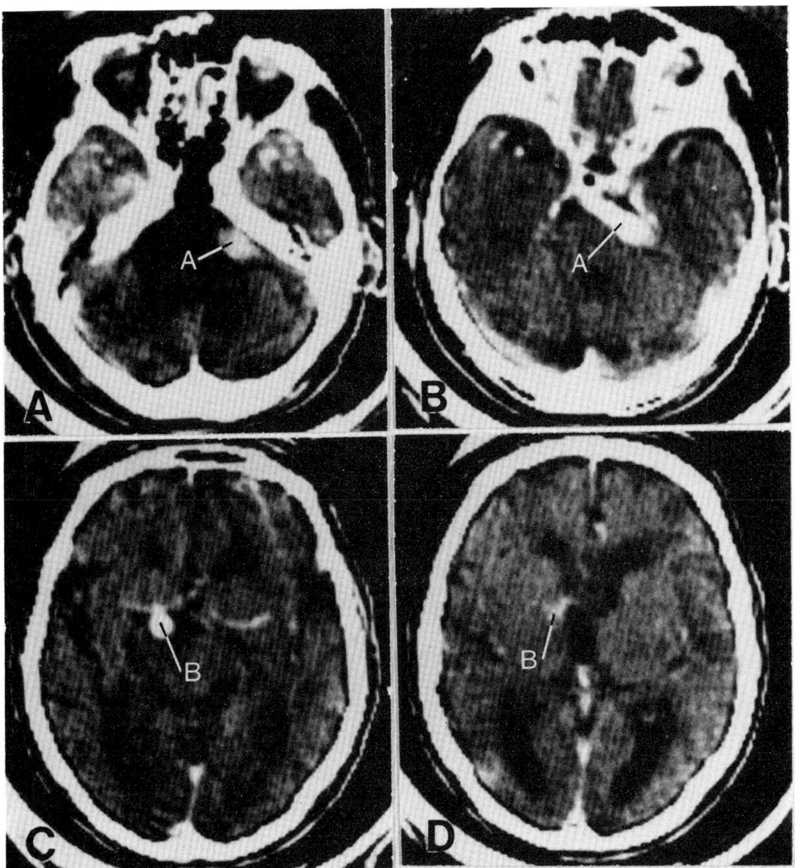

Figure 16-8-1. **Fusiform Basilar Artery Aneurysm with Posterior Cerebral Distribution Infarction.** (Same case as Figures 16-8-2, 3). A four-level post contrast study demonstrates a fusiform aneurysm (A) crossing obliquely in front of the brain stem (*A, B*). In *C,* the tip of the aneurysm (B) mimics a posterior communicating artery aneurysm. A decreased density without contrast enhancement is noted medial to the occipital horn, corresponding to the area of infarction as identified in the pathological specimen (See Figure 16-8-3). *D* demonstrates extension of the tip of the aneurysm (B) slightly lateral to the anterior portion of the third ventricle. Ectatic aneurysms occasionally present as intra-axial lesions due to their tortuosity and ability to slowly indent into the brain stem, and the angle and thickness of the CT section obtained. This case demonstrates the need to obtain multiple overlapping sections to fully demonstrate the anatomy of such lesions. Letters in italics refer to larger letters denoting subdivisions of the illustration. Nonitalicized letters refer to small letters that indicate individual structures in the illustration.

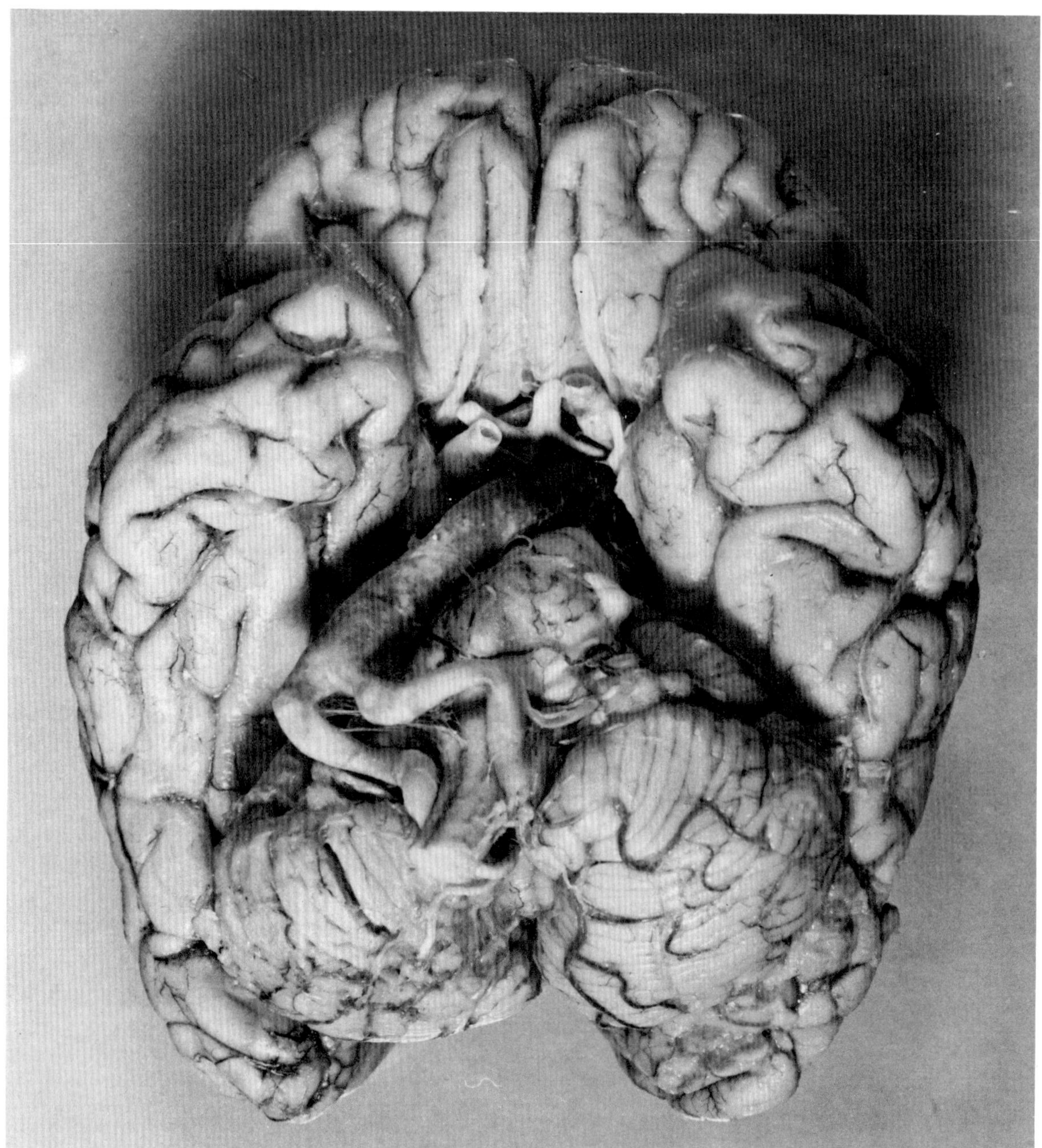

Figure 16-8-2. **Fusiform Aneurysm of Basilar Artery, with Infarction of Left Posterior Cerebral Region of Supply.** Continuation of Figure 16-8-1. View of base of brain. The CT density proved to be a fusiform (in this case, arteriosclerotic) aneurysm of the basilar artery. The vertebral arteries are sclerotic.

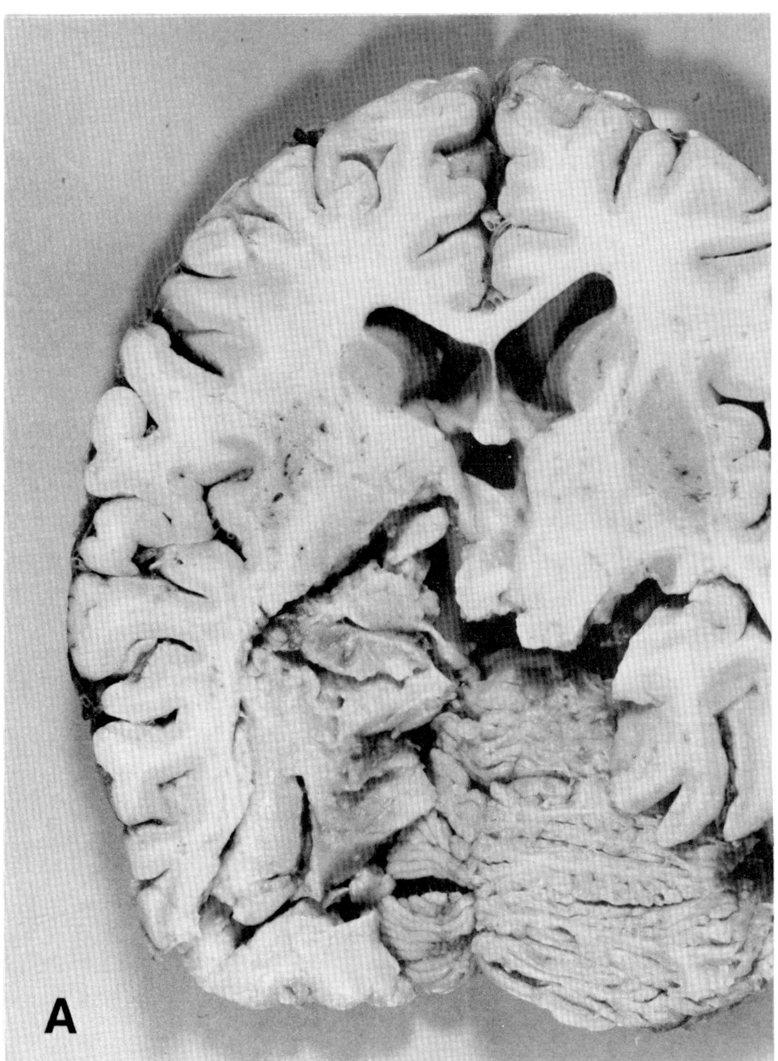

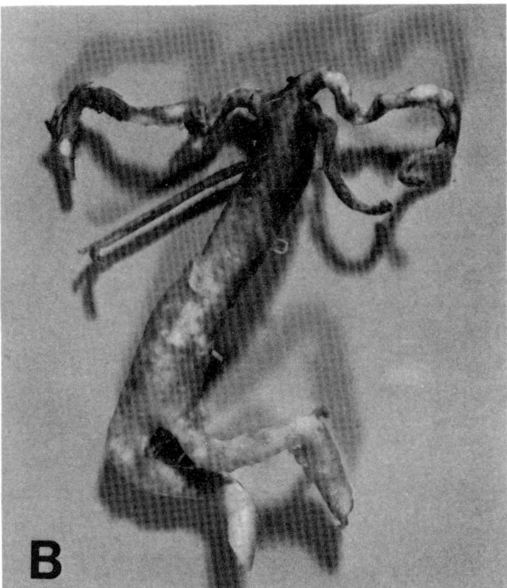

Figure 16-8-3. Continuation of Figure 16-8-2.

A. 15° Axial section. Infarction of left occipital lobe is seen.

B. The removed basilar artery and tributaries, showing the aneurysm. The lumen of the aneurysm was partially occluded by thrombus; the latter extended around into the left posterior cerebral artery, occluding it completely.

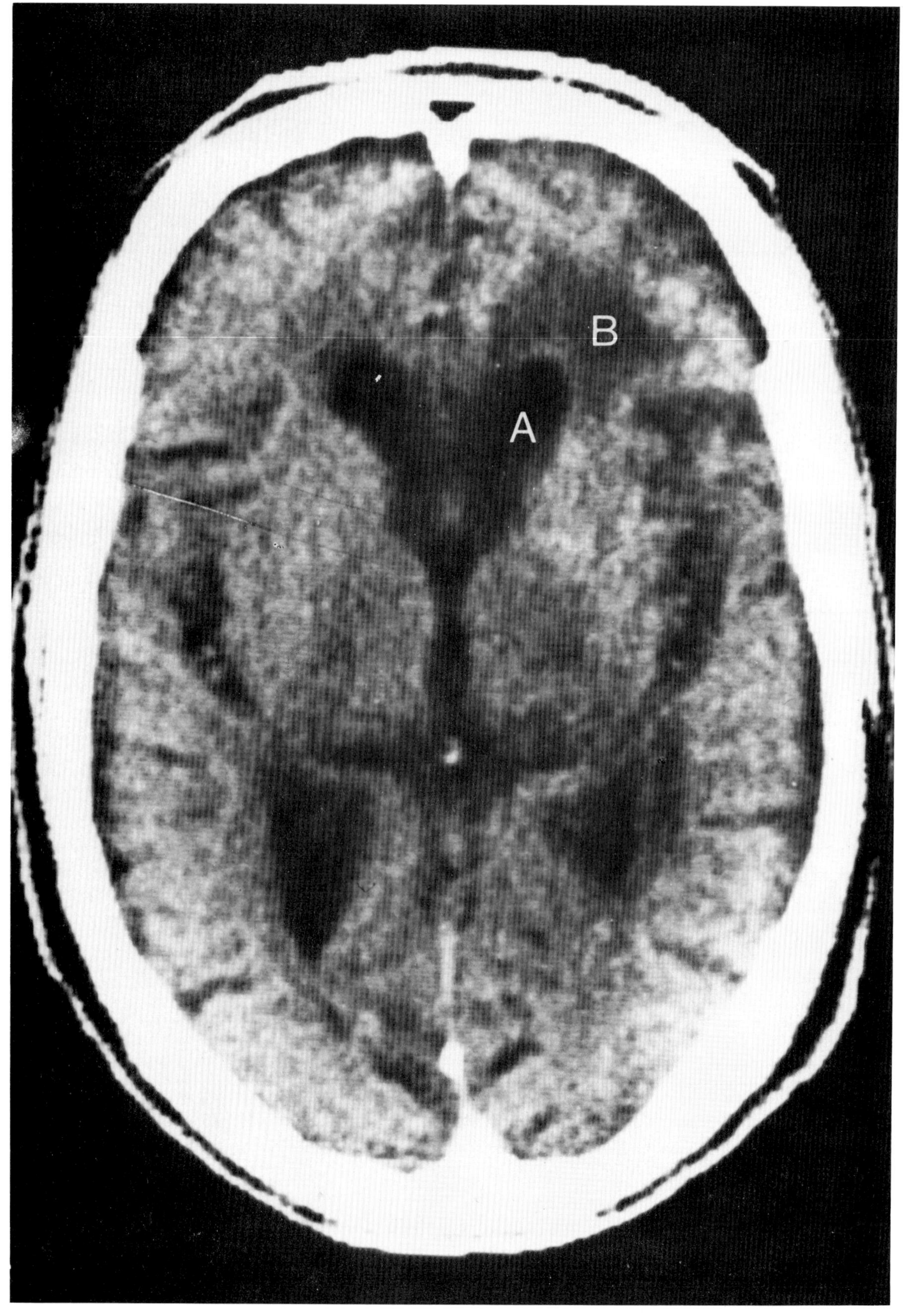
B
A

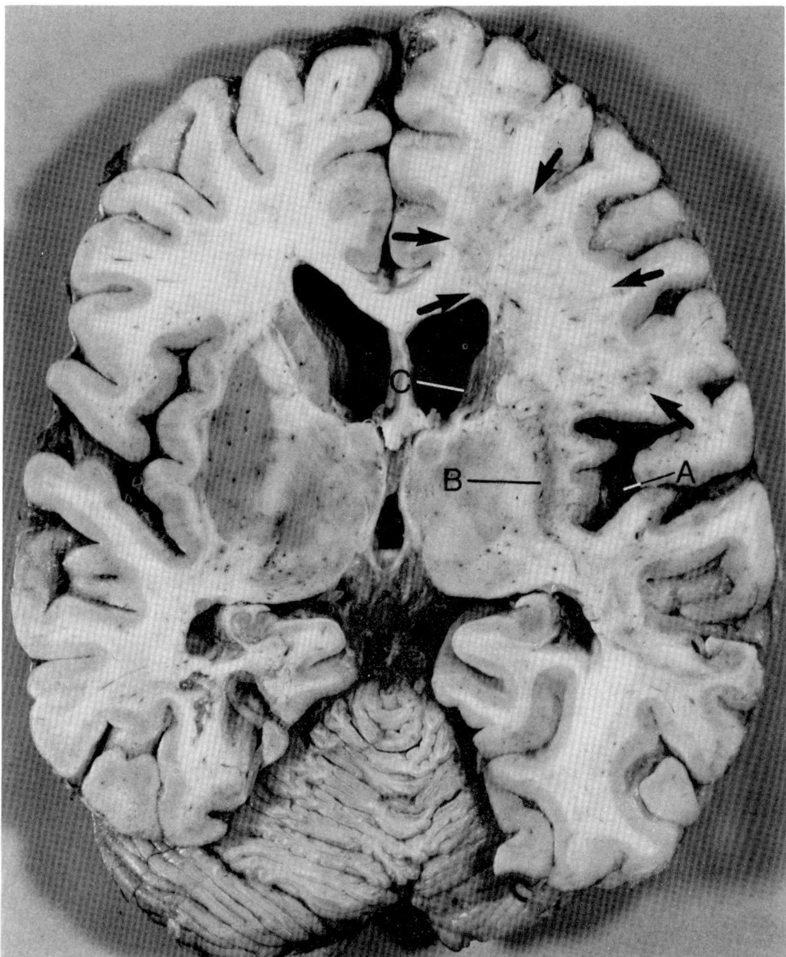

Figure 16-9-2. **Old Infarct, with Incomplete Destruction, of some Structures in the Middle Cerebral Arterial Region of Supply.** Continuation of Figure 16-9-1. *Arrows:* A region of tissue devitalization (although not complete breakdown) for correlation with comparable region in the CT.

Some added structures involved:

A. The suprainsular sulcus is widened. The insula and other underlying tissues are atrophic.

B. Putamen also is atrophic.

C. Head of caudate nucleus. It also shows atrophy, with concave rather than convex ventricular surface and with an appearance of spongification of the cross section surface.

The time of the infarct may be considered as being relatively remote, the status being essentially a residual one.

←

Figure 16-9-1. **Old Infarction.** Same Case as Figure 16-9-2, Computed Tomography. A single noncontrast section demonstrates encasement of the anterior horn of the lateral ventricle (A) by an old infarct (B) due to scar tissue from the latter process. No enhancement was noted in this lesion. This case demonstrates that occasionally "positive" mass effects may be caused by old inactive gliotic lesions.

Chapter Eight

Idiopathic—Miscellaneous

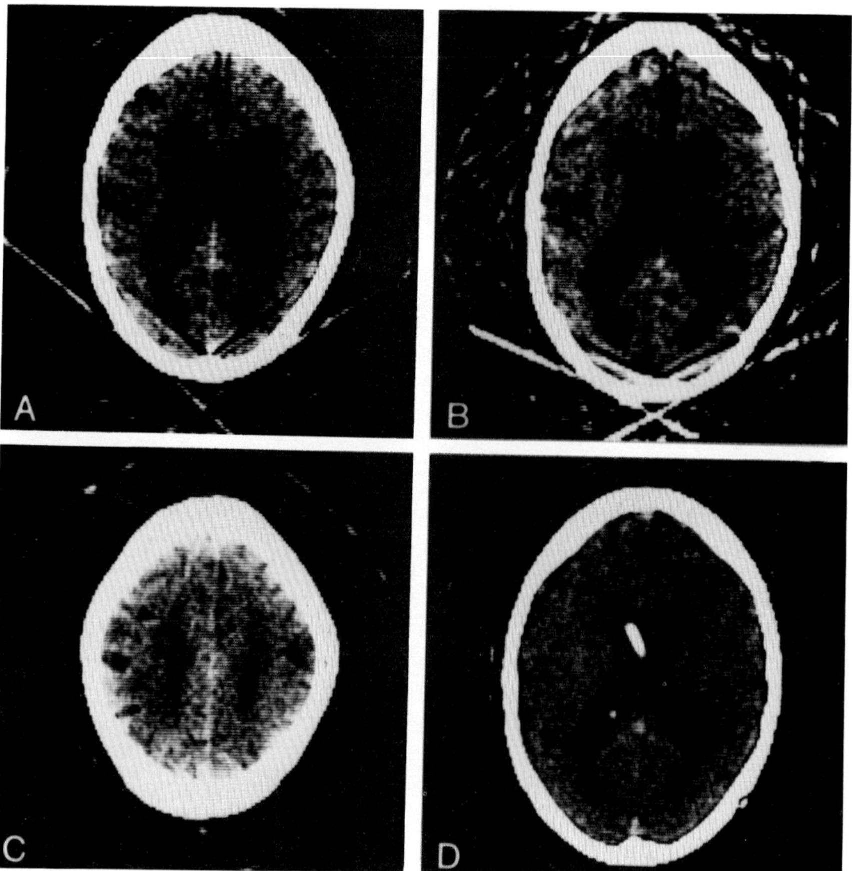

Figure 17-1-1. **CT of Cerebral Pseudoatrophy. A-C.** Various preshunt CT levels demonstrate ventriculomegaly which is suggestive of some degree of hydrocephalus. However, the cortical sulci are quite prominent as well, and the over-all diagnosis could well be severe atrophy. **D.** Same patient as **A-C**, following a ventricular shunt procedure. Note that not only have the ventricles decreased in size, but so have the cortical sulci. This represents communicating hydrocephalus with secondary dilation of sulcal CSF spaces. (Illustrations from *Surgical Neurology,* 10:209, 1978).

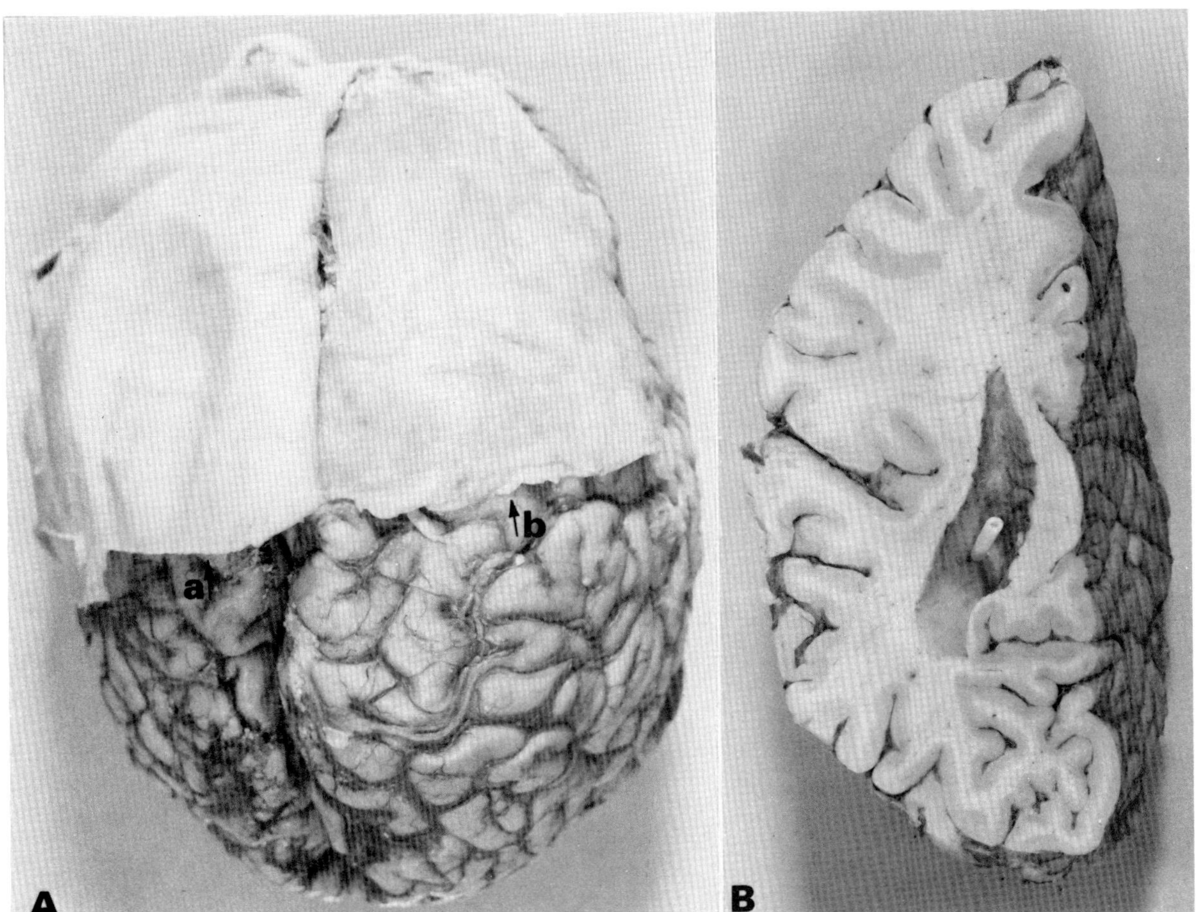

Figure 17-1-2. **Cerebral Pseudoatrophy.** Continuation of Figure 17-1-1.
A. Oblique vertex view of brain with approximately half of the dura removed. The remaining half, covering the right cerebral hemisphere, has been folded back on the left (a). An adventitious subdural membrane remains in place on the right (b).
B. Inferior view of a horizontally sectioned vertex portion of the right cerebral hemisphere. Ventriculostomy tube is in place.
In neither illustration is convolutional atrophy in evidence.

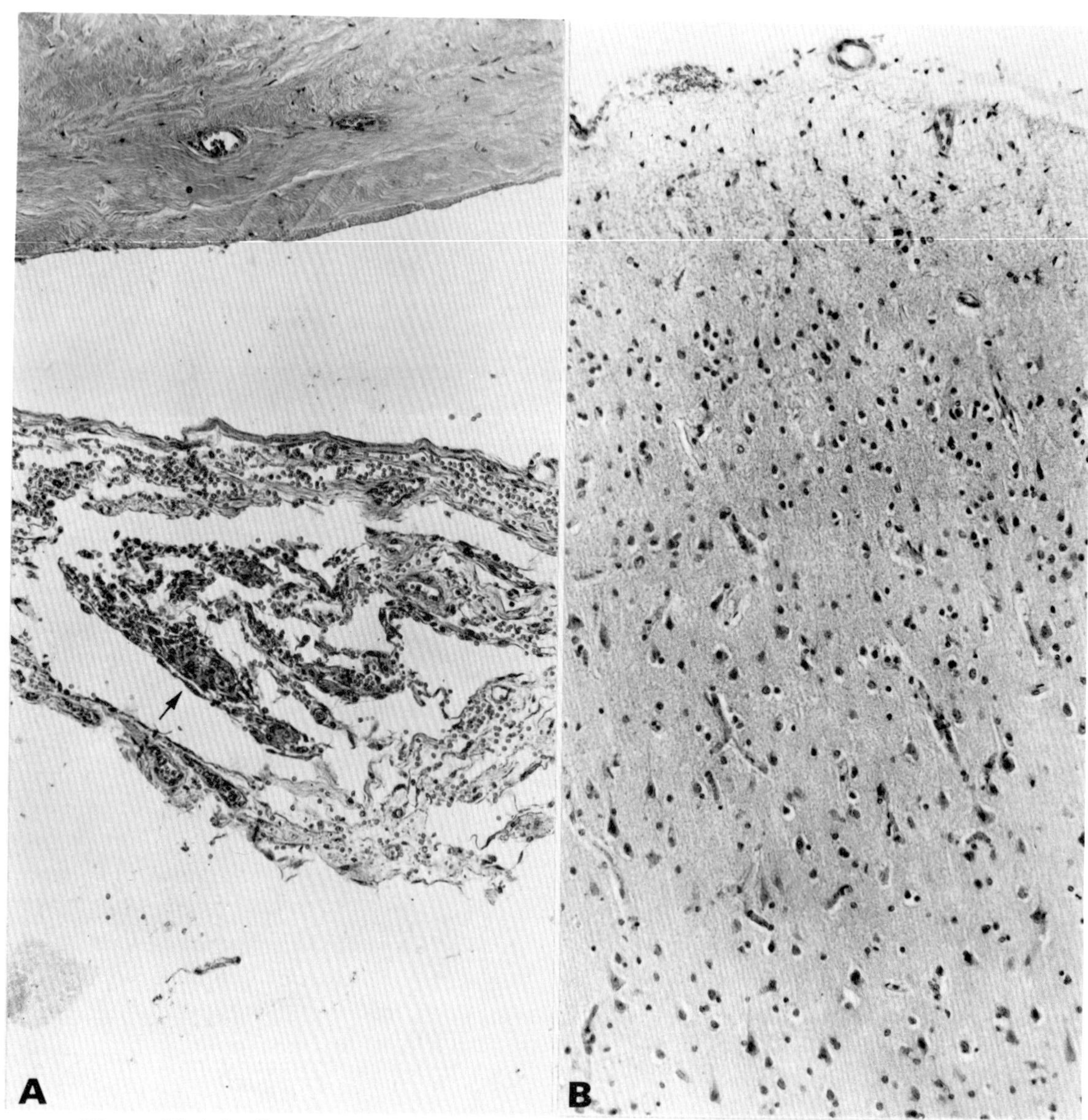

Figure 17-1-3. Continuation of Figure 17-1-2.
A. Microphotograph of meninges. Dura extends across the upper portion of the illustration. The extra membrane extends across the center. An arachnoidal villus is entrapped within the membrane (*arrow*); this has a possible bearing on resistance to reabsorption of CSF.
B. Microphotograph of cerebral cortex. Loss of nerve cells, as might be anticipated in true atrophy, is not in evidence.

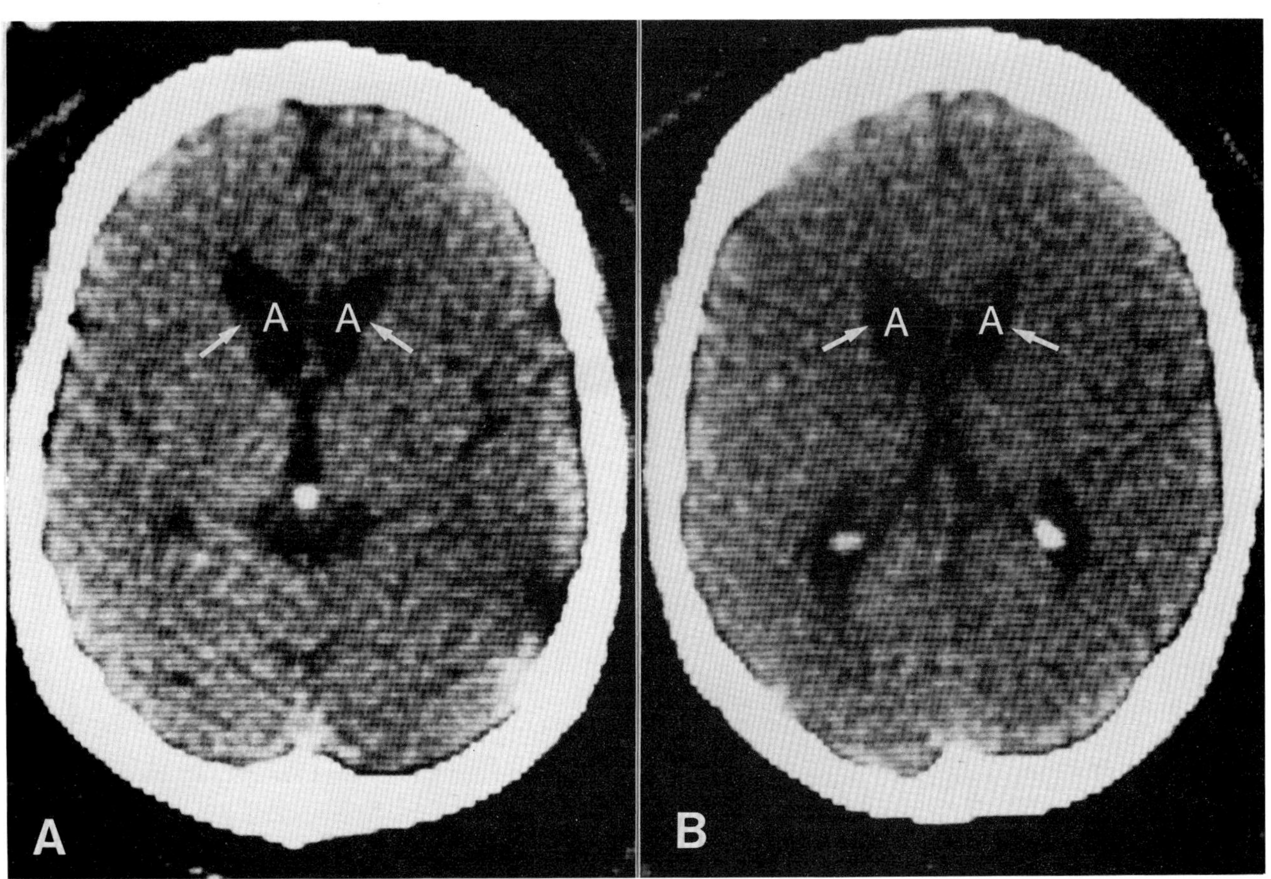

Figure 17-2-1. **Huntington's Chorea.** A noncontrast CT scan demonstrates disproportionate enlargement of the anterior horns of the lateral ventricles (A) with flattening of the caudate impression (*arrows*), compatible with Huntington's chorea.

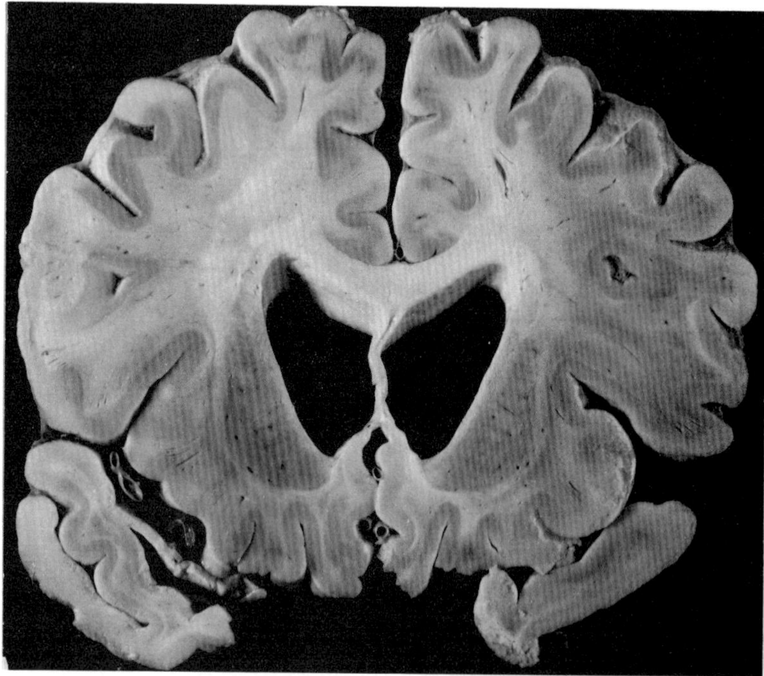

Figure 17-2-2. **Huntington's Chorea.** Continuation of Figure 17-2-1. Coronal section of brain. There is severe atrophy of the caudate nuclei, which can scarcely be identified, and the ventricles are enlarged. There is less severe general convolutional atrophy, with widening of sulci. From Dublin, W. B.: *Fundamentals of Neuropathology,* Ed. II, 1967, Charles C Thomas, Springfield, Illinois.